EXOTIC ANIMAL FORMULARY

D0858550

James W. Carpenter, MS, DVM,
Diplomate ACZM

Ted Y. Mashima, DVM, Diplomate ACZM

David J. Rupiper, DVM

Contributor
James K. Morrisey, DVM,
Diplomate ABVP (Avian)

Second Edition

W.B. Saunders Company
A Harcourt Health Sciences Company
The Curtis Center
Independence Square West
Philadelphia, Pennsylvania 19106, USA

Library of Congress Cataloging-in-Publication Data

Carpenter, James W. (James Wyman)
  Exotic animal formulary / James W. Carpenter,
Ted Y. Mashima, David J. Rupiper;
contributor, James K. Morrisey.—2nd ed.
    p. cm.
  ISBN 0-7216-8312-6
    1. Veterinary drugs.
    2. Veterinary drugs—Dosage.
    3. Exotic animals. I. Mashima, Ted Y. II. Rupiper,
David J.

SF917 .C27 2001
636.089'514—dc21   00-032964

ISBN 0-7216-8312-6

PREFACE

The purpose of this book is to serve as a quick reference to veterinary clinicians, students, and technicians working with exotic animals. With the explosion in interest in nontraditional animals as companion animals, we believe that there is a need for a "user-friendly," portable exotic animal formulary.

However, this book is intended not to replace existing medical resources or the use of sound medical judgment, but rather to serve as a guide in providing medical care to exotic animals. This book contains a formulary, tables and appendices containing commonly needed information, and a reference section for fish, amphibians, reptiles, birds, sugar gliders, hedgehogs, rodents, rabbits, ferrets, miniature pigs, and primates. The formulary section assumes that the reader has a reasonable understanding of veterinary medicine. For example, drug indications are generally listed only in unique situations. The appendices have been carefully selected to include those topics of major importance in clinical practice.

The selection of species, drugs, and other information used in this reference was based on an extensive review of the literature and on our collective teaching and clinical experience. The book, therefore, is intended not to be all-inclusive, but rather a quick reference for the common questions and medical situations we have encountered in clinical practice.

In summary, we hope that you find this formulary and selected tables and appendices "handy" to use, and that it adds to the quality of the medical care you provide to your exotic animal patients. We would appreciate any suggestions or recommendations that you might have for future editions of this book.

This book is revised, updated, and greatly expanded from our *Exotic Animal Formulary* published by Greystone Publications in 1996.

James W. Carpenter, MS, DVM, Dipl. ACZM
Ted Y. Mashima, DVM, Dipl. ACZM
David J. Rupiper, DVM

ACKNOWLEDGMENTS

The support and encouragement to write this book by the faculty and students of the College of Veterinary Medicine, Kansas State University, and our wives, Terry Carpenter, Julie Mashima, and Dr. Susan Boynton-Rupiper, are gratefully acknowledged. We are indebted to Julie Mashima, Bernie Robe, Eric Klaphake, and Micah Kohles for technical assistance in collecting and tabulating some of the information contained in this book. We also wish to acknowledge Dr. Geoff Pye for writing the sugar glider section, and Dr. Ned Gentz and Ms. Cindy Chard-Bergstrom for updating the wildlife appendices. Some illustrations were provided by Ms. Mal Hoover, and the snake anatomy illustrations were made by Dr. Tripp Stewart. The secretarial assistance provided by Ms. Kathy Merrifield, Ms. Carol Porter, and Ms. Donna Kelly is also greatly appreciated! We also appreciate the assistance of W.B. Saunders Company in doing a quality job in publishing this formulary.

DEDICATION

To my Interns and Residents who have helped me develop and evolve an exciting and challenging Service in Exotic Animal, Wildlife, and Zoo Animal Medicine at the College of Veterinary Medicine, Kansas State University. Their dedication, pursuit of excellence, and encouragement have made the completion of this book a reality.

James W. Carpenter

The authors have attempted to verify and double-check all references, dosages, and other data contained in this book. However, despite these efforts, errors in the original sources or in the preparation of this book may have occurred. All users of this reference, therefore, should empirically evaluate all dosages to determine that they are reasonable prior to use. The authors assume no responsibility for and make no warranty with respect to results obtained from the uses, procedures, or dosages listed, or for any misstatement or error, negligent or otherwise, contained in this book. In addition, the authors do not necessarily endorse specific products, procedures, or dosages reported in this book. Also, the listing of a drug or commercial product in this book does not indicate approval by the FDA or the manufacturer for use in exotic animals.

ABBREVIATIONS

d	day
EpiCe	epicoelomic
h, hr	hour
IA	intra-articular
ICe	intracoelomic
IM	intramuscularly
IO	intraosseous
IP	intraperitoneally
IPPV	intermittent positive-pressure ventilation
IT	intratracheally
IV	intravenously
IU	international units
kg	kilogram
L	liter
LRS	lactated Ringer's solution
mg	milligram
min	minute
mo	month
PD	pharmacologic data
PO	orally
prn	as needed
q	every
SC	subcutaneously
wk	week

About the Authors

James W. Carpenter, MS, DVM, Diplomate ACZM, is a Professor at the College of Veterinary Medicine, Kansas State University, where he heads the Exotic Animal, Wildlife, and Zoo Animal Medicine Service. He has been a clinical and research veterinarian for 25 years in the field of exotic animal, wildlife, and zoo animal medicine and is the author of over 135 scientific papers and book chapters. Dr. Carpenter was the Editor of the *Journal of Zoo and Wildlife Medicine* (1987-1992) and Chair of its Editorial Board (1992-1997), and is currently Editor-in-Chief, *Journal of Avian Medicine and Surgery*; Chairman of the Editorial Board of the *Journal of Avian Medicine and Surgery* and on the Editorial Board of *Seminars in Avian and Exotic Pet Medicine*; Chairman, Wildlife Scientific Advisory Board, Morris Animal Foundation; and President, American Association of Zoo Veterinarians.

Ted Y. Mashima, DVM, Diplomate ACZM, completed an Internship in Exotic Animal, Wildlife, and Zoo Animal Medicine at Kansas State University in 1993, and a Residency in Zoological Medicine at North Carolina State University in 1996. He has published scientific papers on a variety of areas in zoological medicine, and served as the Projects Director for the National Association of Physicians for the Environment, Bethesda, Maryland (1996-1999). He is an Associate Director, Center for Government and Corporate Veterinary Medicine, Virginia-Maryland Regional College of Veterinary Medicine, College Park, Maryland. Dr. Mashima also serves on the Board of Directors for the Alliance of Veterinarians for the Environment.

David J. Rupiper, DVM, a private practitioner working almost exclusively with birds at the East Petaluma Animal Hospital, Petaluma California, is a leading authority on avian medicine and surgery. He has published scientific papers on avian medicine and parasitology and has lectured at veterinary conferences and at a local college.

About the Contributor

James K. Morrisey, DVM, Diplomate ABVP (Avian), completed an Internship in Exotic Animal, Wildlife, and Zoo Animal Medicine at Kansas State University in 1996, and a Residency in Avian and Exotic Pet Medicine at The Animal Medical Center, New York, New York, in 1998. He served as an Instructor in Zoological Medicine in 1998-1999 at the School of Veterinary Medicine, University of Wisconsin. Dr. Morrisey is currently a clinician at The Animal Medical Center.

CONTENTS

SECTION II. SELECTED APPENDICES

—

Fish

Amphibians

Reptiles

Birds

Sugar Gliders

Hedgehogs

Rodents

Rabbits

Ferrets

Miniature Pigs

Primates

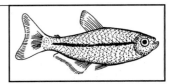

Table 1. Antimicrobial and antifungal agents used in fish [a-d]

Agent	Dosage	Comments
Amikacin	5 mg/kg IM q12h[11]	
Amoxicillin	40-80 mg/kg/day in feed × 10 days[9] 25 mg/kg PO q12h[13]	Rarely indicated in aquarium fish because few pathogens are gram +
Ampicillin	50-80 mg/kg/day in feed × 10 days[9]	Rarely indicated in aquarium fish because few pathogens are gram +
Aztreonam (Azactam, Squibb)	100 mg/kg IM, IP q48h × 15 days[5]	*Aeromonas salmonicida*; used by koi hobbyists
Chloramphenicol	50 mg/kg PO, IM once, then 25 mg/kg q24h[13] 20-40 mg/kg IM, IP q48h × 15 days[5] 20-50 mg/kg IP q7d × 2 treatments[9]	*Aeromonas salmonicida* in goldfish
Enrofloxacin	2.5-5.0 mg/L × 5 hr bath q24h8 × 5-7 days[5] 0.1% feed × 10-14 days[5] 5-10 mg/kg PO q24h × 10-14 days[5] 5-10 mg/kg IM, IP q48h[8] × 15 days[5] 5 mg/kg PO, IM, IP q24h[13]	Red pacu/PD[8]; change 50-75% of water between treatments Oral or injectable form can be given orally Red pacu/PD[8]
Erythromycin	— 100 mg/kg PO, IM q24h × 7-10 days[13] 50-100 mg/kg PO q24h × 10 days[5]	Commonly sold as tank treatment for aquarium fish; not recommended because of toxicity to nitrifying bacteria[9]
Florfenicol (Nuflor, Schering Plough)	40-50 mg/kg PO, IM, IP q12-24h[13]	

3

Table 1. Antimicrobial and antifungal agents used in fish (cont.)

Agent	Dosage	Comments
Flumequine	50-100 mg/L × 3 hr bath[9]	Quinolone; gram-negative bacteria; freshwater fish at pH 6.8-7.2; decreased uptake in hard water; increase dose for marine fish
	10 mg/kg q24h in feed × 10 days[9]	
	30 mg/kg IM, IP[9]	High antibiotic levels for several days when given IM
Formalin	All doses based on volumes of 100% formalin (= 37% formaldehyde)	Mycotic infections on eggs; don't treat within 24 hr of hatching; caution: carcinogenic; do not use if highly toxic white precipitates are present; some fish are very sensitive; test on small number first, monitor for piping and pale color; increased toxicity in soft, acid water and at high temperature; treat with vigorous aeration because of oxygen depletion; toxic to plants
	1-2 ml/L bath, up to 15 min[9]	
	0.23 ml/L bath up to 60 min[9]	
Furazolidone	1-10 mg/L tank water for > 24 hr[9]	Nitrofuran; caution: carcinogenic; toxic to scaleless fish; absorbed from water; drug inactivated in bright light
	50-100 mg/kg q24h in feed × 10-15 days[9]	
Gentamicin	2.5 mg/kg IM q72h[13]	Nephrotoxic; substantial risk in species for which dosages have not been determined[10]
Iodine, potentiated (Betadine, Purdue Frederick)	Topical to wound, rinse immediately[9]	Do not use solutions combined with detergent (eg, Betadine scrub)
Itraconazole (Sporanox, Janssen)	1-5 mg/kg q24h in feed q1-7d[13]	Systemic mycoses
Kanamycin sulfate (Kantrex, Adothecon)	50-100 mg/L × 5 hr bath q72h × 3 treatments[5]	Change 50-75% of water between treatments; absorbed from water
	50 mg/kg q24h in feed[9]	
	20 mg/kg IP q3d × 14 days[9]	Toxic to some fish

4

Table 1. Antimicrobial and antifungal agents used in fish (cont.)

Agent	Dosage	Comments
Ketoconazole	2.5-10.0 mg/kg PO, IM, IP[13]	Systemic mycoses
Malachite green (zinc-free)	—	Freshwater fish/mycotic infections; caution: mutagenic, teratogenic; toxic to some fish species and to fry; increased toxicity at higher temperatures and lower pH; stains objects, especially plastic; toxic to plants
	100 mg/L topical to skin lesions[9]	
	0.1 mg/L tank water q3d × 3 treatments[9]	Remove residual chemical with activated carbon after last treatment
	50-60 mg/L × 10-30 sec bath[9]	
	1 mg/L × 30-60 min bath[9]	Use 2 mg/L if pH high
	10 mg/L × 10-30 min bath[9]	Freshwater fish eggs
	0.5 mg/L × 1 hr bath[9]	Freshwater fish eggs
Methylene blue	2 mg/L tank water q48h, up to 3 treatments[9]	Preventing infections of freshwater eggs; toxic to nitrifying bacteria; stains many objects; toxic to plants
Miconazole (Monistat, Janssen)	10-20 mg/kg PO, IM, IP[13]	Systemic mycoses
Naladixic acid (Neg Gram, Sanofi Winthrop)	13 mg/L × 1-4 hr bath, repeat prn[9] 5 mg/kg PO, IM q24h[13]	Quinolone; gram-negative bacteria
Neomycin	66 mg/L tank water q3d, up to 3 treatments[9]	Commonly sold as tank treatment for aquarium fish; toxic to nitrifying bacteria; keep fish densities low

Table 1. Antimicrobial and antifungal agents used in fish (cont.)

Agent	Dosage	Comments
Nifurpirinol	1-2 mg/L × 5 min - 6 hr bath[9] 0.1 mg/L tank water q24h × 3-5 days[9] 4-10 mg/kg in feed q12h × 5 days[9] 0.45-0.90 mg/kg q24h × 5 days[9]	Nitrofuran; caution: carcinogenic; toxic to scaleless fish; absorbed from water; drug inactivated in bright light
Nitrofurazone	100 mg/L × 30 min bath[9] Add > 2 mg/L tank water q24h × 5-10 days[9] 20 mg/L × 5 hr bath q24h × 5-7 days[5]	Nitrofuran; caution: carcinogenic; toxic to scaleless fish; absorbed from water; drug inactivated in bright light; water soluble formulations preferred Change 50-75% of water between treatments
Oxolinic acid	25 mg/L × 15 min bath q12h × 3 days[9] 1 mg/L tank water × 24 hr[9] 10 mg/kg q24h in feed × 10 days[9] 5-25 mg/kg PO q24h[13]	Quinolone; gram-negative bacteria; decreased uptake in hard water; better uptake pH < 6.9 Up to 30 mg/kg/day in seawater
Oxytetracycline	10-50 mg/L × 1 hr bath[9] 10-100 mg/L tank water[9] 100 mg/L × 1 hr bath[13] 400 mg/L × 1 hr bath[13]	Surface bacterial infections; yellow-brown foam may develop in treatment water Higher doses in hard water; if fish still sick, retreat on day 3 after 50% water change; drug light sensitive; keep tank covered to prevent photo-inactivation; drug turns dark brown when decomposing: change 50% of water immediately Freshwater fish Marine fish

Table 1. Antimicrobial and antifungal agents used in fish (cont.)

Agent	Dosage	Comments
Oxytetracycline (continued)	20-50 mg/L × 5-24 hr bath q24h × 5-7 days[5]	Change 50-75% of water between treatments
	7 mg/g feed, q24h × 10 days[14]	
	55-83 mg/kg/day in feed × 10 days[9]	
	20 mg/kg PO q8h[13]	
	50 mg/kg PO q24h × 10 days[5]	
	70 mg/kg PO q24h × 10-14 days[14]	
	25-50 mg/kg IM, IP[9]	Produces high levels for several days when given IM
	10 mg/kg IM q24h[13]	
	25 mg/kg IM, IP q24h × 5-7 days[5]	
Potassium permanganate	1000 mg/L × 10-40 sec bath[9] 5 mg/L × 30-60 min bath[9]	Freshwater fish/skin and gill bacterial infections; toxic in water with high pH; do not mix with formalin; can be toxic in goldfish[11]
Sarafloxacin (Saraflox, Abbott)	10-14 mg/kg PO q24h × 10 days[13]	Fluoroquinolone
Silver sulfadiazine cream (Silvadine, Marion Merrill Dow)	Topical q12h[7]	External bacterial infection; keep lesion out of water 30-60 sec following application; keep gills submerged
Sulfadimethoxine/ ormetoprim (Romet, Hoffman-LaRoche)	50 mg/kg/day in feed × 5 days[9] Medicated brine shrimp	Available as a powder to add to feed and as medicated feed Place brine shrimp nauplii (larvae) in 3 mg/L seawater x 4 hr, rinse in seawater with brine shrimp net, then feed immediately to fish; may also work with adult brine shrimp and other live feeds[9]

Table 1. Antimicrobial and antifungal agents used in fish (cont.)

Agent	Dosage	Comments
Trimethoprim/sulfa	20 mg/L × 5-12 hr bath q24h × 5-7 days[5] 0.2% feed × 10-14 days[5] 30 mg/kg PO q24h × 10-14 days[5]	Change 50-75% of water between treatments
Triple antibiotic ointment (polymyxin B sulfate/bacitracin/ neomycin sulfate)	Topical q12h[5]	External bacterial infection; keep lesion out of water 30-60 sec following application; keep gills submerged

[a] Not to be used in fish for human consumption.
[b] Preferable to treat single fish of a species to determine toxicity.
[c] Tank treatment: When treating the fishes' resident aquarium, disconnect activated carbon filtration to prevent drug removal. Many drugs adversely affect the nitrifying bacteria, so water quality should be monitored closely (especially ammonia and nitrite concentrations). Always keep water well aerated and monitor fish closely. Perform water changes and reconnect filtration to remove residual drug following treatment. Discard carbon following drug removal.
[d] Bath treatment: Remove fish from resident aquarium and place in container with known volume of water and concentration of therapeutic agent. Watch closely for signs of toxicity, eg, listing and dyspnea. Always keep water well aerated.

Table 2. Antiparasitic agents used in fish [a-d]

Agent	Dosage	Comments
Acetic acid, glacial	2 ml/L × 30-45 sec bath[6]	Trematode, crustacean ectoparasites; safe for goldfish; may be toxic to smaller tropical fish
Chloroquine diphosphate	10 mg/L tank water, once[9]	*Amyloodinium ocellatum*; monitor for 21 days, retreat prn; use activated carbon to remove drug if no relapse
Copper sulfate	—	Marine fish/ protozoan, trematode ectoparasites; copper levels must be assessed with a commercial kit, and adjusted as needed; toxic to gill tissue; immunosuppressive; extremely toxic to invertebrates and many plants; copper removed by activated carbon
	100 mg/L × 1-5 min bath[2]	Prepare stock solution of 1 mg/ml (1 g $CuSO_4 \cdot 5H_2O$ in 250 ml distilled water)
	Maintain free ion levels at 0.25-1.0 mg/L × 24-48 hr bath[2]	
	Maintain free ion levels at 0.15-0.2 mg/L tank water, until therapeutic effect[9]	
	Maintain copper levels at 0.2 mg/L tank water × 14-21 days[14]	Citrated copper sulfate; prepare stock solution of 1 mg/ml (3 g $CuSO_4 \cdot 5H_2O$ and 2 g citric acid monohydrate in 750 ml distilled water)[2]
Difluorobenzuron (Dimilin, Union Carbide)	0.01 mg/L tank water × 48 hr q6d × 3 treatments[11]	Crustacean ectoparasites; inhibits chitin synthesis; drug persists in water long-term; marketed for control of terrestrial insects
Dimethyl phosphonate	—	See trichlorphon
Fenbendazole	2 mg/L tank water q7d × 3 treatments[9] 0.2% feed × 3 days, repeat in 14-21 days[6]	Nonencysted gastrointestinal nematodes

Table 2. Antiparasitic agents used in fish (cont.)

Agent	Dosage	Comments
Fenbendazole (continued)	2.5 mg/g feed × 2-3 days, repeat in 14 days[14]	
	50 mg/kg PO q24h × 2 days, repeat in 14 days[14]	
	Medicated brine shrimp	Place live brine shrimp in 400 mg fenbendazole per 100 ml water x 15-20 min, immediately before feeding to fish; feed 2 consecutive days and repeat in 14 days[14]
Formalin	—	Formalin combination follows
	All doses based on volumes of 100% formalin (= 37% formaldehyde)	Protozoan, trematode, crustacean ectoparasites; caution: carcinogenic; do not use if highly toxic white precipitates are present; some fish are very sensitive: test on small number first, monitor for piping and pale color; increased toxicity in soft, acid water and at high temperature; treat with vigorous aeration because of oxygen depletion; toxic to plants
	0.125-0.25 ml/L, up to 60 min bath, repeat q24h × 2-3 days prn[9]	When using maximum dose, treat q3d
	0.015-0.025 ml/L tank water[9]	For *Ichthyophthirius*, use 0.025 ml/L tank water q48h x 3 treatments; change up to 50% of water on alternate days
	0.4 ml/L up to 1 hr bath q3d, up to 3 treatments[11]	Soft water
	0.5 ml/L up to 1 hr bath q3d, up to 3 treatments[11]	Hard water
	2 ml/L up to 1 hr bath q3d, up to 3 treatments[11]	Marine water
Formalin (F)/ malachite green (M)	(F) 0.025 ml/L /(M) 0.1 mg/L tank water q48h × 3 treatments[9]	Combination synergistic for *Ichthyophthirius*; change up to 50% water on alternate days

Table 2. Antiparasitic agents used in fish (cont.)

Agent	Dosage	Comments
Freshwater	3-15 min bath, repeat q7d prn[9] 4-5 min bath[6]	Marine fish/ectoparasites; aerate well; monitor closely; some small fish are sensitive
Hydrogen peroxide (3%)	17.5 ml/L × 4-10 min bath, once[2]	Ectoparasites; monitor closely; may be harmful to smaller fish
Ivermectin	—	Do not use; neurologic signs and death at therapeutic doses[2]
Levamisole	1-2 mg/L × 24 hr bath[2] 50 mg/L × 2 hr bath[2] 4 g/kg feed q7d × 3 treatments[2] 10 mg/kg PO q7d × 3 treatments[2] 11 mg/kg IM q7d × 2 treatments[2]	Internal nematodes, especially larval External trematodes
Malachite green	— 100 mg/L topical to skin lesions[9] 0.1 mg/L tank water q3d x 3 treatments[9] 50-60 mg/L x 10-30 sec bath[9] 1 mg/L × 30-60 min bath[9]	See formalin for combination Freshwater fish/ protozoan ectoparasites; prepare stock solution of 3.7 mg/ml (1.4 g malachite green in 380 ml water); caution: mutagenic, teratogenic; toxic to some fish species (eg, tetras) and fry; increased toxicity at higher temperatures and lower pH; toxic to plants; stains objects especially plastic; remove residual chemical with activated carbon after last tank treatment Use 2 mg/L if pH high
Mebendazole	100 mg/L × 10 min - 2 hr bath[2] 1 mg/L × 24 hr bath[2] 20 mg/kg PO q7d × 3 treatments[13]	Monogenean trematodes Monogenean trematodes Gastrointestinal nematodes; do not administer to brood fish: embryotoxic and teratogenic

11

Table 2. Antiparasitic agents used in fish (cont.)

Agent	Dosage	Comments
Methylene blue	1-3 mg/L tank water[9]	Freshwater fish/ectoparasites; not recommended because of poor efficacy; toxic to nitrifying bacteria; stains objects; toxic to plants
Metronidazole	6.6 mg/L tank water q24h × 3 days[9] 25 mg/L tank water q48h × 3 treatments[9]	*Hexamita* and other internal flagellates; some external flagellates; poorly soluble in water: dissolve before adding to water or feed; change water between tank treatments
	25 mg/kg q24h in feed × 5-10 days[9]	Equivalent to 0.25% in feed at 1% BW/day
	100 mg/kg q24h in feed × 3 days[9]	Equivalent to 1% in feed at 1% BW/day
	6.25-18 mg/g feed × 5 days[14]	
	50 mg/kg PO q24h × 5 days[2]	
	Medicated brine shrimp	Place live brine shrimp in 625 mg metronidazole per 100 ml water x 15-20 min, immediately before feeding to fish; feed 5 consecutive days[14]
Piperazine	10 mg/kg q24h in feed × 3 days[9]	Nonencysted gastrointestinal nematodes; equivalent to 0.1% in feed at 1% BW/day
Potassium permanganate	1000 mg/L × 10-40 sec bath[9] 100 mg/L × 5-10 min bath[9] 5 mg/L × 30-60 min bath[9]	Freshwater fish/ protozoan crustacean ectoparasites; toxic in water with high pH; do not mix with formalin; can be toxic in goldfish[11]
Praziquantel	5-10 mg/L × 3-6 hr bath, repeat in 7 days[6]	Monogenean trematode ectoparasites, cestodes; aerate water well; some marine fish sensitive; toxic to *Coryodoras* catfish

Table 2. Antiparasitic agents used in fish (cont.)

Agent	Dosage	Comments
Praziquantel (continued)	2-10 mg/L up to 4 hr bath[14]	Monitor closely for lethargy incoordination, loss of equilibrium
	5-12 mg/g feed × 3 days[14]	
	5 mg/kg feed q7d, up to 3 treatments[13]	
	5 mg/kg in feed, IP, repeat in 14-21 days[6]	Cestodes, some internal digenean trematodes
	50 mg/kg PO once[9]	Adult cestodes; gavage or give 0.5% in feed at 1% BW/day
	Medicated brine shrimp	Place live brine shrimp in 400 mg praziquantel per 100 ml water x 15-20 min, immediately before feeding to fish; feed 3 consecutive days[14]
Pyrantel pamoate	10 mg/kg in feed, once[13]	Gastric nematodes
Salt (sodium chloride)	—	Freshwater fish/protozoan trematode ectoparasites; seawater or artificial seasalts preferred; seawater is approximately 30-35 g/L; use only nonionized table/ rock salts; some anticaking agents in solar salts are highly toxic; species sensitivity is highly variable (many catfish sensitive); may be toxic to plants
	1-5 g/L tank water, indefinitely[9]	Prophylaxis or treatment of ectoparasites
	10-30 g/L up to 30 min bath[9]	With salt-sensitive or weak fish use lower dosage and repeat in 24 hr
	30-35 g/L × 4-5 min bath[6]	
Thiabendazole	10-25 mg/kg in feed, repeat in 10 days[13]	Gastric nematodes; anorexia may be seen (more severe at higher doses), generally resolves within 2-4 days
	66 mg/kg PO, once[13]	

13

Table 2. Antiparasitic agents used in fish (cont.)

Agent	Dosage	Comments
Trichlorfon (dimethyl phosphonate)	—	Caution: organophosphate, neurotoxic, avoid inhalation and skin contact; aerate water well; especially toxic to larval fish and tetras; liquid form marketed for cattle is convenient to dispense
	0.5 mg/L tank water q10d × 3 treatments[6]	Crustacean ectoparasites; change 20-30% of water 24-48 hr following each treatment
	0.25 mg/L tank water[9]	Freshwater fish/ use 0.5 mg/L tank water if > 27°C (80°F); treat q3d x 2 treatments for *Dactylogyrus* and other oviparous monogeneans; treat q7d x 4 treatments for anchor worms; single treatment will usually suffice for other copepods, other monogeneans, *Argulus*, leeches
	0.5-1.0 mg/L tank water[9]	Marine fish/ treat q3d x 2 treatments for oviparous monogeneans; use 1 mg/L q48h x 3 treatments for turbellarians; single treatment will usually suffice for copepods (except sea lice), other monogeneans, *Argulus*, leeches

[a] Not to be used in fish for human consumption.

[b] Preferable to treat single fish of a species to determine toxicity.

[c] Tank treatment: When treating the fishes' resident aquarium, disconnect activated carbon filtration to prevent drug removal. Many drugs adversely affect the nitrifying bacteria, so water quality should be monitored closely (especially ammonia and nitrite concentrations). Always keep water well aerated and monitor fish closely. Perform water changes and reconnect filtration to remove residual drug following treatment. Discard carbon following drug removal.

[d] Bath treatment: Remove fish from resident aquarium and place in container with known volume of water and concentration of therapeutic agent. Watch closely for signs of toxicity, eg, listing and dyspnea. Always keep water well aerated.

14

Table 3. Chemical restraint/anesthetic agents used in fish [a-c]

Agent	Dosage	Comments
Atipamezole (Antisedan, Pfizer)	0.2 mg/kg IM[3]	Reversal agent for medetomidine
Benzocaine	—	Not sold as fish anesthetic in US; available from chemical supply companies; do not use topical anesthetic products marketed for mammals; prepare stock solution in ethanol (poorly soluble in water); store in dark bottle at room temperature
	15-40 mg/L bath[9]	Transport sedation
	50-500 mg/L bath[9]	Anesthesia
	1 g/L spray[9]	Large fish/ anesthesia; spray onto gills with an aerosol pump sprayer
Butorphanol (Torbugesic, Fort Dodge)	0.05-0.10 mg/kg IM[13]	Analgesia, post-operative
Carbon dioxide	—	Euthanasia: bubble gas through water until no breathing > 10 min; other agents preferred[9]
Clove oil (eugenol)	40-120 mg/L bath[6]	Stock solution: 100 mg/ml of ethanol by diluting 1 part clove oil with 9 parts 95% ethanol (poorly soluble in water); over-the-counter preparation available at most pharmacies contains approximately 1 g eugenol per ml of clove oil; recovery may be prolonged
Ethanol	1.0-1.5% bath[3]	Anesthetic levels difficult to , control resulting in overdose; not recommended
	> 3% bath[3]	Euthanasia; other agents preferred
Halothane	0.5-2.0 ml/L bath or vaporize then bubble in water[3]	Anesthetic levels difficult to control, resulting in overdose; not recommended
Isoflurane	0.5-2.0 ml/L bath or vaporize then bubble in water[3]	Anesthetic levels difficult to control, resulting in overdose; not recommended

Table 3. Chemical restraint/anesthetic agents used in fish (cont.)

Agent	Dosage	Comments
Ketamine	—	Ketamine combination follows
	66-88 mg/kg IM[12]	Immobilization for short procedures; complete recovery can take > 1 hr
Ketamine (K)/ medetomidine (M)	(K) 1-2 mg/kg / (M) 0.05-0.1 mg/kg IM[3]	Immobilization; reverse (M) with atipamezole 0.2 mg/kg IM
Lidocaine	—	Local anesthetic; use cautiously in small fish; do not exceed 1-2 mg/kg total dose[3]
Medetomidine		See ketamine for combination
Metomidate (Marinil, Wildlife Pharmaceuticals)	—	Not currently available in US; stock solution: 10 g/L; store stock in dark container; some fish turn very dark transiently; gouramis may be sensitive; contraindicated in cichlids in water of pH < 5
	0.06-0.20 mg/L water[12]	Transport sedation
	0.5-1.0 mg/L water[3]	Light sedation
	2.5-5.0 mg/L water[3]	Heavy sedation
	5-10 mg/L bath[3]	Anesthesia; some species require 10-30 mg/L bath
	2.5-5.0 mg/L bath induction; 0.2-0.3 mg/L maintenance[12]	Marine fish/anesthesia
	1-10 mg/L bath induction; 0.1-1.0 mg/L maintenance[12]	Freshwater fish/anesthesia
MS-222	—	See tricaine methanesulfonate
Quinaldine sulfate (Current Research Laboratories)	50-100 mg/L bath induction; 15-60 mg/L maintenance[3]	Anesthesia; not sold as fish anesthetic in US; stock solution: 10 g/L, buffer the acidity by adding sodium bicarbonate to saturation; store stock in dark container; shelf-life of stock extended by refrigeration or freezing; aerate water to prevent hypoxemia; drug not metabolized, excreted unchanged; euthanasia: keep in solution > 10 min after breathing stops

Table 3. Chemical restraint/anesthetic agents used in fish (cont.)

Agent	Dosage	Comments
Sodium bicarbonate	30 g/L bath[9]	Euthanasia; generates CO_2; use when other agents unavailable; keep in solution > 10 min after breathing stops
Sodium bicarbonate tablets (Alka-Seltzer, Bayer)	2 tablets/ 0.5-1.0 L bath[1]	Euthanasia; generates CO_2; use when other agents unavailable; keep in solution > 10 min after breathing stops
Pentobarbital	60 mg/kg IP[9]	Euthanasia
Tricaine methanesulfonate (MS-222; Finquel, Argent)	50-100 mg/L bath induction; 50-60 mg/L maintenance[12] 100-200 mg/L bath induction; 50-100 mg/L maintenance[3]	Anesthesia; stock solution: 10 g/L, buffer the acidity by adding sodium bicarbonate to saturation; store stock in dark container; shelf-life of stock extended by refrigeration or freezing; stock that develops an oily film should be discarded; aerate water to prevent hypoxemia; narrower margin of safety in young fish, and soft, warm water; euthanasia: keep in solution > 10 min after breathing stops
	15-50 mg/L water[3]	Sedation
	1 g/L spray[9]	Large fish/ anesthesia; spray onto gills with an aerosol pump sprayer

[a] Not to be used in fish for human consumption.
[b] Preferable to treat single fish of a species to determine toxicity.
[c] Aerate water during anesthetic procedures. Dissolved oxygen concentrations should be maintained between 6 and 10 ppm.

Table 4. Miscellaneous agents used in fish [a-c]

Agent	Dosage	Comments
Atropine	0.1 mg/kg IM, IP, IV[11]	Organophosphate, chlorinated hydrocarbon toxicity
Carbon, activated	75 g/40 L tank water[9]	Removal of medications and other organics from water; usually added to filter system; discard after 2 wk; 75 g ≈ 250 ce dry volume
Carp pituitary extract	5 mg/kg IM, repeat in 6 hr[13]	Dose when combined with human chorionic gonadotropin (20 IU/kg); hormone to stimulate release of eggs; does not cause eggs to mature: do not administer unless eggs are mature
Chlorine/chloramine neutralizer	Use as directed	See sodium thiosulfate
Dexamethasone	1-2 mg/kg IM, IP[13]	Adjunct to treatment of shock, trauma, chronic stress syndromes
	2 mg/kg IP, IV q12h[6]	Chlorine toxicity; may improve prognosis
Doxapram	5 mg/kg IP, IV[11]	Respiratory depression
Epinephrine (1:1000)	0.2-0.5 ml IM, IP, IV, IC[11]	Cardiac arrest
Furosemide	2-5 mg/kg IM q12-72h[13]	Diuretic; ascites, generalized edema
Haloperidol	0.5 mg/kg IM[13]	Dopamine blocking agent; use with LRH-A to stimulate release of eggs
Human chorionic gonadotropin (hCG)	30 IU/kg IM, repeat in 6 hr[13]	Hormone to stimulate release of eggs; does not cause eggs to mature: do not administer unless eggs are mature
	20 IU/kg IM, repeat in 6 hr[13]	Dose when combined with carp pituitary extract (5 mg/kg)
Hydrocortisone	1-4 mg/kg IM, IP[13]	Adjunct to treatment of shock, trauma, chronic stress syndromes
Hydrogen peroxide (3%)	0.25 ml/L water[9]	Acute environmental hypoxia; see oxygen

Table 4. Miscellaneous agents used in fish (cont.)

Agent	Dosage	Comments
LRH-A	2 μg/kg IM, then 8 μg/kg 6 hr later[13]	Synthetic luteinizing hormone analog; stimulates release of eggs; does not cause eggs to mature: do not administer unless eggs are mature; in species that do not respond to LRH-A alone, administer with haloperidol or reserpine with the first injection of LRH-A
Nitrifying bacteria	Use as directed for commercial products Add material (e.g. floss, gravel) from a tank with an active biological filter and healthy fish to new tank[9]	Seed or improve development of biological filtration to detoxify ammonia and nitrate; numerous commercial preparations; do not expose products to extreme temperatures; use before expiration date
Oxygen (100%)	Fill plastic bag with O_2 containing $1/3$ vol of water[6]	Acute environmental hypoxia, common with transportation; close bag tightly with rubberband; keep fish in bag until normal swimming and respiratory behavior
Reserpine	50 mg/kg IM[13]	Dopamine blocking agent; use with LRH-A to stimulate release of eggs
Salt (sodium chloride)	1-3 g/L tank water[4] 3-5 g/L tank water[9]	Freshwater fish/ prevention of stress-induced mortality; seawater or artificial seasalts preferred; use only noniodized table/rock salts; some anticaking agents in solar salts are highly toxic; highly variable species sensitivity to salt (many catfish sensitive); may be toxic to plants
	Add chloride to produce at least a 6:1 ratio (w/w) of $Cl:NO_2$ ions[9]	Treatment of nitrite toxicity; amount of Cl^- needed (mg/L) = [6 x (NO_2^- in water)] - (Cl^- in water); table/rock salt = 60% Cl, artificial sea salts = 55% Cl

Table 4. Miscellaneous agents used in fish (cont.)

Agent	Dosage	Comments
Sodium thiosulfate	Use as directed for chlorine/chloramine neutralizers 10 mg/L tank water[6] 10 g neutralizes chlorine (up to 2 mg/L) from 1000 L water[6] 100 mg/L tank water[11]	Active ingredient in numerous chlorine/chloramine neutralizers; chlorine and chloramine are common additions to municipal water supplies and are toxic to fish; ammonia released by detoxification of chloramine is removed by functioning biological filter (see nitrifying bacteria) or chemical means (see zeolite) Chlorine exposure
Zeolite (clinoptilite; Ammonex, Argent)	Use as directed 20 g/L tank water[9]	Ion-exchange resin that exchanges ammonia for sodium ions; clinoptilite is an active form of zeolite; used to reduce or prevent ammonia toxicity

[a]   Not to be used in fish for human consumption.
[b]   Preferable to treat single fish of a species to determine toxicity.
[c]   Bath treatment: Remove fish from resident aquarium and place in container with known volume of water and concentration of therapeutic agent. Watch closely for signs of toxicity, eg, listing and dyspnea. Always keep water well aerated.

Appendix 1. Literature cited—Fish

1. Gratzek JB, Shotts EB, Dawe DL. Infectious diseases and parasites of freshwater ornamental fish. In: Gratzek JB, Matthews FR (eds). *Aquariology: The Science of Fish Health Management*. Tetra Press, Morris Plains, NJ, 1992. Pp 227-274.

2. Harms CA. Treatments for parasitic diseases of aquarium and ornamental fish. *Sem Avian Exotic Pet Med* 5:54-63, 1996.

3. Harms CA. Anesthesia in fish. In: Fowler ME, Miller RE (eds). *Zoo & Wild Animal Medicine: Current Therapy 4*. WB Saunders Co, Philadelphia, 1999. Pp 158-163.

4. Lewbart GA. Emergency pet fish medicine. In: Bonagura JD (ed). *Kirk's Current Veterinary Therapy XII: Small Animal Practice*. WB Saunders Co, Philadelphia, 1995. Pp 1369-1374.

5. Lewbart GA. Antibiotic use in ornamental fish. *Proc Am Assoc Zoo Vet/Am Assoc Wildl Vet Joint Conf*: 362-365, 1998.

6. Lewbart GA. Emergency and critical care of fish. *Vet Clin N Am: Exotic Anim Pract* 1:233-249, 1998.

7. Lewbart GA. Koi medicine and management. *Suppl Comp Contin Educ Pract Vet* 20, 3(A):5-12, 1998.

8. Lewbart G, Vaden S, Deen J, et al. Pharmacokinetics of enrofloxacin in the red pacu (*Colossoma brachypomum*) after intramuscular, oral and bath administration. *J Vet Pharmacol Therap* 20:124-128, 1997.

9. Noga EJ. *Fish Disease: Diagnosis and Treatment*. Mosby, St. Louis, 1996.

10. Reimschuessel R, Chamie SJ, Kinnel M. Evaluation of gentamicin-induced nephrotoxicosis in toadfish. *J Am Vet Med Assoc* 209:137-139, 1996.

11. Stoskopf MK. Appendix V: chemotherapeutics. In: Stoskopf MK (ed). *Fish Medicine*. WB Saunders Co, Philadelphia, 1993. Pp 832-839.

12. Stoskopf MK. Anesthesia of pet fishes. In: Bonagura JD (ed). *Kirk's Current Veterinary Therapy XII: Small Animal Practice*. WB Saunders Co, Philadelphia, 1995. Pp 1365-1369.

13. Stoskopf MK. Fish pharmacotherapeutics. In: Fowler ME, Miller RE (eds). *Zoo & Wild Animal Medicine: Current Therapy 4*. WB Saunders Co, Philadelphia, 1999. Pp 182-189.

14. Whitaker BR. Preventive medicine programs for fish. In: Fowler ME, Miller RE (eds). *Zoo & Wild Animal Medicine: Current Therapy 4*. WB Saunders Co, Philadelphia, 1999. Pp 163-181.

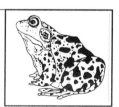

Table 5. Antimicrobial agents used in amphibians [a,b]

Agent	Dosage	Comments
Amikacin	5 mg/kg SC, IM, ICe q24[37]-48h[7,20,34]	Most species; may be used in combination with piperacillin[37]
	5 mg/kg IM q36h[17]	Bullfrogs/PD
Carbenicillin	100 mg/kg SC, IM, q72h[7]	
	200 mg/kg SC, IM, ICe q24h[20]	
Chloramphenicol	50 mg/kg SC, IM, ICe q12-24h[7,20]	
	20 mg/L bath[20]	Change daily
Ciprofloxacin	500 mg/75 L (6.7 mg/L) bath[37]	May be used when large numbers of animals require treatment; always conduct clinical sampling prior to treatment
Doxycycline (Vibramycin, Pfizer)	10-50 mg/kg PO q24h[23]	African clawed frogs/chlamydiosis
Enrofloxacin	5-10 mg/kg PO, SC, IM q24h[17,20,34]	Most/PD (bullfrogs)[17]
Gentamicin	2-4 mg/kg IM q72h × 4 treatments[12]	Salamanders, frogs, toads/*Aeromonas hydrophila* (red leg)
	2.5 mg/kg IM q72h[26]	Salamanders (ie, *Necturus*)/PD; can be administered in dorsal lymph sac of anurans;[7] more frequent dosing may be needed if temperature > 4°C (39.2 °F)
	3 mg/kg IM q24h @ 22.2 °C (72 °F)[27]	Leopard frogs/PD; at higher temperatures, serum concentrations will be lower
	1.3 mg/L × 1 hr bath q24h × 7 days[12,23]	Bacterial dermatoses; can be toxic
	Topical to eyes[33]	All/ocular infections; dilute to 2 mg/ml
Isoniazid	12.5 mg/L bath[23]	Mycobacteriosis
Nifurpirinol (Furanace, Dainippon)	250 mg/38 L × 1 hr bath q24h[12]	Salamanders, frogs, toads/*Aeromonas hydrophila* (red leg)

Table 5. Antimicrobial agents used in amphibians (cont.)

Agent	Dosage	Comments
Nitrofurazone	10-20 mg/L bath to effect[20]	Change daily
Oxytetracycline	25 mg/kg SC, IM q24h[20]	Most species
	50 mg/kg PO q12-24h[20,34]	Most species
	50 mg/kg IM q48h[17]	Bullfrogs/PD;[17] especially useful in cases of chlamydiosis (use up to 30 days)[37]
	100 mg/L × 1 hr bath[34]	Most species
	1 g/kg feed × 7 days[20]	
Piperacillin	100 mg/kg SC, IM q24h[23,34]	Anaerobes; may be used in combination with amikacin[37]
Potassium permanganate	200 mg/L × 5 min bath[20]	
Silver sulfadiazine (Silvadine Cream 1%, Marion)	Topical q24h[5]	Antibiotic cream
Sulfadiazine	132 mg/kg PO q24h[20]	
Sulfamethazine	1 g/L bath to effect[20]	Change daily
Tetracycline	167 mg/kg (5 mg/30 g) PO q12h × 7 days[12]	Salamanders, frogs, toads/ *Aeromonas hydrophila* (red leg)
	50 mg/kg PO q12h[7]	Salamanders, frogs, toads
	150 mg/kg PO × 5-7 days[31]	Salamanders, frogs, toads
Trimethoprim/sulfa	3 mg/kg PO, SC, IM q24h[7]	

[a] Water baths containing antibiotics are generally unreliable and less preferable than parenteral administration.

[b] SC can be administered in dorsal lymph sac of anurans.[8]

26

Table 6. Antifungal agents used in amphibians

Agent	Dosage	Comments
Benzalkonium chloride	2 mg/L × 1 hr bath q24h[20,23,32]	Saprolegniasis
	1:4,000,000 bath[20]	Saprolegniasis; change water 3x/wk
Ketoconazole	10 mg/kg PO q24h[20]	
	Topical[9]	Terrestrial species
Malachite green	0.15-0.20 mg/L × 1 hr bath q24h[12,34]	Salamanders, frogs, toads/ cutaneous mycoses (*Saprolegnia, Phialophora*); caution: mutagenic, teratogenic; potentially toxic
Mercurochrome	4 mg/L water × 1 hr bath q24h[32]	Saprolegniasis
Methylene blue	2-4 mg/L bath to effect[7,20]	Tadpoles/reduces mortality in newly hatched tadpoles
	4 mg/L bath × 1 hr bath q24h[32]	Saprolegniasis
Miconazole	5 mg/kg ICe q24h × 14-28 days[34]	Systemic mycoses
Potassium permanganate	1:5000 water × 5 min bath q24h[4]	Salamanders, frogs, toads/ cutaneous mycoses (*Saprolegnia, Phialophora*)
Tolnaftate (Tinavet Cream 1%, Schering)	Topical[12]	Salamanders, frogs, toads/ cutaneous mycoses (*Saprolegnia, Phialophora*)

Table 7. Antiparasitic agents used in amphibians [a,b]

Agent	Dosage	Comments
Acriflavin	0.025% bath × 5 days[20]	Protozoa
	500 mg/L × 30 min bath[30]	Protozoa
Benzalkonium chloride	2 mg/L × 1 hr bath q24h to effect[30]	Protozoa
Copper sulfate	500 mg/L × 2 min bath q24h to effect[20]	Some protozoa
Fenbendazole	—	Fenbendazole combinations follow
	30-50 mg/kg PO[8]	GI nematodes
	50 mg/kg PO q24h × 3-5 days, repeat in 14-21 days[35]	Resistant nematode infections
	50-100 mg/kg PO,[19,23,34] repeat in 2-3 wk prn	Most species/GI nematodes
	100 mg/kg PO,[28] repeat in 14 days	GI nematodes
Fenbendazole (F)/ ivermectin (I)	(F) 100 mg/kg PO on day 1, then (I) 0.2 mg/kg PO on days 2,11[28]	GI nematodes
Fenbendazole (F)/ metronidazole (M)	(F) 100 mg/kg PO, repeat in 10-14 days/ (M) 10 mg/kg PO q24h for 5 days[28]	Concurrent GI nematodes and protozoa
Formalin (10%)	1.5 ml/L × 10 min bath q48h to effect[20]	Monogenic trematodes
Ivermectin	0.2-0.4 mg/kg PO, SC, repeat q14d prn[8]	Nematodes, including lungworms; mites
	2 mg/kg topical to thorax,[20,34] repeat in 2-3 wk	Especially useful for small specimens[35] and *Rana* sp.
Levamisole	10 mg/kg topical,[35] IM,[7] repeat in 2 wk	Nematodes, including lungworms
	12 mg/L bath × 4 days[11]	African clawed frogs/cutaneous nematodes (*Capillaria*); use ≥ 4.2 L of tank water/frog

Table 7. Antiparasitic agents used in amphibians (cont.)

Agent	Dosage	Comments
Levamisole (continued)	100-300 mg/L × 24 hr bath, repeat in 1-2 wk[35]	Nematodes, including subcutaneous nematodes in aquatic amphibians; water soluble form is available through aquaculture supply companies
	100 mg/L × ≤ 72 hr bath[35]	Resistant nematodes
Malachite green	0.15 mg/L × 1 hr bath q24h to effect[20]	Protozoa; caution: mutagenic, teratogenic; potentially toxic
Metronidazole	—	See fenbendazole combinations
	10 mg/kg PO q24h × 5-10 days[28,35]	Protozoa; for unfamiliar or sensitive species
	50 mg/kg PO q24h × 3-5 days[35]	Confirmed cases of amoebiasis and flagellate overload
	100 mg/kg PO q3d[9]	Protozoa
	100-150 mg/kg PO, repeat in 2-3 wk or prn[20,31,34,35]	Protozoa (ie, *Entamoeba, Hexamita, Opalina*)
	500 mg/100 g feed × 3-4 treatments[7,20]	Ciliates
	0.05 ml of 1.008 mg/ml on dorsum q24h × 3 days[18]	Fire-bellied toads (1.8 g)/ protozoa; rinse 1 hr after treatment; results in absorption of 23 mg/kg BW of metronidazole
	50 mg/L × 24 hr bath[23,35]	Aquatic amphibians/protozoa
Oxfendazole	5 mg/kg PO[31]	GI nematodes
Oxytetracycline	25 mg/kg SC, IM q24h[30]	Protozoa
	50 mg/kg PO q12h[30]	Protozoa
	1 g/kg feed × 7 days[30]	Protozoa
Paromomycin (Humatin, Parke Davis)	50-75 mg/kg PO q24h[34]	GI protozoa
Piperazine	50 mg/kg PO, repeat in 2 wk[12]	Salamanders, frogs, toads/ GI nematodes (ie, *Oxsomatium*)

Table 7. Antiparasitic agents used in amphibians (cont.)

Agent	Dosage	Comments
Potassium permanganate	7 mg/L × 5 min bath q24h to effect[20,30]	Ectoparasitic protozoa
Praziquantel	8 mg/kg PO, SC, IM,[13] repeat in 2 wk	Trematodes, cestodes
	8-24 mg/kg PO[28]	Trematodes, cestodes
	10 mg/L × 3 hr bath[34]	Trematodes, cestodes
Salt (sodium chloride)	4-6 g/L bath[20]	Ectoparasitic protozoa
	6 g/L × 5-10 min bath q24h x 3-5 days[30]	Ectoparasitic protozoa
	25 g/L × 10 min bath[13]	Ectoparasitic protozoa
Sulfadiazine	132 mg/kg q24h[30]	Coccidiosis
Sulfamethazine	1 g/L bath[30]	Coccidiosis; change daily to effect
Tetracycline	50 mg/kg PO q12h[30]	Protozoa
Thiabendazole	50-100 mg/kg PO,[12,23] repeat in 2 wk prn	Salamanders, frogs, toads/GI nematodes (ie,*Ophidascaris*)
	100 mg/L bath, repeat in 2 wk[32]	Verminous (capillariid) dermatitis
Trimethoprim/sulfa	3 mg/kg PO, SC, IM q24h[30]	Coccidiosis

[a] Baths are for aquatic species.
[b] SC can be administered in dorsal lymph sac of anurans.

Table 8. Chemical restraint/anesthetic/analgesic agents used in amphibians [a]

Agent	Dosage	Comments
Benzocaine (Sigma Chemical)	—	Anesthesia; not sold as fish anesthetic in US; available from chemical supply companies; do not use topical anesthetic products marketed for mammals prepare stock solution in ethanol; (poorly soluble in water); store in dark bottle at room temperature
	50 mg/L bath to effect[8]	Larvae/dissolve in ethanol first
	200-300 mg/L bath to effect[8]	Frogs, salamanders/dissolve in ethanol first
	200-500 mg/L bath[6]	Dissolve in acetone first
Buprenorphine (Buprenex, Reckitt & Colman)	0.01-0.03 mg/kg SC, IM[2]	Analgesia; dosage not determined,[9] but assumed to be similar to that in select mammals[2]
Butorphanol (Torbugesic, Fort-Dodge)	0.2-0.4 mg/kg IM[22]	Analgesia; dosage not determined,[9] but assumed to be similar to that in mammals
Diazepam	—	See ketamine combination
Halothane	4-5% to effect[8]	Terrestrial species/induction chamber
	Bubbled into water to effect[23]	Aquatic species
	5%[3]	Terrestrial species/euthanasia; induction chamber
Isoflurane	—	Anesthesia; induction chamber; inhalant of choice
	3-5% induction, 1-2% maintenance[22]	Terrestrial species
	0.28 ml/100 ml bath[29]	Induce in closed container
	Bubbled into water to effect[23]	Aquatic species
	Topical application of liquid isoflurane[29]	*Bufo* sp. (0.015 ml/g BW),[29] African clawed frog (0.007 ml/g BW)[29]/induce in closed container; once induced, remove excess from animal

31

Table 8. Chemical restraint/anesthetic/analgesic agents used in amphibians (cont.)

Agent	Dosage	Comments
Isoflurane (continued)	Topical mixture of isoflurane (3.0 ml), KY jelly (3.5 ml), and water (1.5 ml)[29,36]	*Bufo* sp. (0.035 ml/g BW),[29] African clawed frog (0.025 ml/g BW)[29]/induce in closed container; once induced, remove excess from animal
	5%[3]	Terrestrial species/euthanasia; induction chamber
Ketamine	—	May have long induction and recovery times; does not provide good analgesia so may not be suited for major surgical procedures;[29] other agents preferred; ketamine combination follows; see lidocaine
	10-50 mg/kg SC, IM[6]	Most species
	75-100 mg/kg IM[36]	Surgical plane of anesthesia; use lower dosage (30 mg/kg) for sedation
	50-150 mg/kg SC, IM[8]	Most species
Ketamine (K)/ diazepam (D)	(K) 20-40 mg/kg/ (D) 0.2-0.4 mg/kg IM[22]	Variable results
Lidocaine 1-2%	Local infiltration[14]	All/local anesthesia; with or without epinephrine; 2% lidocaine in combination with ketamine has been used for minor surgeries;[22] use with caution
Methoxyflurane	0.5-1.0 ml in 1 L container (cotton soaked)[14]	Induction in 2 min; surgical anesthesia maintained for about 30 min; recovery within 7 hr; not recommended because of potential of overdose[22]
Pentobarbital sodium	40-50 mg/kg IP[22]	Frogs, toads/seldom used; other agents preferred; can also administer in dorsal lymph sac; anesthesia and recovery are prolonged
	60 mg/kg ICe,[3] IV	Euthanasia; ICe is preferred route; can also be administered in lymph sacs in anurans

Table 8. Chemical restraint/anesthetic/analgesic agents used in amphibians (cont.)

Agent	Dosage	Comments
Propofol (Rapinovet, Pitman-Moore; Depriван, Zeneca)	10-30 mg/kg ICe[36]	Pilot study in White's tree frogs/ use the lower dosage for sedation or light anesthesia; induction within 30 min; recovery in 24 hr
Tiletamine/ zolazepam (Telazol, Fort Dodge)	10-20 mg/kg IM[22]	Results variable between species; recovery rapid; not suitable as single anesthetic agent for anurans[15]
Tricaine methanesulfonate (MS-222) (Finquel, Argent)	—	Anesthesia; stock solution: 10 g/L, buffer the acidity by adding sodium bicarbonate to saturation or bath solutions can be buffered to a pH of 7.0-7.1 with Na_2HPO_4 (34 ml of Na_2HPO_4:2 L of 1 g/L MS-222 solution) and aerated with 100% O_2 if possible;[5] store stock in dark container; shelf-life of stock extended by refrigeration or freezing; stock that develops an oil film should be discarded; aerate water to prevent hypoxemia; overdosing with MS-222 can readily occur; following bath, place terrestrial amphibians on moist towel or in very shallow water to recover;[7] some species can be induced at much lower concentrations than listed here;[29] in some cases, anesthesia can be maintained by dripping a dilute solution of this drug (100-200 mg/L) over the skin or by covering animal with a paper towel moistened with the anesthetic[29]
	1 g/L bath to effect[10,29]	Most gill-less adult species (unless very large)/induction; maintenance at 100-200 mg/L[29]
	100-200 mg/L bath to effect[29]	Larvae/induction; less may be required for maintenance
	200-500 mg/L bath to effect[8]	Tadpoles, newts/induction in 15-30 min
	0.5-2.0 g/L bath to effect[8]	Frogs, salamanders/induction in 15-30 min

33

Table 8. Chemical restraint/anesthetic/analgesic agents used in amphibians (cont.)

Agent	Dosage	Comments
Tricaine methanesulfonate (continued)	2-3 g/L bath to effect[29]	Toads/induction; takes 15-30 min
	50-200 mg/kg SC, IM, ICe[8,10]	Most species; may be irritating administered SC, IM (neutral solution is preferred)[10]
	100-200 mg/kg ICe[25]	Leopard frogs
	100-400 mg/kg ICe[25]	Bullfrogs
	10 g/L bath[3]	Euthanasia; can be administered ICe or in lymph sacs

a   SC can be administered in dorsal lymph sac in anurans.

Table 9. Hormones used in amphibians [a]

Agent	Dosage	Comments
Gonadotropin-releasing hormone (GnRH)	0.1 mg/kg SC, IM, repeat prn[20]	Induction of ovulation in those non-responsive to PMSG or hCG; administer to females 8-12 hr before males
Human chorionic gonadotropin (hCG)	50-100[8] to 300[20] IU SC, IM	For mating or release of sperm in males; follow with GnRH in 8-24 hr
	250-400 IU SC, IM[8]	African clawed frogs, axolotls, etc/induction of ovulation; may be used with PMSG and/or progesterone
Pregnant mare serum gonadotropin (PMSG)	50 IU SC, IM[8]	African clawed frogs, axolotls, etc/induction of ovulation; administer 600 IU hCG IM, SC 72 hr later[20]
Progesterone	1-5 mg SC, IM[8]	African clawed frogs, axolotls, etc/used in addition to PMSG or hCG for induction of ovulation

a SC can be administered into the dorsal lymph sac of anurans.

Table 10. Miscellaneous agents used in amphibians [a]

Agent	Dosage	Comments
Amphibian Ringer's solution (ARS)	6.6 g NaCl, 0.15 g KCl, 0.15 g $CaCl_2$, and 0.2 g $NaHCO_3$ in 1 L water[9]	For treating hydrocoelom and subcutaneous edema in septic animals; place animal in shallow ARS bath until stabilized ($\approx$ 24 hr or more); may need to wean animal off ARS by placing it in gradually more dilute solutions[37]
Calcium gluconate	100-200 mg/kg SC[9]	Nutritional hypocalcemia
Cyanoacrylate surgical adhesive (Vet Bond, 3M)	Topical on wounds[9]	Produces a seal for aquatic and semiaquatic species
Dexamethasone	1.5 mg/kg SC, IM[33]	Vascularizing keratitis
Emeraid-II (Lafeber) and Repto-Min (Tetra Sales)	<2% BW PO q24h[34]	Nutritional support; generally gavaged
Hill's Feline A/D (Hill's)	PO[9]	Nutritional support; mix 1:1 with water; generally gavaged
Laxative (Laxatone, Evsco)	PO[9]	Laxative, especially for intestinal foreign bodies
Orabase (Colgate)	Topical on wounds[9]	Protective water-resistant ointment; antibiotics can be incorporated into the ointment[9]
Vitamin B1	25 mg/kg feed fish[20]	Deficiency resulting from thiaminase-containing fish
Vitamin E (alpha-tocopherol)	200 IU/kg feed[20]	Deficiency resulting from improperly stored feed fish
Waltham Feline Concentration (Waltham)	PO[9]	Nutritional support; mix 120 ml with 40-80 ml water; generally gavaged

[a] SC can be administered into the dorsal lymph sac of anurans.

35

Appendix 2. Physiological and hematologic values of amphibians [a,1,8]

Measurement	Leopard frog (Rana pipiens) ♂♂	Leopard frog (Rana pipiens) ♀♀	American bullfrog (Rana catesbeiana)	Grass frog (Rana temporria)	Edible frog (Rana esculenta)	Cuban tree frog (Hyla septentrionalis)	African clawed frog (Xenopus laevis)	Mud-puppy (Necturus maculatus)	Tiger salamander (Ambystoma tigrinum)
Body wt (g)	25-42	25-46	225-306	—	—	28-35	—	—	35
RBC ($10^3/\mu l$)	227-767	174-701	450	461	308	—	566	20	1657
PCV (%)	19-52	16-51	39-42	—	—	20-24	—	21	40
Hgb (g/dl)	3.8-14.6	2.7-14.0	9.3-9.7	14.34	9.7	5.6-6.8	14.86	4.6	9.4
MCV (fl)	722-916	730-916	—	—	—	—	—	10,070	—
MCH (pg)	182-221	182-238	—	—	—	—	—	2160	—
MCHC (g/dl)	22.7-26.8	19.9-27.7	21.1-25.9	—	—	25-31	—	22	—
Blood volume (ml/100 g body wt)	—	—	3.1-3.6	—	—	7.2-7.8	—	—	—
WBC ($10^3/\mu l$)	3.1-22.2	2.8-25.9	—	14.4	6.1	—	8.2	—	4.6
Early stages (%)	—	—	—	1.5	1.0	—	0.7	—	—
Neutrophils (%)	—	—	—	6.5±1.0	8.8±2.1	—	8.0±1.1	—	—
Eosinophils (%)	—	—	—	14.5±2.9	19.4±1.3	—	?	—	—
Basophils (%)	—	—	—	24.2±2.2	16.6±1.3	—	8.5±1.4	—	—
Monocytes (%)	—	—	—	0.8	1.3	—	0.5	—	—
Plasmocytes (%)	—	—	—	0.4	1.0	—	0.2	—	—
Lymphocytes (%)	—	—	—	68.5±2.9	52.0±3.3	—	65.3±2.7	—	—
Thrombocytes ($10^3/\mu l$)	—	—	—	20.8	16.3	—	17.1	—	—

[a] Hematology is presently of limited diagnostic value because of the lack of normal data and the wide variation in hematologic and biochemical values according to sex, season, and state of hydration.

Appendix 3. Literature cited—Amphibians

1. Anver MR, Pond CL. Biology and diseases of amphibians. In: Fox JG, Cohen BJ, Loew FM (eds). *Laboratory Animal Medicine*. Academic Press, Orlando, FL, 1984: 427-447.

2. Bennett A. Personal communication. 1999.

3. Burns RB, McMahan W. Euthanasia methods for ectothermic vertebrates. In: Bonagura JD (ed). *Kirk's Current Veterinary Therapy XII: Small Animal Practice*. WB Saunders Co, Philadelphia, 1995:1379-1381.

4. Campbell TW. Amphibian husbandry and medical care. In: Rosenthal KL (ed). *Practical Exotic Animal Medicine* (Compendium Collection). Veterinary Learning Systems, Trenton, NJ, 1997:65-68.

5. Carpenter JW. Personal communication. 1999.

6. Cooper JE. Anesthesia of exotic animals. *Anim Technol* 35:13-20, 1984.

7. Crawshaw GJ. Medical care of amphibians. *Proc Am Assoc Zoo Vet*: 155-165, 1989.

8. Crawshaw GJ. Amphibian medicine. In: Fowler ME (ed). *Zoo & Wild Animal Medicine: Current Therapy 3*. WB Saunders Co, Philadelphia, 1993. Pp 131-139.

9. Crawshaw GJ. Amphibian emergency and critical care. *Vet Clin N Am: Exotic Anim Pract* 1:207-231, 1998.

10. Downes H. Tricaine anesthesia in amphibia: a review. *Bull Assoc Rept Amph Vet* 5:11-16, 1995.

11. Iglauer F, Willmann F, Hilken G, et al. Anthelmintic treatment to eradicate cutaneous capillariasis in a colony of South African clawed frogs (*Xenopus laevis*). *Lab Anim Sci* 47:477-482, 1997.

12. Jacobson E, Kollias GV, Peters LJ. Dosages for antibiotics and parasiticides used in exotic animals. *Compend Contin Educ Pract Vet* 5:315-324, 1983.

13. Jenkins JR. A formulary for reptile and amphibian medicine. *Proc Fourth Annu Avian/Exotic Anim Med Symp*, University of California, Davis, CA: 24-27, 1991.

14. Johnson JH. Anesthesia, analgesia and euthanasia of reptiles and amphibians. Proc Am *Assoc Zoo Vet*: 132-138, 1991.

15. Letcher J. Evaluation of use of tiletamine/zolazepam for anesthesia of bullfrogs and leopard frogs. *J Am Vet Med Assoc* 207:80-82, 1995.

16. Letcher J, Glade M. Efficacy of ivermectin as an anthelmintic in leopard frogs. *J Am Vet Med Assoc* 200:537-538, 1992.

17. Letcher J, Papich M. Pharmacokinetics of intramuscular administration of three antibiotics in bullfrogs (*Rana catesbeiana*). *Proc Assoc Rept Amph Vet/Am Assoc Zoo Vet*: 79-93, 1994.

18. Mombarg M, Claessen H, Lambrechts L, Zwart P. Quantification of percutaneous absorption of metronidazole and levamisole in the fire-bellied toad (*Bombina orientalis*). *J Vet Pharmacol Therap* 15:433-436, 1992.

19. Poynton SL, Whitaker BR. Protozoa in poison dart frogs (*Dentrobatidae*): Clinical assessment and identification. *J Zoo Wildl Med* 25:29-39, 1994.

20. Raphael BL: Amphibians. *Vet Clin N Am: Small Anim Pract* 23:1271-1286, 1993.

21. Schaeffer DO. Anesthesia and analgesia in nontraditional laboratory animal species. In: Kohn DF, Wixson SK, White WJ, Benson GJ (eds). *Anesthesia and Analgesia in Laboratory Animals*. Academic Press, New York, 1997: 337-378.

22. Schumacher J. Reptiles and amphibians. In: Lumb WV, Jones EW (eds). 2nd ed. *Veterinary Anesthesia*. Williams & Wilkins, Philadelphia, 1996. Pp 670-685.

23. Stein G. Reptile and amphibian formulary. In: Mader DR (ed). *Reptile Medicine and Surgery*. WB Saunders Co, Philadelphia, 1996. Pp 465-472.

24. Stetter MD, Raphael B, Indiviglio F, Cook RA. Isoflurane anesthesia in amphibians: comparison of five application methods. *Proc Am Assoc Zoo Vet*: 255-257, 1996.

25. Stoskopf MK. Pain and analgesia in birds, reptiles, amphibians, and fish. *Invest Ophthalmol Visual Sci* 35:775-780, 1994.

26. Stoskopf MK, Arnold J, Mason M. Aminoglycoside antibiotic levels in the aquatic

salamander (*Necturus necturus*). *J Zoo Anim Med* 18:81-85, 1987.

27. Teare JA, Wallace RS, Bush M. Pharmacology of gentamicin in the leopard frog (*Rana pipiens*). *Proc Am Assoc Zoo Vet*: 128-131, 1991.

28. Whitaker BR. Developing an effective quarantine program for amphibians. *Proc N Am Vet Conf*: 764-765, 1997.

29. Whitaker BR, Wright KM, Barnett SL. Basic husbandry and clinical assessment of the amphibian patient. *Vet Clin N Am: Exotic Anim Pract* 2:265-290, 1999.

30. Willette-Frahm M, Wright KM, Thode BC. Select protozoan diseases in amphibians and reptiles. *Bull Assoc Rept Amph Vet* 5:19-29, 1995.

31. Williams DL. Amphibians. In: Beynon PH, Cooper JE (eds). *Manual of Exotic Pets*. British Small Animal Veterinary Association, Gloucestershire, UK, 1991. Pp 261-271.

32. Williams DL. Amphibian dermatology. In: Bonagura JD (ed). *Kirk's Current Veterinary Therapy XII: Small Animal Practice*. WB Saunders Co, Philadelphia, 1995:1375-1379.

33. Williams DL, Whitaker BR. The amphibian eye - a clinical review. *J Zoo Wildl Med* 25:18-28, 1994.

34. Wright KM. Amphibian husbandry and medicine. In: Mader DR (ed). *Reptile Medicine and Surgery*. WB Saunders Co, Philadelphia, 1996. Pp 436-459.

35. Wright KM. Treating parasites in amphibians. *Proc N Am Vet Conf*: 772, 1997.

36. Wright KM. Anesthesia of amphibians. *Proc N Am Vet Conf*: 823, 1998.

37. Wright KM. Treating the septic amphibian. *Proc N Am Vet Conf*: 824-825, 1998.

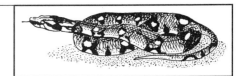

Table 11. Antimicrobial agents used in reptiles [a, b]

Agent	Dosage	Comments
Acyclovir (Zovirax, Burroughs-Wellcome)	80 mg/kg PO q24h × 10 days[108]	Tortoises/antiviral (ie, herpes virus dermatitis)
	Topical (5% ointment)[168] q12h	Tortoises/antiviral (ie, herpes virus dermatitis)
Amikacin	—	Potentially nephrotoxic; maintain hydration; frequently used with a penicillin or cephalosporin
	5 mg/kg IM, then 2.5 mg/kg q72h[131]	Snakes/PD (gopher snakes); house at high end of optimum temperature range during treatment; use 1 mg/kg for blood pythons and 2 mg/kg for black-headed and rock pythons[142]
	3 mg/kg q72h SC, IM[101]	Pythons/PD (ball pythons)
	5 mg/kg IM, then 2.5 mg/kg q72h[7,65]	Lizards
	5 mg/kg IM q24h[7]	Lizards
	5 mg/kg IM q48h[35]	Chelonians/PD (gopher tortoises)
	5 mg/kg IM, then 2.5 mg/kg q72h[135]	Chelonians
	2.5-3.0 mg/kg IM q72h x 5 treatments[198]	Sea turtles
	2.25 mg/kg IM q72h[93]	Crocodilians/PD (alligators)
	50 mg/10 ml saline × 30 min nebulization q12h[148]	Most species/pneumonia
	12.5 mg/7.5 ml DMSO q12-24h topical × 3-4 wk[184]	For deep local penetration; abscesses involving bone
Amoxicillin	22 mg/kg PO q12-24h[69]	Use with an aminoglycoside
	10 mg/kg IM q24h[193]	Use with an aminoglycoside
Ampicillin	—	May be used with an aminoglycoside
	3-6 mg/kg PO, SC, IM q12-24h[67,69]	Most species

41

Table 11. Antimicrobial agents used in reptiles (cont.)

Agent	Dosage	Comments
Ampicillin (continued)	10 mg/kg SC, IM q12h[98] or 20 mg/kg SC, IM q24h[20,184]	Most species, including chameleons
	20 mg/kg IM q24h[135,154]	Chelonians
	6 mg/kg IM q12h[94]	Chelonians/ulcerative shell disease
	50 mg/kg IM q12h[88,183]	Tortoises/preliminary study
Carbenicillin	400 mg/kg IM q24h[115]	Snakes/PD
	400 mg/kg SC, IM q24h[7]	Lizards/may be used with an aminoglycoside (administer at different time of day)
	400 mg/kg IM q48h[116]	Chelonians/PD (*Testudo* spp)
	200-400 mg/kg IM q48h[135,154]	Chelonians/may be used with an aminoglycoside; may cause skin sloughing in desert tortoises
Cefotaxime	20-40 mg/kg IM q24h[69,154]	May be used with an aminoglycoside
	100 mg/10 ml saline × 30 min nebulization q12h[148]	Most species/pneumonia
Ceftazidime (Taxidime, Eli Lilly)	20 mg/kg SC, IM, IV q72h[7,91,114]	Most species/PD (snakes); especially effective against gram-negative (ie, *Pseudomonas*); q24-48h in chameleons[187]
	20 mg/kg IM, IV q72h[191]	Sea turtles
Ceftiofur	2.2 mg/kg IM q48h[193]	Snakes
	2.2 mg/kg IM q24h[193]	Turtles
	4 mg/kg IM q24h[69]	Tortoises/respiratory infection
Cefuroxime (Zinacef, Glaxo Wellcome)	50 mg/kg IM q48h[3]	Most species
	100 mg/kg IM q24h[54,69]	Most species, including snakes/ may be used with an aminoglycoside
Cephalexin	20-40 mg/kg PO q12h[193]	Most species

42

Table 11. Antimicrobial agents used in reptiles (cont.)

Agent	Dosage	Comments
Cephaloridine	10 mg/kg SC, IM q12h[67]	Most species
Cephalothin	20-40 mg/kg IM q12h[69]	Most species
Cephazolin	20 mg/kg SC, IM q24h[130]	Most species/burns
Cephoperazone (Cefobid, Roerig)	100 mg/kg IM q96h[181]	Snakes/PD (ground snakes)
	125 mg/kg IM q24h[181]	Lizards/PD (tegus)
Chloramphenicol	—	Most species/public health concern; may result in permanent pigmentation change in chameleons given IM; may cause bone marrow suppression in water snakes;[109] because it is bacteriostatic, it has limited usefulness in reptiles
	40 mg/kg PO, SC, IM q24h, or 20 mg/kg PO, SC, IM q12h[88,94,97,135,154]	Most species/20 mg/kg may be given q24h in larger crocodilians
	40 mg/kg SC q24h[33]	Snakes/PD (gopher snakes)
	50 mg/kg SC q12-72h[40,89,92]	Snakes/PD; q12h in indigo, rat, king snakes; q24h in boids, moccasin snakes; q48h in rattlesnakes; q72h in red-bellied water snakes
	Topical ophthalmic ointment[94]	Most species
Chlorhexidine (Nolvasan 2%, Fort Dodge)	Topical 0.05% aqueous solution or ointment[36]	All species/topical disinfection; infectious stomatitis
	1:30 aqueous solution[24]	Most species/topical disinfection; infectious stomatitis; middle ear infection flush in box turtles
	1:10 aqueous solution, irrigation q24h[137]	Lizards/periodontal disease (irrigation of gingival pockets)
	1:10 dilution, soak 1 hr q12h[94]	Lizards, snakes/in conjunction with antibiotic therapy; soak at 27-30 °C (81-86 °F)

Table 11. Antimicrobial agents used in reptiles (cont.)

Agent	Dosage	Comments
Chlorhexidine (Nolvasan Wound Cleanser) (continued)	Topical[9]	Chelonians/shell infections
Chlortetracycline	200 mg/kg PO q24h[3]	Most species
Ciprofloxacin	10 mg/kg PO q48h[54] 11 mg/kg PO q48-72h[108]	Most species Pythons/PD (reticulated pythons)
Clarithromycin (Biaxin, Abbott)	15 mg/kg PO q48-72h[99,201]	Tortoises/PD (desert tortoises); upper respiratory tract disease (mycoplasmosis)
Clindamycin	2.5-5.0 mg/kg PO q12h[67] 5 mg/kg PO q24h[193]	Most species/gram + and anaerobes Most species
Dihydrostrepto-mycin	5 mg/kg IM q12-24h[69,193]	Most species/maintain hydration
Doxycycline (Vibramycin, Pfizer)	5-10 mg/kg PO q24h × 10-45 days[3,69,97] 10 mg/kg PO q24h[205] 50 mg/kg IM, then 25 mg/kg q72h[88,183]	Most species/respiratory infection (ie, mycoplasmosis); may use nystatin concurrently to prevent secondary yeast infections[142] Tortoises Tortoises
Enrofloxacin (Baytril, Bayer)	5-10 mg/kg q24h PO, SC, IM, ICe[3] 5 mg/kg PO, IM q24h[136] 10 mg/kg IM q5d[83] 6.6 mg/kg IM q24h, or 11 mg/kg IM q48h[108]	Most species/IM administration is painful and may result in tissue necrosis and sterile abscesses; may cause skin discoloration or tissue necrosis if given SC Lizards/PD (green iguanas); marked pharmacokinetic variability with PO administration may make IM more suitable in critically ill animals Monitors/PD (savannah monitors); preliminary data Pythons/PD (reticulated pythons); *Pseudomonas*

Table 11. Antimicrobial agents used in reptiles (cont.)

Agent	Dosage	Comments
Enrofloxacin (continued)	10 mg/kg IM q48h[206]	Snakes/PD (Burmese pythons); *Pseudomonas*
	10 mg/kg IM, then 5 mg/kg q48h[206]	Snakes/PD (Burmese pythons)
	5 mg/kg IM q24-48h[88,160]	Chelonians and most other reptiles/PD (gopher tortoises); hyperexcitation, incoordination, diarrhea reported in a Galapagos tortoise[38]
	5 mg/kg IM q12-24h[166]	Chelonians/PD (star tortoises); q12h for *Pseudomonas* and *Citrobacter*; q24h for other bacteria
	5 mg/kg IM q48h[198]	Sea turtles
	10 mg/kg IM q24h[183]	Chelonians/PD (Hermann's tortoises)
	5 mg/kg IV q36h[78]	Crocodilians/PD (alligators); mycoplasmosis
	1-3 ml (50 mg/250 ml sterile water) nasal flush/nostril q24-48h[97]	Upper respiratory infection; use until no discharge; use concurrently with parenteral antibiotics
	11.4 mg/7.5 ml DMSO topical q12-24h × 3-4 wk[184]	For deep local penetration; abscesses involving bone
Gentamicin	—	Nephrotoxicity has been reported especially in snakes; maintain hydration; commonly used with a penicillin or cephalosporin
	2.5 mg/kg IM q72h[33,34]	Snakes/PD (gopher snakes)
	2.5-3.0 mg/kg IM, then 1.5 mg/kg q96h[80]	Snakes/PD (blood pythons)
	3 mg/kg IM q>96h[10]	Turtles/PD (eastern box turtles); lower dose may be more appropriate
	5 mg/kg IM q72h[135,154]	Chelonians

Table 11. Antimicrobial agents used in reptiles (cont.)

Agent	Dosage	Comments
Gentamicin (continued)	6 mg/kg IM q72-96h[165]	Turtles/PD (red-eared sliders)
	2-4 mg/kg IM q72h[94]	Tortoises
	1.75-2.25 mg/kg IM q72-96h[88,93]	Crocodilians/PD (alligators); respiratory infection
	10-20 mg/15 ml saline × 30 min nebulization q12h[74]	Most species/pneumonia; acetylcysteine may be added
	40 mg/l ml DMSO/8 ml saline, nebulization[205]	Tortoises
	Topical ophthalmic ointment[94] or drops	Most species/superficial ocular infection; lesions in oral cavity[127]
Gentamicin/ betamethasone ophthalmic drops (Gentocin Durafilm, Schering-Plough)	1-2 drops to eye q12-24h[99]	Tortoises/upper respiratory infections; may also be given as a reverse nasal flush q48-72h or intranasal q12-24h
Kanamycin	10-15 mg/kg IM, IV q24h (or in divided doses)[67]	Most species/avoid in cases of dehydration or renal or hepatic dysfunction; maintain hydration
Lincomycin	5 mg/kg IM q12-24h[54] 10 mg/kg PO q24h[54]	Most species/wound infection; potentially nephrotoxic; maintain hydration
Metronidazole	20 mg/kg PO q24h × ≥7 days[90]	Most species/anaerobes; dose range 12.5-40.0 mg/kg[67]
	20 mg/kg PO q24-48h[112]	Iguanas/PD; use q24h for resistant anaerobes
	20 mg/kg PO q48h[111]	Snakes/PD (yellow rat snakes)
	50 mg/kg PO q24h × 7-14 days[108]	Most species/may be administered concurrently with amikacin for broader spectrum; because of potential side effects at this dose, a lower dose may be prudent[108]
Neomycin	10 mg/kg PO q24h[54]	Most species
Oxytetracycline	6-10 mg/kg PO, IM, IV q24h[54,67]	Most species/may produce local inflammation at injection site

Table 11. Antimicrobial agents used in reptiles (cont.)

Agent	Dosage	Comments
Oxytetracycline (continued)	5-10 mg/kg IM q24h[99]	Tortoises/upper respiratory tract infection (mycoplasmosis)
	10 mg/kg PO q24h[158]	Alligators
	10 mg/kg IM q7d[79]	Crocodilians/PD (alligators); mycoplasmosis
	10 mg/kg IV q>96h[78]	Crocodilians/PD (alligators); mycoplasmosis; dosage interval may be as long as q10d
Penicillin, benzathine	10,000 units/kg IM q48-96h[67]	Most species/frequency dependent on temperature; may be used with an aminoglycoside
Penicillin G	10,000-20,000 IU/kg SC, IM, IV, ICe q8-12h[67]	Most species/infrequently used
Piperacillin (Pipracil, Lederle)	50-100 mg/kg IM q24h[67]	Most species/broad-spectrum bactericidal agent; maintain hydration; may use with an aminoglycoside
	100-200 mg/kg IM q24-48h[98,184]	Most species (including chameleons)/can be administered SC in most species
	50 mg/kg IM, then 25 mg/kg q24h[193]	Snakes
	100 mg/kg IM q48h[81]	Snakes/PD (blood python)
	100 mg/10 ml saline × 30 min nebulization q12h[148]	Most species/pneumonia; acetylcysteine may be added
Polymyxin B, neomycin, bacitracin cream	Topical[158]	All species
Povidone-iodine solution (0.05%) or ointment	Topical[158]	All species/can soak in 0.005% aqueous solution ≤ 1 hr q12-24h
Silver sulfadiazine cream (Silvadene, Marion)	Topical q24-72h[128,158]	All species/broad-spectrum antibacterial for skin (ie, wounds burns) or oral cavity; dressing is generally not necessary

Table 11. Antimicrobial agents used in reptiles (cont.)

Agent	Dosage	Comments
Streptomycin	10 mg/kg IM q12-24h[67]	Potentially nephrotoxic; maintain hydration; avoid in cases of dehydration or renal or hepatic dysfunction
Sulfadiazine	25 mg/kg PO q24h[193]	Maintain hydration
Sulfadimethoxine	90 mg/kg IM, then 45 mg/kg q24h[67]	Potentially nephrotoxic; maintain hydration
Tetracycline	10 mg/kg PO q24h[94]	Most species/seldom used
Ticarcillin (Ticar, SmithKline Beecham)	50-100 mg/kg IM q24h[67]	Most species/maintain hydration
Tobramycin (Nebcin, Lilly)	—	Potentially nephrotoxic; maintain hydration; potentiated by ß-lactams
	2.5 mg/kg IM q24-72h[3,69]	Most species
	2.5 mg/kg IM q72h[187]	Chameleons/more frequent administrations have been reported[98]
	10 mg/kg IM q24h[54]	Chelonians/can be given q48h in tortoises
Trimethoprim/ sulfadiazine	—	Maintain hydration; parenteral form must be compounded
	15-25 mg/kg PO q24h[193]	Most species
	20-30 mg/kg PO, SC, IM q24-48h[108]	Most species
	30 mg/kg IM q24h × 2 days, then q48h[7,89,135]	Most species; also administered PO or SC
Trimethoprim/ sulfamethoxazole	10-30 mg/kg PO q24h[67]	Most species/maintain hydration
Tylosin	5 mg/kg IM q24h × 10-60 days[69,94]	Most species/mycoplasmosis

a Because reptiles are ectothermic, pharmacokinetics of drugs are influenced by ambient temperature. Antimicrobial therapy should be conducted at the upper end of the patient's preferred optimum temperature zone.
b See Appendix 83 for antimicrobial combination therapies, some of which are commonly used in reptiles.

Table 12. Antifungal agents used in reptiles

Agent	Dosage	Comments
Amphotericin-B	0.5-1.0 mg/kg IV, ICe q24-72h × 14-28 days[54]	Most species/aspergillosis
	1.0 mg/kg IT q24h × 2-4 wk[96]	Most species/respiratory infection; dilute with water or saline
	0.5 mg/kg IV q48-72h[67]	Most species/nephrotoxic; can use in combination with ketoconazole; administer slowly
	5 mg/150 ml saline × 1 hr nebulization q12h × 7 days[87]	Most species/pneumonia
Chlorhexidine (Nolvasan 2%, Fort Dodge)	20 ml/gal water bath[202]	Lizards/dermatophytosis
Clotrimazole (Veltrim, Haver-Lockhart; Otomax, with gentamicin and betamethasone, Schering-Plough)	Topical[168]	Most species/dermatitis; may bathe q12h with dilute organic iodine prior to use
Fluconazole	5 mg/kg PO q24h[202]	Lizards/dermatophytosis
Griseofulvin	20-40 mg/kg PO q72h × 5 treatments[168]	Most species/dermatitis; limited success
Itraconazole	23.5 mg/kg PO q24h[68]	Lizards/PD (spiny lizards); following a 3-day treatment, a therapeutic plasma concentration persists for 6 days beyond peak concentration; treatment interval was not determined
Ketoconazole	—	May use antibiotics concomitantly to prevent bacterial overgrowth; may use concurrently with thiabendazole
	15-30 mg/kg PO q24h × 2-4 wk[69]	Most species
	25 mg/kg PO q24h × 3 wk[88]	Snakes, turtles
	15-30 mg/kg PO q24h × 2-4 wk[135,155]	Chelonians/PD (gopher tortoises); systemic infection

Table 12. Antifungal agents used in reptiles (cont.)

Agent	Dosage	Comments
Ketoconazole (continued)	50 mg/kg PO q24h × 2-4 wk[193]	Crocodilians
Malachite green	0.15 mg/L water × 1 hr bath × 14 days[54]	Dermatitis
Miconazole (Monistat-Derm, Ortho)	Topical[168]	Most species/dermatitis; may bathe q12h with dilute organic iodine prior to use
Nystatin	100,000 IU/kg PO q24h × 10 days[87]	Most species/enteric yeast infections; limited success
Thiabendazole	50 mg/kg PO q24h × 2 wk[94]	Chelonians/pneumonia; dermatitis; may use concurrently with ketoconazole
Tolnaftate 1% cream (Tinactin, Schering-Plough)	Topical q12h prn[3]	Most species/dermatitis; may bathe q12h with dilute organic iodine prior to use

Table 13. Antiparasitic agents used in reptiles

Agent	Dosage	Comments
Albendazole	50 mg/kg PO[193]	Most species/ascarids
Carbaryl powder (5%)	Topical q7d prn[7]	Most species, primarily snakes/mites; apply sparingly; may rinse after 1-5 min; must treat environment concurrently; alternatively, dust empty cage lightly, place animal in cage for 24 hr, then bathe animal and wash cage
Chloroquine	125 mg/kg PO q48h × 3 treatments[193]	Tortoises/hemoprotozoa
Dimetridazole (Emtryl, Rhone-Poulenc, Canada)	100 mg/kg PO, repeat in 2 wk,[89] or 40 mg/kg PO q24h × 5-8 days[139]	Snakes (except milk and indigo)/amoebae, flagellates; not available in US
	40 mg/kg PO, repeat in 2 wk[89]	Milk and indigo snakes/amoebae, flagellates
Emetine	0.5 mg/kg SC, IM q24h × 10 days[3]	Most species/amoebae, trematodes; higher doses (2.5-5.0 mg/kg) have been reported;[109] avoid use in debilitated animals
Fenbendazole	—	Drug of choice for nematodes; may have an antiprotozoan effect;[106] can be given percloacally or use powdered form on food in tortoises[84]
	25 mg/kg PO q7d for up to 4 treatments[107]	All species
	50-100 mg/kg PO, repeat q14d prn[7,87,89,135]	All species/use 25 mg/kg in ball pythons
	50 mg/kg PO q24h × 3-5 days[70]	All species
	50 mg/kg PO q24h × 3 days or 100 mg/kg PO q14-21d[205]	Tortoises
	100 mg/kg PO q48h × 3 treatments; repeat the 3 treatments in 3 wk[24,142]	Turtles/lower dose (25 mg/kg) has also been recommended[104]

Table 13. Antiparasitic agents used in reptiles (cont.)

Agent	Dosage	Comments
Fipronil (0.25%) (Frontline, Merial)	Spray or wipe over q7-10d[57]	Most species/mites, ticks; beware of reactions to alcohol carrier; use with caution; use in reptiles needs further evaluation[36]
Ivermectin	0.2 mg/kg PO, SC, IM, repeat in 2 wk[7,88,200]	Snakes (except indigo), lizards (except skinks)[30]/nematodes, mites; caution: do not use in chelonians (may be toxic)[197] and crocodilians;[106] colored animals may have skin discoloration at injection site; rarely, adverse effects have been observed in chameleons, possibly associated with breakdown of parasites;[7] do not use within 10 days of diazepam and tiletamine/zolazepam; can dilute with propylene glycol; narrower range of safety than fenbendazole; rare deaths and occasional nervous system signs, lethargy, or inappetence have been reported (especially in lizards)[106]
	5[3,107]-10 mg[107]/L water topical q4-5d up to 4 wk[107]	Snakes, lizards/mites; spray on skin and in cage; some wash cage out 15 min later, others let cage dry before replacing reptile; some recommend ivermectin spray for the animal and a pyrethroid or larval inhibitor for the environment;[106] do not use in chelonians, indigo snakes, skinks, and crocodilians
Levamisole (Levasole 13.65%, Mallinckrodt)	5-10 mg/kg SC, ICe, repeat in 2 wk[108] (5 mg/kg in chelonians;[135] 10 mg/kg in lizards,[7] snakes[87])	Most species/nematodes (including lungworms); very narrow range of safety; main advantage is that it can be administered parenterally; avoid concurrent use with chloramphenicol; avoid use in debilitated animals; low dose may stimulate depressed immune system; can be used IM, but less effective
	10-20 mg/kg SC, IM, ICe[96]	Most species, including turtles

Table 13. Antiparasitic agents used in reptiles (cont.)

Agent	Dosage	Comments
Mebendazole	20-100 mg/kg PO, repeat in 14 days[57]	Most species/strongyles, ascarids
Metronidazole	—	Protozoan (ie, flagellates, amoebae) overgrowth; may stimulate appetite; may cause seizures if overdosed;[109] for small patients, injectable form administered PO may be preferable; oral liquid is not available in US, but can be compounded
	25-40 mg/kg PO on days 1, 3 or q24h for up to 1 wk[107]	Most species
	40-125 mg/kg PO, repeat in 10-14 days[96,98]	Most species/q72h x 5-7 treatments for amoebae
	100 mg/kg PO q3d × 2-3 wk[9]	Most species
	100 mg/kg PO, repeat in 2 wk[7,88-90]	Most species (except uracoan rattler, milk, tricolor king, and indigo snakes)
	125-250 mg/kg PO, repeat in 2 wk[67,154]	Most species/recommend using lower end of dose range
	40 mg/kg PO, repeat in 2 wk[89]	Uracoan rattler, milk, tricolor king, and indigo snakes
	40-60 mg/kg PO q7-14d × 2-3 treatments[187]	Chameleons
	40-200 mg/kg PO, repeat in 2 wk[144]	Geckos/ocular lesions (40 mg/kg) and subcutaneous lesions (200 mg/kg) caused by *Trichomonas*
	50 mg/kg PO q24h × 3-5 days or 100 mg/kg PO q14-21d[205]	Chelonians (tortoises)/use the lower dosage for severe cases
Milbemycin	0.25-0.50 mg/kg SC[21] prn	Chelonians/nematodes; parenteral form is not commercially available in US; fenbendazole preferred

Table 13. Antiparasitic agents used in reptiles (cont.)

Agent	Dosage	Comments
Milbemycin (continued)	0.5-1.0 mg/kg PO[21] prn	Chelonians/nematodes; fenbendazole preferred
Nitrofurazone	25.5 mg/kg PO[199]	Most species/coccidia; seldom used
Olive oil	Coat q7d[7]	Most species, especially small, delicate lizards/mites; wash animal with mild soap (and rinse well) the next day; messy to use; environment must be treated
Oxfendazole (Benzelmin, Fort Dodge)	68 mg/kg PO, repeat in 14-28 days prn[57]	Most species/nematodes
Paromomycin (Humatin, Parke Davis)	35-100 mg/kg PO q24h × ≤4 wk[67,87,200]	Most species/amoebae
	300-360 mg/kg PO q48h × 14 days[157]	Lizards (gila monsters)/ cryptosporidia
	300-800 mg/kg PO q24h[42] prn	Geckos/cryptosporidia; reduced clinical signs; does not eliminate organism
	100 mg/kg PO q24h × 7 days, then 2 ×/wk × 3 mon[46]	Snakes/cryptosporidia; reduced clinical signs and oocyte shedding; does not eliminate the organism
Permethrin (10%) (Permectrin II, Boehringer Ingelheim)	Topical, repeat in 10 days[22]	Most species/mites; a pyrethroid; safer than pyrethrins; use with care; dilute to a 1% solution and apply lightly via spray bottle in a well ventilated enclosure (with water bowl removed for 24 hr); blot off excess; administer in conjunction with environmental control
Piperazine	40-60 mg/kg PO, repeat in 2 wk[3]	Most species/nematodes
	50 mg/kg PO, repeat in 2 wk[94]	Crocodilians

Table 13. Antiparasitic agents used in reptiles (cont.)

Agent	Dosage	Comments
Praziquantel (Droncit, Mobay)	8 mg/kg PO, SC, IM, repeat in 2 wk[7,89,98]	Most species/cestodes, trematodes; doses >8 mg/kg have shown potential for treating pentastomids;[109] higher dosages have been administered PO[4,20]
Pyrantel pamoate (Nemex-2, Pfizer)	5 mg/kg PO, repeat in 2 wk[67]	Most species/nematodes
Pyrethrin spray (0.09%)	Topical q7d × 2-3 treatments	Most species/use water-based sprays labeled for kittens and puppies; apply with cloth; can also spray cage, wash out after 30 min; use sparingly and with caution; pyrethroids are safer (see permethrin, resmethrin)
Quinacrine (Atabrine, Winthrop)	19-100 mg/kg PO q48h × 2-3 wk[199]	Most species/some hematozoa
Quinine sulfate	75 mg/kg PO q48h × 2-3 wk[199]	Most species/some hematozoa; toxic at >100 mg/kg q24h; ineffective against exoerythrocytic forms
Resmethrin spray or shampoo (Durakyl, DVM Pharmaceuticals)	Topical[133], repeat prn q≥10d	Most species/mites; a pyrethroid; safer than pyrethrins; use with care; spray (0.35%) or shampoo entire animal, then rinse off immediately in running, tepid water; protect eyes (other than snakes) with 1 drop of mineral oil; lightly spray environment, wipe off in 5-10 min
Spiramycin (Spirasol, May and Baker)	160 mg/kg PO q24h × 10 days[45,46]	Snakes/cryptosporidia; may reduce clinical signs and oocyte shedding; does not eliminate organism
Sulfadiazine, sulfamerazine	25 mg/kg PO q24h × 3 wk[7,94,199]	Snakes, lizards/coccidia; avoid in cases of dehydration or renal dysfunction
	50 mg/kg PO q24h × 3 days, off 3 days, on 3 days[103]	Most species/avoid in cases of dehydration or renal dysfunction

55

Table 13. Antiparasitic agents used in reptiles (cont.)

Agent	Dosage	Comments
Sulfadiazine, sulfamerazine (continued)	75 mg/kg PO, then 45 mg/kg q24h × 5 days[67,199]	Most species/coccidia
Sulfadimethoxine (Albon, Roche)	—	Coccidia; avoid in cases of dehydration or renal dysfunction
	50 mg/kg PO q24h × 3-5 days, then q2d prn[103,110]	Most species
	90 mg/kg PO, IM, IV, then 45 mg/kg q24h × 5-7 days[69,87,199]	Most species
Sulfadimidine (33% solution)	1 oz/gal drinking water × 10 days[199]	Most species/coccidia
	0.3-0.6 mg/kg PO q24h × 10 days[199]	Most species/coccidia; alternatively, 0.3-0.6 mg/kg, then 0.15-0.30 mg/kg q24h x 2-10 days
Sulfamethazine	75 mg/kg PO, IM, IV, then 40 mg/kg q24h × 5-7 days[3,69,87]	Most species/coccidia
	50 mg/kg PO q24h × 3 days, off 3 days, on 3 days[103]	Most species/coccidia
	25 mg/kg PO, IM q24h × 7-21 days[3,199]	Snakes/coccidia
Sulfamethoxydiazine	80 mg/kg SC, IM, then 40 mg/kg q24h × 4 days[199]	Most species/coccidia
Sulfaquinoxaline	75 mg/kg PO, then 40 mg/kg q24h × 5-7 days[87]	Most species/coccidia
Thiabendazole	50-100 mg/kg PO, repeat in 2 wk[67,89]	Most species/nematodes; fenbendazole preferred
Trimethoprim/sulfa	30 mg/kg IM q24h × 2 days, then 15 mg/kg q48h × 5-14 days[199]	Most species/coccidia; may be administered SC[142]

Table 13. Antiparasitic agents used in reptiles (cont.)

Agent	Dosage	Comments
Trimethoprim/sulfa (continued)	30 mg/kg PO q24h × 7 days, or 15 mg/kg PO q12h × 7 days[97]	Most species/coccidia
	30 mg/kg PO q24h × 2 days, then q48h × 3 wk[7,199]	Most species/coccidia
	30-60 mg/kg PO q24h × 2 mon[3]	Snakes/use in treatment of cryptosporidia is of questionable value; may be toxic at this dosage
Vapona No-Pest Strip (Shell Chemical)	6 mm strip/10 ft[3] × 3-5 days; 2.5 cm[2] in perforated plastic film container × 2-5 days[67,69]	Most species/mites; use with caution; prevent contact with animals (ie, place strip above cage); avoid in cases of renal or hepatic dysfunction; remove water container; some recommend not to use continuously (expose 2-3 hr, 2-3 x/wk for 3-4 wk);[103] because of its toxicity and availability of safer alternatives, use is discouraged
Water	Bathe × 30 min[126]	Snakes, lizards/mites; use lukewarm water; safe, but not very effective; does not kill mites on head

Table 14. Chemical restraint/anesthetic/analgesic agents used in reptiles

Agent	Dosage	Comments
Acepromazine	0.05-0.25 mg/kg IM[97]	Most species/can be used as a preanesthetic with ketamine
	0.1-0.5 mg/kg IM[145,153]	Most species/preanesthetic; reduce by 50% if used with barbiturate
Alphaxalone/ alphadolone (Saffan, Glaxcovet Labs)	6-9 mg/kg IV, or 9-15 mg/kg IM[117]	Most species/good muscle relaxation; variable results; drug requires more evaluation; may have violent recovery;[12] don't use within 10 days of DMSO treatment; not available in US
	9 mg/kg IV, intracardiac[145]	Snakes/induction 5 min; good muscle relaxation; variable results; minimal effect if administered IM
	15 mg/kg IM[145]	Lizards, chelonians/induction 35-40 min; duration 15-35 min; good muscle relaxation; variable results
	24 mg/kg ICe[72]	Chelonians (red-eared sliders)/ surgical anesthesia with good relaxation
Atipamezole (Antisedan, Pfizer)	5 × medetomidine dose IM, IV[57,180]	Medetomidine reversal
Atropine	0.01-0.04 mg/kg SC, IM,[23] IV,[67] ICe[176]	Most species/preanesthetic; bradycardia; rarely indicated; generally use only in profound or prolonged bradycardia[176]
Buprenorphine (Buprenex, Reckitt & Colman)	0.005-0.02 mg/kg IM q24-48h[75]	Analgesia
	0.01 mg/kg IM[118]	Analgesia
Butorphanol (Torbugesic, Fort Dodge)	—	Butorphanol combination follows; see ketamine for combinations
	0.4-1.0 mg/kg SC, IM[176]	Analgesia; sedation; preanesthetic; 0.2 mg/kg IM used experimentally in tortoises[75]
	0.05 mg/kg IM q24h × 2-3 days[125]	Lizards (iguanas)

Table 14. Chemical restraint/anesthetic/analgesic agents used in reptiles (cont.)

Agent	Dosage	Comments
Butorphanol (continued)	1.0-1.5 mg/kg SC, IM[176]	Lizards/administer 30 min prior to isoflurane for smooth, shorter induction
Butorphanol (B)/ midazolam (M)	B) 0.4 mg/kg/ (M) 2 mg/kg IM[17]	Preanesthetic; administer 20 min before induction
Carprofen (Rimadyl, Pfizer)	1-4 mg/kg PO, SC, IM, IV q24h[118]	Analgesia; non-steroidal anti-inflammatory
Chlorpromazine	0.1-0.5 mg/kg IM[67]	Most species/preanesthetic; not commonly used
	10 mg/kg IM[12]	Chelonians/preanesthetic
Diazepam	—	Diazepam combination follows; see ketamine for combinations
	—	Muscle relaxation; give 20 min prior to anesthesia; potentially reversible with flumazenil
	2.5 mg/kg IM, IV[169]	Most species/seizures
	0.2-0.8 mg/kg IM[176]	Snakes/used in conjunction with ketamine for anesthesia with muscle relaxation
	2.5 mg/kg PO[170]	Iguanas/reduce anxiety which often leads to aggression
	0.2-1.0 mg/kg IM[176]	Chelonians/used in conjunction with ketamine for anesthesia with muscle relaxation
Diazepam (D)/ succinylcholine (S)	(D) 0.2-0.6 mg/kg IM, followed in 20 min (S) 0.14-0.37 mg/kg IM[182]	Alligators
Disoprofol	5-15 mg/kg IV to effect[29]	All species/anesthesia; similar characteristics to propofol; not available in US

59

Table 14. Chemical restraint/anesthetic/analgesic agents used in reptiles (cont.)

Agent	Dosage	Comments
Doxapram	5 mg/kg IM, IV[17] q10min prn 4-12 mg/kg IM, IV[176]	Respiratory stimulant; reduces recovery time; reported to partially "reverse" effects of dissociatives[120] Respiratory stimulant
Etorphine (M-99, Wildlife Pharmaceuticals)	0.3-2.75 mg/kg IM[117] 0.3-0.5 mg/kg IM[145]	Crocodilians, chelonians/very potent narcotic; crocodilians: induction 5-30 min, duration 30-180 min; chelonians: induction 10-20 min, duration 40-120 min; not very effective in reptiles other than the alligator;[153] poor relaxation; adequate for immobilization and minor procedures; requires an antagonist; limited use because of expense and legal restrictions
Flumazenil (Romazicon, Roche)	1 mg/20 mg of zolazepam[120]	Crocodilians/reversal
Flunixin meglumine	0.1-0.5 mg/kg IM q12-24h[118] 1-2 mg/kg IM q24h × 2 treatments[29,188]	Analgesia; use for maximum of 3 days Lizards/postsurgical analgesia; see Table 17
Gallamine (Flaxedil, American Cyanamid)	0.4-1.25 mg/kg IM[14] 0.6-4.0 mg/kg IM[121] 0.7 mg/kg IM[147] 1.2-2.0 mg/kg IM[66]	Crocodiles/results in flaccid paralysis, but no analgesia; larger animals require the lower dosage; reverse with neostigmine; use in alligators questionable; unsafe in alligators at $\geq$ 1.0 mg/kg[153]
Glycopyrrolate (Robinul-V, Robins)	0.01 mg/kg SC,[23] IM, IV[17]	Most species/preanesthetic; for excess oral or respiratory mucus; rarely indicated; generally use only in profound or prolonged bradycardia; may be preferable to atropine[67]
Halothane	3-4% induction, 1.5-2.0% maintenance[23,67]	Most species/isoflurane preferred; in lizards, in particular, use lowest concentration needed

Table 14. Chemical restraint/anesthetic/analgesic agents used in reptiles (cont.)

Agent	Dosage	Comments
Hyaluronidase (Wydase, Wyeth)	25 IU/dose SC[120]	Crocodilians/combine with premedication, anesthetic, or reversal drugs to accelerate SC absorption
Isoflurane	3-5% induction,[96] 1.0-3.0% maintenance[1,30]	Most species/inhalation anesthetic of choice in reptiles; induction 6-20 min; recovery 30-60 min; not as smooth in reptiles as compared to other animals; intubation and intermittent positive pressure ventilation advisable; may preanesthetize with low dose of propofol, ketamine, etc
Ketamine	—	Ketamine combinations follow
	—	Muscle relaxation and analgesia may be marginal; prolonged recovery with higher doses; larger reptiles require lower dose than smaller reptiles; painful at injection site; safety is questionable in debilitated patients; avoid use in cases with renal dysfunction; snakes may be permanently aggressive after ketamine anesthesia;[12] generally recommended to be used only as a preanesthetic prior to isoflurane for surgical anesthesia
	22-44 mg/kg SC, IM[12-14]	Most species/sedation
	55-88 mg/kg SC, IM[13,14]	Most species/surgical anesthesia; induction 10-30 min; recovery 24-96 hr
	10 mg/kg SC, IM q30 min[23]	Most species/maintenance of anesthesia; recovery 3-4 hr
	20-60 mg/kg IM, or 5-15 mg/kg IV[97]	Most species/muscle relaxation improved with diazepam 2-5 mg/kg[43]
	20-60 mg/kg SC, IM[23,100]	Snakes/sedation; induction 30 min, recovery 2-48 hr

61

Table 14. Chemical restraint/anesthetic/analgesic agents used in reptiles (cont.)

Agent	Dosage	Comments
Ketamine (continued)	60-80 mg/kg IM[30]	Snakes/light anesthesia; intermittent positive pressure ventilation may be needed at the high dose
	5-10 mg/kg IM[176]	Lizards/decreases the incidence of breath-holding during chamber induction
	20-30 mg/kg IM[65]	Lizards/sedation (ie, facilitates endotracheal intubation); preanesthetic; requires lower dose than other reptiles
	30-50 mg/kg SC, IM[23,100]	Lizards/sedation; variable results
	20-60 mg/kg IM[82,100,153]	Chelonians/sedation; induction 30 min; recovery $\geq$ 24 hr; potentially dangerous in dehydrated and debilitated tortoises
	25 mg/kg IM, IV[198]	Sea turtles/sedation; used at higher doses (50-70 mg/kg), recovery times may be excessively long and unpredictable; combination of ketamine and acepromazine gives a more rapid induction and recovery
	38-71 mg/kg ICe[203]	Green sea turtles/anesthesia; induction 2-10 min; duration 2-10 min; recovery <30 min
	60-90 mg/kg IM[100,145]	Chelonians/light anesthesia; induction <30 min; recovery hr to days; requires higher doses than most other reptiles
	20-40 mg/kg SC, IM, ICe (sedation), to 40-80 mg/kg (anesthesia)[120]	Crocodilians/induction <30-60 min; recovery hr to days; in larger animals, 12-15 mg/kg may permit tracheal intubation[176]
Ketamine (K)/ butorphanol (B)	(K) 10-30 mg/kg/ (B) 0.5-1.5 mg/kg IM[176]	Chelonians/minor surgical procedures (ie, shell repair)
	See (K) dosages/ (B) $\leq$1.5 mg/kg IM[176]	Snakes/anesthesia with improved muscle relaxation

62

Table 14. Chemical restraint/anesthetic/analgesic agents used in reptiles (cont.)

Agent	Dosage	Comments
Ketamine (K)/ diazepam (D)	(K) 60-80 mg/kg[145]/ (D) 0.2-1.0 mg/kg IM[176]	Chelonians/anesthesia; muscle relaxation
	See (K) dosages/ (D) 0.2-0.8 mg/kg IM[176]	Snakes/anesthesia with improved muscle relaxation
Ketamine (K)/ medetomidine (M)	—	Reverse medetomidine with atipamezole
	(K) 10 mg/kg/ (M) 0.1-0.3 mg/kg IM[56]	Most species
	(K) 5-10 mg/kg IM/ (M) 0.10-0.15 mg/kg IM, IV[77]	Lizards (iguanas)
	(K) 3-8 mg/kg/ (M) 0.025-0.080 mg/kg IV[122]	Giant tortoises (Aldabra)
	(K) 5 mg/kg/ (M) 0.05 mg/kg IM[151]	Tortoises (gopher)/light anesthesia; tracheal intubation; inconsistent results
	(K) 5-10 mg/kg IM/ (M) 0.10-0.15 mg/kg IM, IV[77]	Tortoises (small-medium)
	(K) 7.5 mg/kg/ (M) 0.075 mg/kg IM[151]	Tortoises (gopher)/anesthesia; tracheal intubation
	(K) 10-20 mg/kg IM/ (M) 0.15-0.30 mg/kg IM, IV[77]	Turtles (fresh water)
Ketamine (K)/ midazolam (M)	(K) 20-40 mg/kg/ (M) ≤2 mg/kg IM[19]	Chelonians/sedation; muscle relaxation
	(K) 60-80 mg/kg[145]/ (M) ≤2 mg/kg IM[176]	Chelonians/anesthesia; muscle relaxation
Ketamine (K)/ propofol (P)	(K) 25-30 mg/kg IM/ (P) 7 mg/kg IV[161]	Chelonians/administer propofol ≈70-80 min post-ketamine; see propofol
Ketoprofen (Ketofen, Fort Dodge)	2 mg/kg SC, IM q24h[118]	Analgesia

Table 14. Chemical restraint/anesthetic/analgesic agents used in reptiles (cont.)

Agent	Dosage	Comments
Lidocaine (0.5-2.0%)	Local or topical[176]	Local analgesia; infiltrate to effect (ie, 0.01 ml 2% lidocaine used for local block for IO catheter placement in iguanas);[15] often used in conjunction with chemical immobilization
Medetomidine (Dormitor, Pfizer)	—	See ketamine for combinations
	—	Produces poor to no immobilization alone; reversible with atipamezole
	0.10-0.15 mg/kg IM[17]	Most species
	0.15 mg/kg IM[180]	Crocodilians/sedation; incomplete immobilization; bradycardia, bradypnea
Meloxicam	0.1-0.2 mg/kg PO q24h[118]	Analgesia (orthopedic pain); not available in US
Meperidine (Demerol, Winthrop-Breon)	5-10 mg/kg IM q12-24h[75]	Analgesia; no noticeable effect in snakes, even at 200 mg/kg[12]
	2-4 mg/kg ICe[3]	Nile crocodiles/analgesia
Methohexital (Brevital, Eli Lilly)	5-20 mg/kg SC,[14] IV[67]	Most species/induction 5-30 min, recovery 1-5 hr; use at 0.125-0.5% concentration; much species variability; decrease dose 20-30% for young animals; avoid use in debilitated animals
	9-10 mg/kg SC,[149] ICe	Colubrids/induction ≥ 22 min, recovery 2-5 hr; does not produce soft tissue irritation seen with other barbiturates; may need to adjust dosage in snakes with large amounts of fat
Methoxyflurane	3-4% induction, 1.5-2.0% maintenance[67]	Not commonly used
Metomidate	10 mg/kg IM[57,174]	Snakes/profound sedation; not available in US

Table 14. Chemical restraint/anesthetic/analgesic agents used in reptiles (cont.)

Agent	Dosage	Comments
Midazolam (Versed, Roche)	—	See butorphanol, ketamine for combinations; potentially reversible by flumazenil
	2 mg/kg IM[12,14]	Most species/preanesthetic; increases the efficacy of ketamine; effective in snapping turtles, notin painted turtles[14]
	1.5 mg/kg IM[152]	Turtles (red-eared sliders)/sedation; onset 5.5 min; duration 82 min; recovery 40 min; much individual variability
Morphine	0.5-4.0 ICe[180]	Crocodilians/analgesia
Neostigmine (Neostigmine, Squibb)	0.063 mg/kg IV[121]	Crocodiles/gallamine reversal; may cause emesis and lacrimation; fast 24-48 hr before use; effects enhanced if combined with 75 mg hyaluronidase per dose when administered SC, IM
	0.03-0.25 mg/kg[121] IM	
	0.07-0.14 mg/kg[147] IM	
Oxymorphone	0.025-0.10 mg/kg IV[67]	Some species/analgesia; avoid in cases with hepatic or renal dysfunction; no noticeable effect in snakes, even at 1.5 mg/kg[12]
	0.5-1.5 mg/kg IM[67]	
	0.05-0.2 mg/kg SC, IM q12-48h[75]	Some species/analgesia
Pentazocine (Talwin, Upjohn)	2-5 mg/kg IM q6-24h[75]	Analgesia
Pentobarbital	15-30 mg/kg ICe[145]	Snakes/induction 30-60 min; duration ≥ 2 hr; prolonged recovery (risk of occasional fatalities); venomous snakes require twice as much as nonvenomous snakes;[12] avoid use in lizards
	10-18 mg/kg ICe[145]	Chelonians
	7.5-15.0 mg/kg ICe, or 8 mg/kg IM[12,145]	Crocodilians

Table 14. Chemical restraint/anesthetic/analgesic agents used in reptiles (cont.)

Agent	Dosage	Comments
Pethidine	20 mg/kg IM q12-24h[118]	Analgesia; not available in US
Prednisolone	2-5 mg/kg PO, IM[118]	Analgesia (chronic pain)
Proparacaine (Ophthaine, Fort Dodge)	Topical to eye[129]	Desensitizes surface of eye; ineffective in animals with spectacles
Propofol (Rapinovet, Pitman-Moore; Deprivan, Zeneca)	—	See ketamine for combination
	—	Anesthesia; rapid, smooth induction; may give 15-25 min anesthesia and restraint in most species; rapid, excitement-free recovery; must be administered (slowly) IV (no inflammation if goes perivascularly); may be administered IO; dosages may be reduced by as much as 50% in premedicated (ie, ketamine) animals; may get apnea and bradycardia; intubation and assisted ventilation generally required; considered by many to be parenteral agent of choice for inducing anesthesia
	5-10 mg/kg IV, intra-cardiac[5,174]	Snakes
	3-5 mg/kg IV, IO[76,77]	Lizards (ie, iguanas)/intubation and minor diagnostic procedures; may need to give an additional increment in 3-5 min; less cardiopulmonary depression than occurs with higher doses
	5-10 mg/kg IO,[18] IV	Iguanas/the higher dose is recommended for induction for short duration procedures or intubation
	10 mg/kg IV, IO[18,57]	Lizards, snakes/0.25 mg/kg/min may be given for maintenance[11]
	2 mg/kg IV[17]	Giant tortoises

Table 14. Chemical restraint/anesthetic/analgesic agents used in reptiles (cont.)

Agent	Dosage	Comments
Propofol (continued)	12-15 mg/kg IV[52]	Chelonians/lower dosages (5-10 mg/kg IV[176]) may be used; 1 mg/kg/min may be given for maintenance[176]
	10-15 mg/kg IV[120]	Crocodilians/duration 0.5-1.5 hr; maintain on gas anesthetics; experimental IM with hyaluronidase[128]
Sevoflurane (Ultane, Abbott)	prn[76]	Most species/anesthesia; rapid induction and recovery
Succinylcholine (Anectine, Burroughs Wellcome)	—	No analgesia; narrow margin of safety; intermittent positive pressure ventilation generally required; paralysis occurs in 5-30 min; avoid if exposed to organo-phosphate parasiticides within last 30 days; administer minimal amount required to perform procedure
	0.25-1.0 mg/kg IM[96]	Most species
	0.75-1.0 mg/kg IM[23]	Large lizards
	0.1-1.0 mg/kg IM[98]	Chameleons
	0.5-1.0 mg/kg IM[24]	Box turtles/induction 20-30 min
	0.25-1.5 mg/kg IM[153,154]	Chelonians/induction 15-30 min; recovery 45-90 min; facilitates intubation
	0.4-1.0 mg/kg IM[153]	Alligators/rapid onset; 3-5 mg/kg in smaller animals have been used[13]
	0.5-2.0 mg/kg IM[14,100]	Crocodilians/variable induction and recovery periods
Thiopental	19-31 mg/kg IV[203]	Green sea turtles/anesthesia; induction 5-10 min; recovery <6 hr; erratic anesthesia

Table 14. **Chemical restraint/anesthetic/analgesic agents used in reptiles (cont.)**

Agent	Dosage	Comments
Tiletamine/ zolazepam (Telazol, Fort Dodge)	—	Sedation, anesthesia; severe respiratory depression possible (may need to ventilate);[30] variable results; may have prolonged recovery; use lower end of dose range in heavier species; not generally recommended for reptiles
	4-5 mg/kg SC, IM[14]	Most species/sedation; induction 9-15 min, recovery 1-12 hr; adequate for most non-invasive procedures
	5-10 mg/kg IM[17]	Most species
	3 mg/kg IM[77]	Snakes/facilitates handling and intubation of large snakes; induction 30-45 min; prolongs recovery
	10-30 mg/kg IM,[145] to 20-40 mg/kg IM[96,175]	Snakes, lizards/induction 8-20 min; recovery 2-10 hr; variable results; longer sedation and recovery times at 22 °C than at 30 °C;[194] good sedation in boa constrictors at 25 mg/kg IM;[194] generally need to supplement with inhalation agents for surgical anesthesia; some snakes died at 55 mg/kg
	3.5-14.0 mg/kg IM[145] (generally 4-8 mg/kg)	Chelonians/sedation; induction 8-20 min; does not produce satisfactory anesthesia even at 88 mg/kg[153]
	5-10 mg/kg IM, IV[176]	Large tortoises/facilitates intubation; if light, mask with isoflurane rather than redosing
	2-10 mg/kg IM[176]	Large crocodilians/may permit intubation
	5-10 mg/kg SC, IM, ICe (sedation), 10-40 mg/kg (anesthesia)[120]	Crocodilians

Table 14. Chemical restraint/anesthetic/analgesic agents used in reptiles (cont.)

Agent	Dosage	Comments
Tiletamine/ zolazepam (continued)	15 mg/kg IM[41]	Alligators/induction > 20 min; adequate for minor procedures
Xylazine	—	Infrequently used; variable effects; potentially reversible with yohimbine; preanesthetic for ketamine
	0.10-1.25 mg/kg IM, IV[67]	Most species
	1-2 mg/kg IM[120,153]	Nile crocodiles
Yohimbine (Yobine, Lloyd)	0.1 mg/kg IM[120]	Xylazine reversal

Table 15. Hormones and steroids used in reptiles

Agent	Dosage	Comments
Arginine vasotocin (AVT) (Sigma Chemical)	0.01-1.0 µg/kg IV (preferred), ICe[119] q12-24h × several treatments	Most species/dystocias; administer 30-60 min after Ca lactate/Ca glycerophosphate; more effective in reptiles than oxytocin but not commercially available for use in animals; higher doses have been reported; 0.5 µg/kg commonly recommended
Calcitonin (Miacalcin, Sandoz; Calcimar, Rhone-Poulenc Rorer)	1.5 IU/kg SC q8h × 2-3 wk prn[67] 50 IU/kg IM, repeat in 2 wk[16,193]	Most species (ie, iguanas)/metabolic bone disease (ie, nutritional secondary hyperparathyroidism); administer following Ca supplementation; do not give if hypocalcemic
Dexamethasone	0.60-1.25 mg/kg IM, IV[67] 2-4 mg/kg IM, IV q24h × 3 days[177]	Shock (septic/traumatic) Inflammatory, noninfectious respiratory disease
Dexamethasone NaPO₄	0.10-0.25 mg/kg SC, IM, IV[69]	Shock (septic/traumatic)
Levothyroxine	0.02 mg/kg PO q48h[150]	Tortoises/hypothyroidism; stimulates feeding in debilitated tortoises
Nandrolone (Deca-Durabolin, Orgamon)	1 mg/kg IM q7-28d[53]	Anabolic steroid; reduces protein catabolism; may stimulate erythropoiesis
Oxytocin	— 1-10 IU/kg IM[65,97] 2 IU/kg IM q4-6h × 1-3 treatments[9] 1-5 IU/kg IM,[51] repeat in 1 hr 1-2,[25] 2-20,[69,135] or 10-20[24] IU/kg IM	Dystocias; results are variable; works well in chelonians, less so in snakes and lizards; generally administer 1 hr following Ca administration; use multiple doses with caution Most species/higher end of the range is commonly used; may be repeated Most species Lizards/alternatively, 5 IU/kg by slow IV or IO over 4-8 hr[51] Chelonians
Prednisolone	2-5 mg/kg PO, IM[118]	Analgesia (chronic pain)

Table 15. Hormones and steroids used in reptiles (cont.)

Agent	Dosage	Comments
Prednisolone Na succinate (Solu-Delta Cortef, Pharmacia & Upjohn)	5-10 mg/kg IM, IV,[67] IO[53]	Shock; brain swelling from hyper-thermia; may help reduce nephrocalcinosis
Stanozolol (Winstrol-V, Winthrop)	5 mg/kg IM q7d prn[69]	Most species/anabolic steroid; management of catabolic disease states

Table 16. Nutritional/mineral/fluid support used in reptiles [a]

Agent	Dosage	Comments
Calcium	PO prn	Sources include crushed cuttlebone, oyster shell, Ca lactate, or other commercially available products[109]
Ca carbonate (Rep-Cal, Rep-Cal Labs; Tums, SmithKline Beecham)	PO prn	Most species/Ca supplement
Ca gluconate	10-50 mg/kg IM[96]	Most species/hypocalcemia; dystocia
	100 mg/kg SC, IM, ICe[9,193] q8h[16]	Most species/metabolic bone disease; hypocalcemic muscle tremors; seizures or flaccid paresis in lizards; when patient is stable, switch to oral Ca
	100-200 mg/kg SC, IM[178]	Most species/hypocalcemia, dystocia; lower dose is preferable
Ca gluconate/ borogluconate	10-50 mg/kg IM[3]	Most species/hypocalcemia; hypocalcemic dystocia
Ca glubionate (Neo-Calglucon, Sandoz)	10 mg/kg PO q12-24h[3] prn	Most species/metabolic bone disease; hypocalcemia; dystocia
Ca lactate/Ca glycerophosphate (Calphosan, Glenwood)	1-5 mg/kg SC, IM[3]	Most species/hypocalcemia; hypocalcemic dystocia
	10-25 mg/kg SC, IM[69]	Most species/hypocalcemia; dystocia
	10 mg/kg SC, IM, ICe q24h × 1-7 days[7,16]	Lizards (iguanas)/metabolic bone disease
Crystalloid (nonlactated) solutions (Normo-Sol-R, Ceva; Plasma-Lyte, Baxter)	PO, SC, IV, ICe, EpiCe, IO prn[29]	Fluid therapy; can mix with equal parts 5% dextrose (if patient is hypoglycemic) or 0.45% NaCl for initial rehydration[29]
Dextrose (2.5%, 5.0%)	PO, SC, IV, ICe, EpiCe, IO prn[36]	Fluid therapy; can mix with crystalloid solutions

Table 16. Nutritional/mineral/fluid support used in reptiles (cont.)

Agent	Dosage	Comments
Electrolyte solutions (Pedialyte, Ross; Gatorade, Gatorade Co)	20-30 ml/kg PO q24h[50]	Oral fluid therapy; anorexia
Emeraid II (Lafeber)	20 ml/kg PO[24]	Turtles/nutritional support; starvation
Iodine	2-4 mg/kg PO q24h × 2-3 wk, then q7d[69]	Herbivorous species/iodine deficiency (ie, goiter); use in species maintained on a goitrogenic diet; alternatively, can use a balanced vitamin-mineral mixture or iodized salt (0.5% of feed)[109]
Iron dextran	12 mg/kg IM 1-2 ×/wk × 45 days[195]	Crocodilians/iron deficiency; also used in other species, but dose not established
Lactated Ringer's solution (LRS)	10-25 ml/kg SC, ICe q24h[36]	Fluid therapy; to prevent nephrotoxicity due to aminoglycosides; use extracoelomically in chelonians; use in reptiles is controversial and other fluids may be preferable
Metronidazole	—	May stimulate appetite by affecting bacterial flora or protozoa levels
	12.5-50.0 mg/kg PO[67]	Most species
	50-100 mg/kg PO[98]	Chameleons
Ringer's solution for reptiles	—	Fluid therapy; 1 part LRS, 2 parts 2.5% dextrose/0.45% saline; or, 1 part LRS, 1 part 5% dextrose, 1 part 0.9% saline;[199] to prevent nephrotoxicity due to aminoglycosides; can use epicoelomically in chelonians
	15 (large reptiles) to 25 (small reptiles) ml/kg q24h or divided q12h for maintenance[9]	All species
	10-25 ml/kg ICe q24h[69]	All species
	20 ml/kg q12h[9]	All species/severe dehydration

Table 16. Nutritional/mineral/fluid support used in reptiles (cont.)

Agent	Dosage	Comments
Selenium	0.028 mg/kg IM[3]	Lizards/deficiency; myopathy
Sodium chloride (0.45%)	PO, SC, IV, ICe, EpiCe, IO prn[36]	Fluid therapy; can mix with crystalloid solutions
Vionate (ARC)	500 mg ($^1/_4$ tsp)/kg PO q24h[178]	Most species/vitamin, mineral supplement
Vitamin A (Aquasol A, Armour)	—	Hypovitaminosis A; may have value in infectious stomatitis; overdose may cause epidermal sloughing; for less severe cases (especially in chelonians); oral vitamin A can be supplied via cod liver oil (2 drops 2x/wk) or commercial reptile vitamin products[109]
	2,000 IU/kg PO, SC, IM q7-14d × 2-4 treatments[9,24,30,187]	Most species
	1,000-5,000 IU/kg IM q7-10d × 4 treatments[4,69]	Most species
	200 IU/kg[60] SC, IM	Turtles/hypovitaminosis A; give in conjunction with PO vitamin A (2,000-10,000 IU/kg feed DM)
Vitamins A,D$_3$,E (Vital E-A&D, Schering-Plough)	0.15 ml/kg IM, repeat in 3 wk[97]	Most species/hypovitaminosis A, D$_3$, or E; product contains alcohol and may sting when administered; a product without alcohol can be compounded commercially
	0.3 ml/kg PO, then 0.06 ml/kg q7d × 3-4 treatments[24]	Box turtles/hypovitaminosis A; parenteral use may result in hypervitaminosis A and D; given PO may enhance Ca uptake
Vitamin B complex	5-10 mg/kg SC, IM	Most species/appetite stimulant; hypovitaminosis B
	25 mg thiamine/kg PO q24h × 3-7 days[9]	Most species/appetite stimulant; hypovitaminosis B
Vitamin B$_1$ (thiamine)	25 mg/kg PO q24h prn[169]	Thiamine deficiency (ie, in piscivorous species)
	30 g/kg feed fish PO[69]	Crocodilians/treat or prevent deficiency

Table 16. Nutritional/mineral/fluid support used in reptiles [a] (cont.)

Agent	Dosage	Comments
Vitamin B$_{12}$ (cyanocobalamin)	0.05 mg/kg SC, IM[69]	Lizards, snakes/appetite stimulant
Vitamin C	10-20 mg/kg SC, IM q24h[70,178]	All species/hypovitaminosis C; supportive therapy for bacterial infections; higher doses (ie, 100 mg/kg) may be used for severe burns[142]
	100-250 mg/kg PO q24h[70]	Most species/infectious stomatitis
Vitamin D$_3$	—	Metabolic bone disease; hypocalcemia; herbivores are sensitive to excess; excessive supplementation may result in soft-tissue calcification
	200 IU/kg IM q4wk[109]	Most species
	1,000 IU/kg IM, repeat in 1 wk[27,28,30]	Most species
	200 IU/kg PO, IM q7d[7,16]	Lizards (ie, iguanas)/PO may be safer than IM, but absorption may be poor
Vitamin E	1 IU/kg[61]	Most species/hypovitaminosis E
	25 mg/kg IM[64]	Lizards/hypovitaminosis E (see Vitamins A,D$_3$,E)
Vitamin K$_1$	0.25-0.50 mg/kg IM[97]	Most species/hypovitaminosis K$_1$; coagulopathies

[a] Also see Appendix 6.

Table 17. Miscellaneous agents used in reptiles

Agent	Dosage	Comments
Allopurinol (Zyloprim, Glaxo Wellcome)	10[135]-20[53,162] mg/kg PO q24h	Most species/gout; decreases production of uric acid;[124] long-term therapy; tortoises may respond best
Aluminum hydroxide (Amphogel, Wyeth-Ayerst)	100 mg/kg PO q12-24h[123a]	Hyperphosphatemia (associated with renal disease); decreases intestinal absorption of P; use cautiously in patients with gastric outlet obstruction
Amidotrizoate (Gastrografin, Squibb)	7.5 ml/kg PO[143]	Tortoises/gastrointestinal contrast agent; give via gavage; mean transit times: 2.6 hr at 30.6 °C; 6.6 hr at 21.5 °C
Aminophylline	2-4 mg/kg IM[67]	Bronchodilator
Atropine	0.01-0.04 mg/kg IM, IV q8-24h[142]	Dry up excess mucous secretions with infectious stomatitis
	0.1-0.2 mg/kg IM[97]	Organophosphate toxicity prn
	0.2 mg/kg SC,[169] IM	Respiratory distress associated with excessive secretions
Barium sulfate	5-20 ml/kg PO[37]	Gastrointestinal contrast studies
Cyanoacrylate (tissue glue) (Nexaband, Veterinary Products)	Topical[97]	Hemostasis of bleeding toenails
Cyanoacrylate (Nexaband Spray, Veterinary Products)	Topical[179]	Protects burns, noninfected lesions, surgical sites
Cimetidine	4 mg/kg PO, IM q8-12h[69]	Gastric and duodenal ulceration; esophagitis; gastroesophageal reflux
Cisapride (Propulsid, Janssen)	0.5-2.0 mg/kg PO q24h[193]	Motility modifier; gastrointestinal stasis
Dioctyl Na sulfosuccinate	1-5 mg/kg PO[70]	Most species/constipation; use 1:20 dilution
Doxorubicin, (Adriamycin, Pharmacia)	1 mg/kg IV q7d × 2 treatments, then q14d × 2 treatments, then q21d × 2 treatments[167]	Snakes/chemotherapy for sarcoma (also lymphoma carcinoma, etc); treatment periods variable

Table 17. Miscellaneous agents used in reptiles (cont.)

Agent	Dosage	Comments
Ferric subsulfate powder (Kwik-Stop, ARC)	Topical[97]	Hemostasis (ie, cut toenails); can use a TB syringe with tip cut off as an applicator
Flunixin meglumine	0.1-0.5 mg/kg IM, IV q12-24h × 1-2 days[69,135]	Nonsteroidal anti-inflammatory; antipyretic
	0.5-1.0 mg/kg IM, IV q24-72h[75]	Nonsteroidal anti-inflammatory
	2 mg/kg IM q24h × 2 treatments[188]	Iguanas/analgesia (postsurgery)
Furosemide	5 mg/kg PO, IM, IV q12-24h[69,97]	Diuretic for edema and pulmonary congestion
Hydrochlorothiazide (HydroDiuril, Merck)	1 mg/kg q24-72h[53]	Promotes diuresis; monitor hydration status
Iodine compound (Conray 280, Mallinckrodt)	500 mg/kg IV, IO[53]	Lizards/intravenous urography; take radiographs 0, 5, 15, 30, and 60 min postinjection
Iohexol (240 mg I/ml; Omnipaque, Sanofi Winthrop)	5-20 ml/kg[36]	Gastrointestinal contrast studies; nonionic, organic iodine solution; good alternative to barium;[37] faster transit time than barium; can be diluted 1:1 with water
Lactulose	0.5 ml/kg PO q24h[189]	Lizards/fatty liver disease
Liquid paraffin (medicinal)	20-30 ml (50:50 with electrolyte solution)/kg PO q24h[50]	Constipation; administer via gavage; use cautiously because of risk of regurgitation and aspiration; seldom indicated[36]
Metoclopramide	0.06 mg/kg PO q24h × 7 days[50,193]	Stimulates gastric motility
	1-10 mg/kg PO q24h[205]	Tortoises/stimulates gastric motility
Mineral oil	PO prn	Constipation; use cautiously because of risk of regurgitation and aspiration; seldom indicated[36]
New Skin (Medtech) Oral cleansing product (Maxi-Guard Oragel, Addison Biological)	Topical[169] Topical[187]	Spray-on bandage Stomatitis; periodontitis

Table 17. Miscellaneous agents used in reptiles (cont.)

Agent	Dosage	Comments
Pentobarbital	60[1,32]-100[32] mg/kg IV, ICe	Euthanasia
Polyurethane barrier (Opsite Spray Bandage, Smith and Nephew, Quebec)	Topical[179]	Encourages healing of cutaneous wounds
Potassium chloride	2 mEq/kg IV, IC[16]	Euthanasia; cardioplegic; administer following a euthanasia solution
Probenecid	Not established[124]	Gout; increases uric acid excretion
Silver nitrate	Topical[97]	Hemostasis (ie, cut toenails)
Silver sulfadiazine cream (Silvadene, Marion)	Topical q24-72h[127,158]	Broad-spectrum antibacterial for skin or oral cavity; dressing is generally not necessary
Simethicone (Mylanta Liquid, Johnson & Johnson)	PO prn	Gastrointestinal disturbance (gas)
Sodium bicarbonate	0.5-1.0 mg/kg IV[193]	Hypoxic acidosis post-anesthesia
Sodium hypochlorite (3%)	Disinfectant	Disinfectant for cages, water bowls, etc; rinse well following use
Sucralfate	500-1,000 mg/kg PO q6-8h[67]	Oral, esophageal, gastric, and duodenal ulcers
Sulfinpyrazone	Not established[124]	Gout; increases uric acid excretion
Tegaderm (3M Health Care)	Topical[36]	Wound dressing

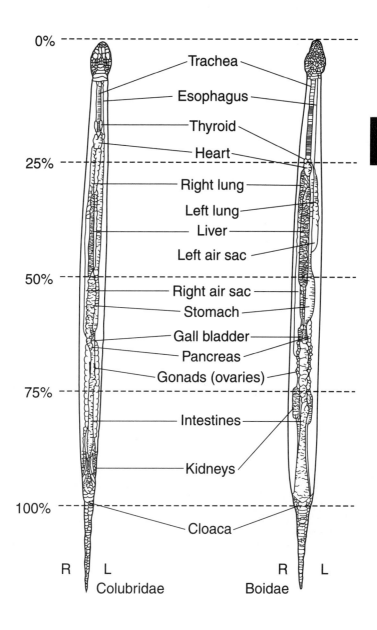

Figure 1. Comparative anatomy of a kingsnake (*Lampropeltis getulus*) (Colubridae) (left) and a common boa (*Boa constrictor*) (Boidae) (right). Positions of organs by percent of body length (nose to vent) are represented on left side of diagram. (Drawings by Tripp Stewart, 1995).

Appendix 4. Hematologic and serum biochemical values of reptiles

Measurements	Boa constrictor (*Boa constrictor*)[39,172]	Ball python (*Python regius*)[102]	Pythons (*Python* spp)[a,172]
Hematology			
PCV (%)	24-40	18 (16-21)	25-40
RBC (10⁶/µl)	1.0-2.5	—	1.0-2.5
Hgb (g/dl)	—	6.7 (5.5-7.9)	—
MCV (fl)	—	—	—
MCH (pg)	—	—	—
MCHC (g/dl)	—	—	—
WBC (10³/µl)	4-10	12.2 (7.9-16.4)	6-12
Heterophils (%)	20-65[b]	62 (56-67)	20-80[b]
Lymphocytes (%)	10-60	14 (7-21)	10-60
Azurophils (%)	—	17 (12-22)	—
Monocytes (%)	0-3	1 (0-1)	0-3
Eosinophils (%)	0-3	—	0-3
Basophils (%)	0-20	1 (0-2)	0-10
Chemistries			
AP (IU/L)	421 (242-652)	106 (96-116)	—
ALT (IU/L)	6 (0-20)	14 (12-16)	—
AST (IU/L)	5-35	33 (15-51)	5-30
Bilirubin, total (mg/dl)	0.3 (0.2-0.4)	—	—
BUN (mg/dl)	<1-10	—	<1-10
Calcium (mg/dl)	10-22	14 (13-14)	10-22
Chloride (mEq/L)	16.8 (14.1-23.7)	—	—
Cholesterol (mg/dl)	118 (104-124)	—	—
Creatine kinase (IU/L)	87 (53-138)	—	—
Creatinine (mg/dl)	<0.1-0.3	—	<0.1-0.3
Glucose (mg/dl)	10-60	29 (28-30)	10-60
LDH (IU/L)	30-300	—	40-300
Magnesium (mEq/L)	—	—	—
Phosphorus (mg/dl)	3.6 (2.6-4.9)	3.0 (2.7-3.4)	—
Potassium (mEq/L)	3.0-5.7	—	3.0-5.7
Protein, total (g/dl)	4.6-8.0	5.2 (5.0-5.6)	5-8
Albumin (g/dl)	—	—	—
Globulin (g/dl)	—	—	—
A:G (ratio)	—	—	—
Sodium (mEq/L)	130-152	—	130-152
Thyroxine (µg/dl)	—	—	—
Uric acid (mg/dl)	1.2-5.8	3.6 (3.2-4.1)	1.2-5.6

Appendix 4. Hematologic and serum biochemical values of reptiles (cont.)

Measurements	Diamond-backed water snake (*Nerodia* sp)[138]	Garter snake (*Thamnophis sirtalis*)[67,146]	Gopher snake (*Pituophis melanoleucus*)[67,132]
Hematology		19-37	
PCV (%)	—	0.71-1.39	25 (15-38)
RBC (10⁶/µl)	—	5.8-11.3	1.09
Hgb (g/dl)	—	264-268	—
MCV (fl)	—	78-86	—
MCH (pg)	—	28-34	—
MCHC (g/dl)	—	—	—
WBC (10³/µl)	—	—	—
Heterophils (%)	—	—	—
Lymphocytes (%)	—	—	—
Monocytes (%)	—	—	—
Eosinophils (%)	—	—	—
Basophils (%)	—	—	—
Chemistries			
AP (IU/L)	69 (27-157)	—	60 (9-133)
ALT (IU/L)	—	—	22 (11-65)
AST (IU/L)	—	—	53 (16-127)
Bilirubin, total (mg/dl)	0.6 (0.3-1.0)	—	—
BUN (mg/dl)	1 (0-3)	5	2 (1-5)
Calcium (mg/dl)	7 (6-8)	3	14.4 (13.0-15.7)
Chloride (mEq/L)	127 (117-131)	130	134 (109-148)
Cholesterol (mg/dl)	—	—	—
Creatine kinase (IU/L)	262 (92-572)	—	—
Creatinine (mg/dl)	0.7 (0.3-1.8)	—	0.3 (0.1-0.6)
Glucose (mg/dl)	33 (4-97)	—	88 (24-129)
LDH (IU/L)	191 (69-538)	—	—
Magnesium (mEq/L)	1.2 (0.9-1.5)	1.5	—
Phosphorus (mg/dl)	1.4 (0.7-2.5)	0.7	4.1 (2.5-5.7)
Potassium (mEq/L)	4.6 (2.8-6.4)	5.9	6.6 (3.6-10.0)
Protein, total (g/dl)	5.8 (4.3-7.6)	4.5	4.3 (2.8-7.3)
Albumin (g/dl)	—	—	1.9 (1.6-2.1)
Globulin (g/dl)	—	—	—
A:G (ratio)	—	—	—
Sodium (mEq/L)	166 (154-175)	152	171 (161-180)
Thyroxine (µg/dl)	—	—	—
Uric acid (mg/dl)	—	—	—

Appendix 4. Hematologic and serum biochemical values of reptiles (cont.)

Measurements	Indigo snake (*Drymarchon corais*)[62]	Yellow rat snake (*Elaphe obsoleta quadrivittata*)[164]
Hematology		
PCV (%)	—	—
RBC (10^6/µl)	—	—
Hgb (g/dl)	—	—
MCV (fl)	—	—
MCH (pg)	—	—
MCHC (g/dl)	—	—
WBC (10^3/µl)	—	—
Heterophils (%)	—	—
Lymphocytes (%)	—	—
Monocytes (%)	—	—
Azurophils (%)	—	—
Eosinophils (%)	—	—
Basophils (%)	—	—
Chemistries		
AP (IU/L)	123 (80-161)	92 (55-130)
ALT (IU/L)	—	18 (7-29)
AST (IU/L)	46 (6-163)	59 (15-103)
Bilirubin, total (mg/dl)	—	—
BUN (mg/dl)	—	—
Calcium (mg/dl)	159 (30-337)	3.6
Chloride (mEq/L)	119 (100-129)	131
Cholesterol (mg/dl)	—	—
Creatine kinase (IU/L)	644 (68-1923)	716 (200-1231)
Creatinine (mg/dl)	—	—
Glucose (mg/dl)	46 (28-89)	198 (15-586)
LDH (IU/L)	313 (13-1055)	203 (86-320)
Magnesium (mEq/L)	—	2.5
Phosphorus (mg/dl)	35 (8-69)	2.5
Potassium (mEq/L)	8.1 (4.3-14.3)	4.9
Protein, total (g/dl)	8.9 (5.9-12.3)	—
Albumin (g/dl)	2.5 (1.7-4.6)	—
Globulin (g/dl)	—	—
A:G (ratio)	—	—
Sodium (mEq/L)	157 (143-170)	162
Thyroxine (µg/dl)	—	—
Uric acid (mg/dl)	8.6 (2.2-17.2)	—

Measurements	Bearded dragon (*Pogona vitticeps*)[47]	Iguanid lizard (*Dipsosaurus dorsalis*)[113]	Green iguana (*Iguana iguana*)[58,67]
Hematology			
PCV (%)	24 (17-28)	—	25-38
RBC (10⁶/µl)	1.1 (0.8-1.8)	—	1.0-1.9
Hgb (g/dl)	—	—	6-10
MCV (fl)	—	—	165-305
MCH (pg)	—	—	48-78
MCHC (g/dl)	—	—	20-38
WBC (10³/µl)	9.4 (5.9-14.3)	—	3-10
Heterophils (%)	—	—	0.35-5.2[e]
Lymphocytes (%)	64 (54-76)	—	0.5-5.5[e]
Monocytes (%)	—	—	0-0.1[e]
Azurophils (%)	3 (0-8)	—	0-1.7[e]
Eosinophils (%)	—	—	0-0.3[e]
Basophils (%)	—	—	0-0.5[e]
Chemistries			
AP (IU/L)	1.6 (1.3-2.1)	14 (4-30)	50-290
ALT (IU/L)	<5-7	13 (3-38)	5-68
AST (IU/L)	63 (14-274)	179 (34-400)	5-52
Bilirubin, total (mg/dl)	1.6 (1.3-2.1)	0.2 (0.1-0.5)	—
BUN (mg/dl)	3 (3-4)	2 (1-5)	—
Calcium (mg/dl)	10 (8-13)	11 (8-30)	8.8-14.0
Chloride (mEq/L)	—	120 (12-155)	117-122
Cholesterol (mg/dl)	—	243 (100-399)	104-333
Creatine kinase (IU/L)	—	4500 (700-14,240)	—
Creatinine (mg/dl)	—	0.5 (0.2-1.8)	—
Glucose (mg/dl)	232 (211-261)	355 (255-575)	169-288
LDH (IU/L)	—	789 (145-2915)	—
Magnesium (mEq/L)	—	—	—
Phosphorus (mg/dl)	—	5.5 (2.8-10.0)	4-6[123a]
Potassium (mEq/L)	—	2.6 (0.4-7.0)	1.3-3.0
Protein, total (g/dl)	2.2 (2.0-2.7)	3.8 (2.4-5.4)	5.0-7.8
Albumin (g/dl)	—	2.3 (1.6-3.0)	2.1-2.8
Globulin (g/dl)	—	1.5 (0.8-2.4)	2.5-4.3
A:G (ratio)	—	1.7 (1.0-2.3)	—
Sodium (mEq/L)	—	164 (137-245)	158-183
Thyroxine (µg/dl)	—	—	—
Triglycerides (mg/dl)	—	—	53-691
Uric acid (mg/dl)	4.5 (2.9-10.0)	5.6 (2.4-13.3)	1.2-2.4

Appendix 4. Hematologic and serum biochemical values of reptiles (cont.)

Measurements	Prehensile-tailed skink (*Corucia* sp)[204]	Box turtle (*Terrapene carolina*)[10]	Red-eared slider (*Trachemys scripta*)[48,67,86]
Hematology			
PCV (%)	35 (24-60)	20-38	29 (25-33)
RBC ($10^6/\mu l$)	1.5 (0.8-1.4)	0.3-0.8	0.3-0.8
Hgb (g/dl)	9.6 (7.4-11.6)	5.0-8.5	8.0
MCV (fl)	263 (152-600)	309-587	310-1000[d]
MCH (pg)	69 (42-111)	79-131	95-308[d]
MCHC (g/dl)	28 (17-56)	25-32	31[d]
WBC ($10^3/\mu l$)	12.4 (3.9-22.4)[c]	7.5	—
Heterophils (%)	37 (16-58)	11	—
Lymphocytes (%)	22 (2-40)	56	—
Monocytes (%)	0.6 (0-6)	9.4	—
Azurophils (%)	—	—	—
Eosinophils (%)	4 (0-18)	—	—
Basophils (%)	15 (4-26)	8	—
Chemistries			
AP (IU/L)	—	—	212 (81-343)
ALT (IU/L)	—	—	—
AST (IU/L)	19 (<4-76)	—	202 (0-419)
Bilirubin, total (mg/dl)	—	—	—
BUN (mg/dl)	—	30	22
Calcium (mg/dl)	13 (11-21)	1.3	14 (14-15)
Chloride (mEq/L)	124 (123-129)	108	102 (97-107)
Cholesterol (mg/dl)	144 (11-252)	—	—
Creatine kinase (IU/L)	210 (27-940)	—	1288 (1093-1483)
Creatinine (mg/dl)	—	—	—
Glucose (mg/dl)	100 (70-122)	36	67 (20-113)
LDH (IU/L)	—	—	3625 (2389-4861)
Magnesium (mEq/L)	—	3.5	2.2
Phosphorus (mg/dl)	3.7 (2.8-6.7)	2.4	4.0 (3.7-4.3)
Potassium (mEq/L)	3.6 (1.4-5.0)	4.7	6.3 (4.3-8.3)
Protein, total (g/dl)	6.5 (5-8)	4.5	5.3 (4.0-6.5)
Albumin (g/dl)	—	—	—
Globulin (g/dl)	—	—	—
A:G (ratio)	—	—	—
Sodium (mEq/L)	158 (145-167)	130	137 (133-140)
Thyroxine ($\mu g/dl$)	—	—	—
Uric acid (mg/dl)	1.6 (<0.3-3.1)	2	1

Appendix 4. Hematologic and serum biochemical values of reptiles (cont.)

Measurements	Desert tortoise (*Gopherus agassizii*)[71,171]	Gopher tortoise (*Gopherus polyphemus*)[196]	Mediterranean tortoises (*Testudo* spp)[67,85,86]
Hematology			
PCV (%)	23-37	23 (15-30)	28-34
RBC ($10^6/\mu l$)	1.2-3.0	0.54 (0.24-0.91)	0.7-1.0
Hgb (g/dl)	6.9-7.7	6.4 (4.2-8.6)	9.1-11.3
MCV (fl)	377-607[d]	—	384-944[d]
MCH (pg)	113-126[d]	—	125-314[d]
MCHC (g/dl)	19-34[d]	—	27-40[d]
WBC ($10^3/\mu l$)	6.6-8.9	15.7 (10-22)	—
Heterophils (%)	35-60[f]	30 (10-57)	—
Lymphocytes (%)	25-50[f]	57 (32-79)	—
Monocytes (%)	0-4[f]	7 (3-13)	—
Eosinophils (%)	0-4[f]	—	—
Basophils (%)	2-15[f]	6 (2-11)	—
Chemistries			
AP (IU/L)	32 (29-35)	39 (11-71)	—
ALT (IU/L)	6.1 (3.8-8.3)	15 (2-57)	—
AST (IU/L)	59 (47-70)	136 (57-392)	—
Bilirubin, total (mg/dl)	—	0.02 (0-0.1)	—
BUN (mg/dl)	46 (30-62)	30 (1-130)	—
Calcium (mg/dl)	10 (9.6-10.3)	12 (10-14)	2.3-4.0
Chloride (mEq/L)	110 (109-112)	102 (35-128)	95-100
Cholesterol (mg/dl)	74 (60-89)	76 (19-150)	—
Creatine kinase (IU/L)	—	160 (32-628)	—
Creatinine (mg/dl)	0.13 (0.12-0.14)	0.3 (0.1-0.4)	—
Glucose (mg/dl)	75 (69-82)	75 (55-128)	78
LDH (IU/L)	25-250	273 (18-909)	—
Magnesium (mEq/L)	2.1 (1.8-2.4)	4.1 (3.3-4.8)	—
Phosphorus (mg/dl)	2.2-4.5	2.1 (1.0-3.1)	—
Potassium (mEq/L)	3.7 (3.5-3.9)	5.0 (2.9-7.0)	4.4-7.8
Protein, total (g/dl)	3.6 (3.4-3.8)	3.1 (1.3-4.6)	6.6
Albumin (g/dl)	1.1 (1.0-1.2)	1.5 (0.5-2.6)	—
Globulin (g/dl)	2.5 (2.3-2.6)	—	—
A:G (ratio)	—	—	—
Sodium (mEq/L)	130-157	138 (127-148)	127
Thyroxine (µg/dl)	—	—	—
Uric acid (mg/dl)	2.2-9.2	3.5 (0.9-8.5)	—

Appendix 4. Hematologic and serum biochemical values of reptiles (cont.)

Measurements	Radiated tortoise (*Tortoise radiata*)[134]	Aldabra tortoise (*Geochelone* sp)[173]	Alligator (*Alligator* sp)[67,195]
Hematology			
PCV (%)	31 (19-45)	17 (11-27)	20-30
RBC (10⁶/µl)	0.5 (0.4-0.7)	0.4 (0.25-0.65)	0.61-1.40
Hgb (g/dl)	6.7 (4.5-8.6)	5.4 (3.2-8.0)	5.9-12.0
MCV (fl)	—	452 (375-537)	327-450
MCH (pg)	—	146 (118-185)	—
MCHC (g/dl)	—	33 (28-40)	27-47
WBC (10³/µl)	4.3 (2.5-5.9)	3.4 (1.0-8.3)	6.4-10.2
Heterophils (%)	2.0 (0.7-3.4)[e]	71 (32-79)	—
Lymphocytes (%)	1.6 (0.4-3.4)[e]	22 (2-40)	—
Monocytes (%)	0.15 (0.03-0.47)[e]	2 (0-8)	—
Eosinophils (%)	0.18 (0.03-0.53)[e]	0.5 (0-7)	—
Basophils (%)	0.34 (0.10-0.94)[e]	2 (0-4)	—
Chemistries			
AP (IU/L)	93 (72-120)	111 (29-182)	—
ALT (IU/L)	—	7 (0-26)	—
AST (IU/L)	73 (42-134)	57 (5-138)	360
Bilirubin, total (mg/dl)	—	0.2 (0-0.3)	—
BUN (mg/dl)	—	33 (21-57)	—
Calcium (mg/dl)	12.2 (10.8-14.4)	12 (6-20)	2.6
Chloride (mEq/L)	97 (92-99)	93 (87-107)	112
Cholesterol (mg/dl)	105 (60-154)	—	—
Creatine kinase (IU/L)	—	—	—
Creatinine (mg/dl)	—	0.1 (0.1-0.2)	—
Glucose (mg/dl)	60 (46-93)	—	45-122
LDH (IU/L)	402 (213-592)	—	7-120
Magnesium (mEq/L)	—	—	1.5
Phosphorus (mg/dl)	3.2 (2.6-4.3)	4.3 (1.6-12.1)	—
Potassium (mEq/L)	5.5 (5.1-5.8)	4.7 (3.2-6.1)	3.8-5.9
Protein, total (g/dl)	4.0 (3.2-5.0)	4.1 (0.6-6.2)	5.1-6.1
Albumin (g/dl)	1.1 (0.8-1.3)	1.5 (0.3-2.6)	1.8
Globulin (g/dl)	2.9	2.6 (0.3-3.6)	—
A:G (ratio)	0.38	—	—
Sodium (mEq/L)	127 (121-132)	133 (129-136)	145
Thyroxine (µg/dl)	—	—	—
Uric acid (mg/dl)	0.3 (0-0.6)	—	1.0-4.1

[a] Includes Burmese (*Python molurus*), ball (*P. regius*), and reticulated (*P. reticulatis*) pythons.
[b] Heterophils and neutrophils.
[c] Includes 22(8-42)% azurophils.
[d] Calculated from data.
[e] Absolute values (10³/µl).
[f] Greatly differing % have also been reported: heterophils, 33±15; lymphocytes, 23±7; monocytes, 11±7; azurophilic monocytes, 2±2; eosinophils, 1±0.5; and basophils, 30±11.[2]

Appendix 5. Environmental, dietary, and reproductive characteristics of reptiles 6,49,55,63,73,95,140,189

| Species | Environmental preference | | Diet[d] | Method of reproduction[e] | Gestation/incubation period (days)[f] |
	Temperature[a-c]	RH (%)			
Snakes					
Boa constrictor (*Boa constrictor*)	28-34 °C (82-93 °F)	50-70	C	V	120-240
Sand boa (*Eryx* sp.)	25-30 °C (77-86 °F)	20-30	C	V	120-180
Burmese (Indian) python (*Python molurus*)	25-30 °C (77-86 °F)	70-80	C	Ov	56-65
Ball (Royal) python (*Python regius*)	25-30 °C (77-86 °F)	70-80	C	Ov	90
Garter snake (*Thamnophis sirtalis*)	22-30 °C (72-86 °F)	60-80	C	V	90-110
King snake (*Lampropeltis getulus*)	23-30 °C (73-86 °F)	50-70	Op/c	Ov	50-60
Chelonians					
Spur-thighed tortoise (*Testudo graeca*)	20-27 °C (68-81 °F)	30-50	H/om	Ov	60
Common box tortoise (*Terrapene carolina*)	24-29 °C (75-84 °F)	60-80	C/f	Ov	50-90

87

Appendix 5. Environmental, dietary, and reproductive characteristics of reptiles (cont.)

| Species | Environmental preference | | Diet[d] | Method of reproduction[e] | Gestation/incubation period (days)[f] |
	Temperature[a-c]	RH (%)			
Desert tortoise (*Gopherus agassizii*)	25-30 °C (77-86 °F)	—	H	Ov	84-120
Red-eared slider (*Trachemys scripta elegans*)	22-30 °C (72-86 °F)	80-90	C	Ov	59-93
Painted turtle (*Chrysemys picta*)	23-28 °C (73-82 °F)	—	H/I/o	Ov	47-99
Musk turtle (*Sternotherus odoratus*)	20-25 °C (68-77 °F)	—	O/i	Ov	60-87
Lizards					
Green iguana (*Iguana iguana*)	29-38 °C (85-100 °F)	60-80	H	Ov	73
Leopard ground gecko (*Eublepharis macularius*)	25-30 °C (77-86 °F)	20-30	I	Ov	55-60
Green anole (*Anolis carolinensis*)	23-29 °C (73-84 °F)	70-80	I/c	Ov	60-90
Jackson's chameleon (*Chamaeleo jacksonii*)	21-27 °C (70-80 °F)	50-70	I	V	90-180

Appendix 5. Environmental, dietary, and reproductive characteristics of reptiles (cont.)

Species	Environmental preference Temperature[a-c]	RH (%)	Method of reproduction[e]	Diet[d]	Gestation/incubation period (days)[f]
Plumed basilisk (Basiliscus plumifrons)	23-30 °C (73-86 °F)	70-80	Ov	C/f	60-64
Water dragon (Physignathus lesueuri)	25-34 °C (77-93 °F)	80-90	Ov	I/om	90
Crocodilian					
American alligator (Alligator mississippiensis)	30-35 °C (86-95 °F)	—	Ov	C/p	62-65

a Temperatures shown are ideal ambient daytime temperature gradients. These should be allowed to fall by approximately 5 °C (9 °F) during the night. "Hot-spot" temperatures should generally be 5 °C (9 °F) greater than the highest temperature shown.

b Preferred day-time temperature range for other commonly housed captive snakes are: rosy boa (Lichanura trivirgata) = 27.0-29.5 °C (80-85 °F); green tree python (Morelia viridis): 24-28 °C (75-82 °F); carpet python (Morelia spilota): 27.0-29.5 °C (80-85 °F); corn snake (Elaphe guttata): 25-30 °C (77-86 °F); yellow rat snake (Elaphe obsoleta): 25-29 °C (77-84 °F); gopher/bullsnake (Pituophis melanoleucus): 25-29 °C (77-84 °F).

c Preferred day-time temperature range for other commonly housed captive lizards are: day gecko (Pheluma sp): 29.5 °C (85 °F); chameleons (montane) (Chamaeleo spp): 21-27 °C (70-80 °F); chameleons (lowland) (Chamaeleo spp): 27-29 °C (80-84 °F); bearded dragon (Pogona vitticeps): 26.7-29.4 °C (80-85 °F); blue-tongued skink (Tiliqua sp): 27.0-29.5 °C (80-85 °F); monitor lizards (Varanus spp): 29-31 °C (84-88 °F); tegus (Tupinambis spp): 27-30 °C (80-86 °F).

d Uppercase letters denote principal dietary requirements: C = carnivorous; F = frugivorous; H = herbivorous; I = insectivorous; O = molluscavorous; Om = omnivorous; Op = ophiophagous; P = piscivorous. Lowercase denotes secondary preference.

e V = viviparous; Ov = oviparous.

f Temperature-dependent

89

Appendix 6. Selected products and guidelines used in force-feeding anorectic or debilitated reptiles [a,b]

Agent	Dosage	Comments
Alfalfa pellets (ie, iguana or rabbit pellets) or powder (Alfalfa Powder, NOW Foods)	Blend (1:2-4) with electrolyte solution or water; 20 ml/kg PO q48h (lizards) to q84h (chelonians)[25,109,186]	Herbivorous lizards, chelonians/administer via gavage; may clog feeding tube; for iguanas, may tube equal volume of water on alternate days until patient is stable and eating;[28,186] soaked pellets can also be hand-fed (especially by owner)
Avian hand-feeding diets (various commercial)	—	Herbivorous reptiles/administer via gavage; for short-term, can use Emeraid II (Lafeber)[25]
Baby foods	Vegetable; blend in with other food sources	Herbivorous lizards, chelonians/administer via gavage; for some species, some fruit baby food can be added
	Meat (small amount); blend in with other food sources	Omnivorous reptiles/administer via gavage
Barley powder (Green Powder, NOW Foods)	Blend with electrolyte solution or water	Herbivorous lizards, chelonians/administer via gavage; higher fiber, lower Ca and P than alfalfa
Dog/cat food, canned (a/d, Hill's; Nutritional Recovery Formula, Eukanuba)	30 ml/kg PO q7-14d[36,105,109]	Carnivorous reptiles/administer via gavage; although low protein (8.5%), some concern over high purine and vitamin A levels (probably OK unless concurrent renal disease); in dehydrated animals, dilute 1:1 with physiological solution, pediatric oral human electrolyte maintenance solution (Pedialyte, Ross), or Gatorade (Gatorade); once stabilized, small whole animals (lubricated with egg white) can be force-fed
Ensure (Ross) (strawberry or vanilla)	Blend 1 can with 1 banana and 1 vitamin tablet (Centrum, Lederle); 20 ml/kg q12-48h PO[8]	Iguanas (others?)/administer via gavage; alfalfa meal (4 Tbs [54 g]) can be added

90

Appendix 6. Selected products and guidelines used in force-feeding anorectic or debilitated reptiles (cont.)

Agent	Dosage	Species/Comments
Electrolyte solutions (Pedialyte, Ross; Gatorade, Gatorade)	15-25 ml/kg PO	Most species (see Table 16)

[a] General guidelines for force-feeding: generally provide nutrition following rehydration of patient; needs may vary with specific disease (ie, low protein with renal disease); force-feeding volumes are frequently started at a low/modest level and gradually brought up to the desired level (for patients with severe disease/cachexia, transition should be very gradual); concurrent to force-feeding and hydrating a patient, highly palatable food items should be provided for voluntary food intake.

[b] Dietary fiber supplements (alfalfa pellets or powder; barley powder; purified cellulose [ie, Solka Floc, James River]) should be an integral part of enteral therapy for herbivorous reptiles.

Appendix 7. Treatment of dystocias in reptiles [a,3,7,31,67,89,119,135,163]

Etiology
- Poor environmental conditions (improper ambient temperature, lack of thermal gradient, lack of suitable nesting area, etc)
- Dietary imbalances (ie, calcium deficiency), malnutrition
- Endocrine imbalances
- Uterine inertia
- Renal disease
- Infections (ie, uterus)
- Anatomic anomalies of the reproductive tract or eggs
- Other (substrate ingestion; over-feeding near oviposition; inadequate exercise)

Diagnosis
- History and clinical signs
- Physical examination (gentle palpation)
- CBC, serum biochemical analysis
- Radiography (chelonian eggs have a calcified outer shell and appear radiographically similar to avian eggs; lizards and snakes generally have soft-shelled eggs with soft tissue density on radiographs)
- Ultrasound

Treatment
- Provide proper environmental conditions (adjust ambient temperature to the preferred body temperature; suitable nesting site; minimal stress)
- Gentle handling
- Warm water soaks x 30-60 min q24h
- Rehydration
- Dextrose (SC, IV, ICe) may be of value in some cases
- Calcium (see Table 16) (low Ca not generally a problem in snakes)
    - Ca lactate/Ca glycerophosphate (Calphosan, Glenwood) (5 mg each/ml): 5 mg/kg SC, IM
    - Ca gluconate (23%): 100-200 mg/kg SC, IM
- Oxytocin[b] (see Table 15)
    - Generally administer 1 hr following Ca administration
    - 1-10 IU/kg IM, ICe in lizards and snakes (results are variable); 2-20 IU/kg IM, ICe for most chelonians; may be repeated in 1 hr
- Arginine vasotocin (Sigma Chemical) (alternative to oxytocin)
    - 0.01-1.0 µg/kg IV (preferred), ICe
    - Appears to be more effective than oxytocin in many reptiles, but it is not commercially available for use in animals
- Lubricate cloaca with water soluble gel
- Manual massage may be useful in some situations
- Salpingostomy may be required

---

[a] Although most reptiles are oviparous, some, including garter snakes, water snakes, boas (not pythons), vipers, Jackson's chameleons, horned toads, and Solomon Island prehensile-tailed skinks are viviparous.

[b] Use only if there is no evidence of obstructive dystocia or of broken eggs.

Appendix 8. Treatment of metabolic bone disease (nutritional secondary hyper-parathyroidism) in the iguana [3,4,7-9,26-28,123,186]

Etiology
- Improper Ca:P ratio; lack of dietary Ca
- Lack of vitamin D_3
- Lack of UVB light in the 290-320 (285-315)[59] nm spectrum
- Other: low ambient temperature; protein deficiency; and, rarely, disease of kidney, small intestines, parathyroid, etc

Clinical signs
- Lethargy, reluctance to move
- Poor appetite or anorexia in advanced cases
- Weight loss or poor weight gain
- Softening of the mandible; shortened/rounded mandible and maxilla; symmetrical swelling of the mandible (fibrous osteodystrophy)
- Fibrous osteodystrophy of the long bones of the legs
- Difficulty in lifting body off ground when walking
- Pathologic fractures
- Ataxia, paresis, or paralysis of the rear legs due to collapsed vertebrae or vertebral luxation
- Osteoporosis
- Less commonly, hypocalcemic muscle fasciculations and, rarely, seizures (both more often in adults than in young)

Diagnosis
- Dietary and environmental history
- Clinical signs
- Physical examination
- Radiography
- Serum Ca generally should be determined, but is usually within normal limits

Treatment
- Provide ambient temperature (with temperature gradient) of 29.5-32.0 °C (85-90 °F) during the day and 24.0-26.5 °C (75-80 °F) at night
  - Focal hot spot should approach ≥37.5 °C (100 °F)
- Improve diet (iguanas are herbivores/folivores, and require high Ca foods)
- Force-feeding (following rehydration) (see Appendix 6)
  - 20 ml/kg q1-2d
  - Vegetable baby foods; blended iguana or rabbit pellets; avian handfeeding formulas; short term use of Emeraid II (Lafeber)
  - Alternatively, force-feed a formula consisting of 1 can strawberry or vanilla human liquid-meal replacement drink (Ensure or Enrich, Ross), 1 banana, and 1 Centrum vitamin tablet (Lederle) blended
  - In addition, pelleted commercial iguana chow can be soaked in water and gently hand-fed (especially by owners)
- Ca supplementation options (see Table 16)
  - Per os (administered in conjunction with parenteral therapy)
    - Ca glubionate (Neo-Calglucon, Sandoz): 10 mg/kg PO q12-24h until patient is gaining weight and consuming adequate Ca (generally 1-3 mo)
    - Sprinkled on food, etc (Ca carbonate; Rep-Cal, Rep-Cal Research Labs; Tums, SmithKline Beecham)

Treatment (cont.)
- ◦ In cases of hypocalcemia, extreme weakness, or when Ca absorption from the
  gastrointestinal tract may be poor, parenteral administration of Ca is indicated
  - • Ca lactate/Ca glycerophosphate (Calphosan, Glenwood) (5 mg each/ml): 10 mg (1
    ml)/kg SC, IM, ICe q24h × 1-7 days
  - • Ca gluconate: 100 mg/kg IM, ICe q8h prn
- • Maintain hydration
  - ◦ Fluid therapy, as needed
  - ◦ Soak in warm water (shallow) for 10-20 min q12-24h to encourage drinking and
    defecation (caution: head may need to be supported; do not leave unattended)
- • Vitamin D_3
  - ◦ 100-1,000 (generally 200) IU/kg IM (can repeat in 1 wk)
  - ◦ 200 IU/kg PO q7d
  - ◦ Best source is UV radiation
- • Calcitonin (Miacalcin, Sandoz; Calcimar, Rhone-Poulenc Rorer) to prevent further transfer
  of Ca from bone to blood.
  - ◦ 50 IU/kg IM q7d × 2 treatments
  - ◦ Ca supplementation should be given prior to and during calcitonin therapy
  - ◦ Serum Ca should be within normal limits prior to calcitonin therapy; if Ca levels cannot
    be determined, administer Ca supplements for 7 days prior to calcitonin
- • Other
  - ◦ Handle gently
  - ◦ Remove climbing branches to prevent injuries

Appendix 9. Selected sources of diets and other commercial products for reptiles [a,b]

Foods and Supplements	
Five Star Diets	800-747-0557
Fluker Farms	800-735-8537
Kaytee	800-529-8331
LM Tropical Magic	800-332-5623
Nektron Rep USA	813-530-3500
Nutri Grow Premium Reptile Diets	800-737-8465
Ocean Nutrition T-Rex	800-275-7186
Pretty Pets	800-356-5020
Rep-Cal	408-356-4289
San Francisco Bay Brand	510-792-7200
Sticky Tongue Farms	909-672-3876
Zoo Med	888-496-6633
ZuPreem	800-345-4767

Live/Frozen Foods for Carnivores		
Bayou Rodents	800-722-6102	Frozen mice, rats
Carolina Mouse Farm	864-944-6192	Frozen mice, rats
Essex Pets	800-336-6423	Frozen mice, rats
G&A Frozen Rodents	718-456-0067	Frozen mice, rats, chicks
The Gourmet Rodent	352-495-9024	Mice, rats
Gretlo Kennel	310-328-2040	Live mice, rats
The Iguana Farm	610-582-7825	Frozen mice
MZ Enterprises	615-687-0757	Quail eggs, chicks, chickens, rabbits
Mice Unlimited	800-642-3469	Live and frozen mice
Mighty Mice	702-658-0921	Live and frozen mice, rats
The Mouse Factory	915-837-7100	Frozen mice, rats
The Mouse Trap	503-824-6423	Frozen mice
Ocean Nutrition	619-336-4728	Frozen mice, rats
Rodent Exchange	203-859-1704	Frozen mice, rats, chicks
Sand Valley Farms	888-811-6423	Mice, rats
Superior Rodents	415-452-3170	Frozen mice, rats
Trans-Pecos Rat	915-837-2928	Frozen rats

Live Foods for Insectivores		
Arbico	800-827-2847	Crickets, waxworms, mealworms, flies
Bassett's	800-634-2445	Crickets, mealworms
Drosophila	800-545-2303	Fruitflies
Fluker Farms	800-735-8537	Crickets, mealworms
Ghann's Cricket Farm	800-476-2248	Crickets, mealworms
Grubco	800-222-3563	Mealworms, crickets, fly larvae, waxworms, superworms
Manchester Farms	800-497-8067	Earthworms, red worms, night-crawlers
Millbrook Cricket Farm	800-654-3506	Crickets, mealworms

Appendix 9. Selected sources of diets and other commercial products for reptiles (cont.)

Live Foods for Insectivores (cont.)		
Nature's Way	800-318-2611	Mealworms, waxworms, fly larvae, crickets
Rainbow Mealworms	800-777-9676	Mealworms, crickets
Ray's Cricket Creek	402-477-1975	Crickets
Sunshine Mealworms	800-322-1100	Crickets, mealworms
Top Hat Cricket	800-638-2555	Crickets, mealworms, waxworms
Lights		
Chromolux	800-788-5781	Incandescent, heat
Duro-Lite	800-688-5826	Fluorescent (Vita-Lite), incandescent, basking, heat
Energy Savers Unlimited	—	Fluorescent, incandescent
MTS Electronics	610-588-6011	Fluorescent
National Biological	800-891-5218	Fluorescent
Reptile Lights	310-784-2770	Fluorescent, incandescent, heat
Zoo Med	888-496-6633	Fluorescent (Reptisun, Iguana Light), heat/basking, incandescent
Heating Devices (also see Lights)		
Clark	405-722-5017	Thermostats
Fluker Farms	800-735-8537	Under-cage heaters
Hagen	—	Under-cage heaters
Helix Controls	619-566-8335	Thermostats, temperature controls, heating systems
JS Technologies	818-353-1577	Thermostats
Ocean Nutrition	619-336-4728	Thermometers
Ram Network	818-345-0484	Ceramic bulb heaters
Zoo Med	888-496-6633	Temperature controls

[a] Many pet stores sell live and frozen food for reptiles, and many of the products listed.
[b] Numerous sources of information were used to compile this table, especially references 36, 156.

Appendix 10. Literature cited—Reptiles

1. _____. Report of the AVMA panel on euthanasia. *J Am Vet Med Assoc* 202:243-249, 1993.

2. Alleman AR, Jacobson ER, Raskin RE. Morphologic and cytochemical characteristics of blood cells from the desert tortoise (*Gopherus agassizii*). *Proc Assoc Amph Rept Vet*: 51-55.

3. Allen DG, Pringle JK, Smith D. *Handbook of Veterinary Drugs*. JB Lippincott Co, Philadelphia, 1993. Pp 534-567.

4. Anderson NL. Diseases of *Iguana iguana*. *Compend Cont Educ Pract Vet* 14:1335-1343, 1992.

5. Anderson NL, Wack RF, Calloway L. Cardiopulmonary effects and efficacy of propofol as an anesthetic agent in brown tree snakes, *Boiga irregularis*. *Bull Assoc Rept Amph Vet* 9:9-15, 1999.

6. Barrie MT. Chameleon medicine. In: Fowler ME, Miller RE (eds). *Zoo & Wild Animal Medicine*: *Current Therapy* 4. WB Saunders Co, Philadelphia, 1999. Pp 200-205.

7. Barten SL. The medical care of iguanas and other common pet lizards. *Vet Clin North Am Small Anim Pract* 23:1213-1249, 1993.

8. Barten SL. Diseases of the green iguana, *Iguana iguana*. *Proc N Am Vet Conf*: 811-814, 1996.

9. Bauck L, Boyer TH, Brown SA, et al. *Exotic Animal Formulary*. American Animal Hospital Association, Lakewood, CO, 1995. Pp 19-36.

10. Beck K, Loomis M, Lewbart G, et al. Preliminary comparison of plasma concentrations of gentamicin injected into the cranial and caudal limb musculature of the eastern box turtle (*Terrapene carolina carolina*). *J Zoo Wildl Med* 26:265-268, 1995.

11. Bennett RA. Personal communication, 1999.

12. Bennett RA. A review of anesthesia and chemical restraint in reptiles. *J Zoo Wildl Med* 22:282-303, 1991.

13. Bennett RA. Current techniques in reptile anesthesia and surgery. *Proc Assoc Rept Amph Vet/Am Assoc Zoo Vet*: 36-44, 1994.

14. Bennett RA. Anesthesia. In: Mader DR (ed). *Reptile Medicine and Surgery*. WB Saunders Co, Philadelphia, 1996. Pp 241-247.

15. Bennett RA. Clinical, diagnostic and therapeutic techniques. *Proc Assoc Rept Amph Vet*: 35-40, 1998.

16. Bennett RA. Management of common reptile emergencies. *Proc Assoc Rept Amph Vet*: 67-72, 1998.

17. Bennett RA. Reptile anesthesia. *Semin Avian Exotic Pet Med* 7:30-40, 1998.

18. Bennett RA, Schumacher J, Hedjazi-Haring K, Newell SM. Cardiopulmonary and anesthetic effects of propofol administered intraosseously to green iguanas. *J Am Vet Med Assoc* 212:93-98, 1998.

19. Bienzle D, Boyd CJ. Sedative effects of ketamine and midazolam in snapping turtles. *J Zoo Anim Med* 23:201-204, 1992.

20. Bishop YM (ed). *The Veterinary Formulary*. 3rd ed. British Veterinary Association and the Royal Pharmaceutical Society, London, 1996. Pp 63-65.

21. Bodri MS, Hruba SJ. Safety of milbemycin (A3-A4 oxime) in chelonians. *Proc Joint Meeting Am Assoc Zoo Vet/Am Assoc Wildl Vet*: 156-157, 1992.

22. Boyer DM. IME - Snake mite (*Ophionyssus natricis*) eradication utilizing permectrin spray. *Bull Assoc Rept Amph Vet* 5:4-5, 1995.

23. Boyer TH. Clinical anesthesia of reptiles. *Bull Assoc Rept Amph Vet* 2:10-13, 1992.

24. Boyer TH. Common problems of box turtles (*Terrapene* spp) in captivity. *Bull Assoc Rept Amph Vet* 2:9-14, 1992.

25. Boyer TH. Emergency care of reptiles. *Semin Avian Exotic Pet Med* 3:210-216, 1994.

26. Boyer TH. Common problems and treatment of green iguanas (*Iguana iguana*). *Bull Assoc Amph Rept Vet* 5: 8-11, 1995.

27. Boyer TH. Metabolic bone disease. In: Mader DR (ed). *Reptile Medicine and Surgery.* WB Saunders Co, Philadelphia, 1996. Pp 385-392.

28. Boyer TH. Diseases of the green iguana. *Proc N Am Vet Conf.* 718-722, 1997.

29. Boyer TH. Emergency care of reptiles. *Vet Clin North Am: Exotic Anim Pract* 1:191-206, 1998.

30. Boyer TH. *Essentials of Reptiles: A Guide for Practitioners.* AAHA Press, Lakewood, CO, 1998.

31. Brown CW, Martin RA. Dystocia in snakes. *Compend Cont Educ Pract Vet* 12:86-92, 1990.

32. Burns RB, McMahan W. Euthanasia methods for ectothermic vertebrates. In: Bonagura JD (ed). *Kirk's Current Veterinary Therapy XII: Small Animal Practice.* WB Saunders Co, Philadelphia, 1995. Pp 1379-1381.

33. Bush M, Smeller JM, Charache PN, et al. Preliminary study of antibiotics in snakes. *Proc Am Assoc Zoo Vet:* 50-54, 1976.

34. Bush M, Smeller JM, Charache P, et al. Biological half-life of gentamicin in gopher snakes. *Am J Vet Res* 39:171-173, 1978.

35. Caligiuri R, Kollias GV, Jacobson E, et al. The effects of ambient temperature on amikacin pharmacokinetics in gopher tortoises. *J Vet Pharmacol Ther* 13:287-291, 1990.

36. Carpenter JW. Personal communication. 1999.

37. Carpenter JW. Radiographic imaging of reptiles. *Proc N Am Vet Conf.* 873-875, 1998.

38. Casares M, Enders F. Enrofloxacin side effects in a Galapagos tortoise (*Geochelone elephantopus nigra*). *Proc Am Assoc Zoo* Vet: 446-448, 1996.

39. Chiodini RJ, Sundberg JP. Blood chemical values of the common boa constrictor (*Constrictor constrictor*). *Am J Vet Res* 43:1701-1702, 1982.

40. Clark CH, Rogers ED, Milton JT. Plasma concentrations of chloramphenicol in snakes. *Am J Vet Res* 46:2654-2657, 1985.

41. Clyde VC, Cardeilhac P, Jacobson E. Chemical restraint of American alligators (*Alligator mississippiensis*) with atracurium or tiletamine-zolazepam. *J Zoo Wildl Med* 25:525-530,1994.

42. Coke RL, Tristan TE. *Cryptosporidium* infection in a colony of leopard geckos, *Eublepharis macularius. Proc Assoc Rept Amph Vet:* 157-163, 1998.

43. Cooper JE. Anaesthesia of exotic animals. *Anim Technol* 35:13-20, 1984.

44. Cooper JE. Physiology (Reptiles). In: Fowler ME (ed). *Zoo & Wildlife Medicine.* 2nd ed. WB Saunders Co, Philadelphia, 1986. Pp 132-135.

45. Cranfield MR, Graczyk TK. An update on ophidian cryptosporidiosis. *Proc Am Assoc Zoo Vet:* 225-230, 1995.

46. Cranfield MR, Graczyk TK. Cryptosporidiosis. In: Mader DR (ed). *Reptile Medicine and Surgery.* WB Saunders Co, Philadelphia, 1996. Pp 359-363.

47. Cranfield M, Graczyk T, Lodwick L. Adenovirus in the bearded dragon, *Pogona vitticeps. Proc Assoc Amph Rept Vet:* 131-132, 1996.

48. Crawshaw GJ. Comparison of plasma biochemical values in blood and blood-lymph mixtures from red-eared sliders, *Trachemys scripta elegans. Bull Assoc Rept Amph Vet* 6:7-9, 1996.

49. Cunningham AA, Gili C. Management in captivity. In: Beynon PH, Lawton MPC, Cooper JE (eds). *Manual of Reptiles.* Iowa State University Press, Ames, IA, 1992 (reprinted 1994). Pp 14-31.

50. Divers SJ. Constipation in snakes with particular reference to surgical correction in a Burmese python (*Python molurus bivittatus*). *Proc Assoc Amph Rept Vet*: 67-69, 1996.

51. Divers SJ. Medical and surgical treatment of pre-ovulatory ova stasis and post-ovulatory egg stasis in oviparous lizards. *Proc Assoc Amph Rept Vet*: 119-123, 1996.

52. Divers SJ. The use of propofol in reptile anesthesia. *Proc Assoc Amph Rept Vet*: 57-59, 1996.

53. Divers SJ. Clinician's approach to renal disease in lizards. *Proc Assoc Rept Amph Vet*: 5-11, 1997.

54. Divers SJ. Empirical doses of antimicrobial drugs commonly used in reptiles. *Exotic DVM Vet Mag*: 23, 1998.

55. Divers SJ. Administering fluid therapy to reptiles. *Exotic DVM Vet Mag* 1:5-10, 1999.

56. Divers SJ. Anesthetics in reptiles. *Exotic DVM Vet Mag*: 7-8, 1999.

57. Divers SJ. Clinical evaluation of reptiles. Vet Clin North Am: *Exotic Anim Pract* 2:291-331, 1999.

58. Divers SJ, Redmayne G, Aves EK. Haematological and biochemical values of 10 green iguanas (*Iguana iguana*). *Vet Rec* 138:203-205, 1996.

59. Donoghue S. Metabolic bone disease in green iguanas and other reptiles. *Proc N Am Vet Conf*: 764-765, 1999.

60. Donoghue S. Nutritional problems of reptiles. *Proc N Am Vet Conf*: 762-764, 1999.

61. Donoghue S, McKeown S. Nutrition of captive reptiles. *Vet Clin North Am: Exotic Anim Pract* 2:69-91, 1999.

62. Drew ML. Hypercalcemia and hyperphosphatemia in indigo snakes (*Drymarchon corais*) and serum biochemical reference values. *J Zoo Wildl Med* 25:48-52, 1994.

63. Dundee HA, Rossman DA. *The Amphibians and Reptiles of Louisiana*. Louisiana State University Press, Baton Rouge, LA, 1989. Pp 270-272.

64. Farnsworth RJ, Brannian RE, Fletcher KC, Klassen S. A vitamin E-selenium responsive condition in a green iguana. *J Zoo Anim Med* 17:42-45, 1986.

65. Faulkner JE, Archambault A. Anesthesia and surgery in the green iguana. Semin Avian Exotic Pet Med 2:103-108, 1993.

66. Fleming GJ. Capture and chemical immobilization of the Nile crocodile (*Crocodylus niloticus*) in South Africa. *Proc Assoc Amph Rept Vet*: 63-66, 1996.

67. Frye FL. Reptile Clinician's Handbook. Krieger Publishing Co, Malabar, FL, 1994.

68. Gamble KC, Alvarado TP, Bennett CL. Itraconazole plasma and tissue concentrations in the spiny lizard (*Sceloporus* sp.) following once-daily dosing. *J Zoo Wildl Med* 28:89-93, 1997.

69. Gauvin J. Drug therapy in reptiles. *Semin Avian Exotic Pet Med* 2:48-59, 1993.

70. Gillespie D. Reptiles. In: Birchard SJ, Sherding RG (eds). *Saunders Manual of Small Animal Practice*. WB Saunders Co, Philadelphia, 1994. Pp 1390-1411.

71. Gottdenker NL, Jacobson ER. Effect of venipuncture sites on hematologic and clinical biochemical values in desert tortoises (*Gopherus agassizii*). *Am J Vet Res* 56:19-21, 1995.

72. Hackenbroich C, Failing K, Axt-Findt U, Bonath KH. Alphaxalone-alphadolone-anaesthesia in *Trachemys scripta elegans* and its influence on respiration, circulation and metabolism. *Proc 2nd Conf Europ Assoc Zoo Wildl Vet*: 431-436, 1998.

73. Harless M, Morlock H. *Turtles-Perspective and Research*. John Wiley & Sons, New York, 1979. Pp 356-366.

74. Hawk CT, Leary SL. *Formulary for Laboratory Animals*. Iowa State University Press, Ames, IA, 1995.

75. Heard DJ. Principles and techniques of anesthesia and analgesia for exotic practice. *Vet Clin North Am:Small Anim Pract* 23:1301-1327, 1993.

76. Heard DJ. Advanced reptile anesthesia and medicine. *Proc Avian Specialty Advanced Prog/Small Mam Rept Prog* (Annu Conf Assoc Avian Vet): 113-119, 1998.

77. Heard DJ. Advances in reptile anesthesia. *Proc N Am Vet Conf*: 770, 1999.

78. Helmick KE, Papich MG, Vliet KA, et al. Preliminary kinetics of single-dose intravenously administered enrofloxacin and oxytetracycline in the American alligator (*Alligator mississippiensis*). *Proc Am Assoc Zoo Vet*: 27-28, 1997.

79. Helmick KE, Papich MG, Vliet KA, et al. Preliminary kinetics of single-dose intramuscularly administered oxytetracycline and orally administered enrofloxacin in the American alligator (*Alligator mississippiensis*). *Proc Joint Conf Am Assoc Zoo Vet/ Am Assoc Wildl Vet*: 274-275, 1998.

80. Hilf M, Swanson D, Wagner R, et al. A new dosing schedule for gentamicin in blood pythons (*Python curtus*): a pharmacokinetic study. *Res Vet Sci* 50:127-130, 1991.

81. Hilf M, Swanson D, Wagner R, et al. Pharmacokinetics of piperacillin in blood pythons (*Python curtus*) and in vitro evaluation of efficacy against aerobic gram-negative bacteria. *J Zoo Wildl Med* 22:199-203, 1991.

82. Holz P, Holz RM. Evaluation of ketamine, ketamine/xylazine, and ketamine/midazolam anesthesia in red-eared sliders (*Trachemys scripta elegans*). *J Zoo Wildl Med* 25:531-537, 1994.

83. Hungerford C, Spelman L, Papich M. Pharmacokinetics of enrofloxacin after oral and intramuscular administration in savanna monitors (*Varanus exanthematicus*). *Proc Am Assoc Zoo Vet*: 89-92, 1997.

84. Innis C. IME - Per-cloacal worming of tortoises. *Bull Assoc Rept Amph Vet* 5:4, 1995.

85. Jackson OF. Chelonians. In: Beynon PH, Cooper JE (eds). *Manual of Exotic Pets*. British Small Animal Veterinary Association, Gloucestershire, UK, 1991. Pp 221-243.

86. Jacobson ER. Evaluation of the reptile patient. In: Jacobson ER, Kollias GV, Jr (eds). *Exotic Animals*. Churchill Livingstone, New York, 1988. Pp 1-18.

87. Jacobson ER. Use of chemotherapeutics in reptile medicine. In: Jacobson ER, Kollias GV, Jr (eds). *Exotic Animals*. Churchill Livingstone, New York, 1988. Pp 35-48.

88. Jacobson ER. Antimicrobial drug use in reptiles. In: Prescott JF, Baggot JD (eds). *Antimicrobial Therapy in Veterinary Medicine*. Iowa State University Press, Ames, IA, 1993. Pp 543-552.

89. Jacobson ER. Snakes. *Vet Clin North Am:Small Anim Pract* 23:1179-1212, 1993.

90. Jacobson ER. Use of antimicrobial therapy in reptiles. In: *Antimicrobial Therapy in Caged Birds and Exotic Pets*. Veterinary Learning Systems Co, Trenton, NJ, 1995. Pp 28-37.

91. Jacobson ER. Bacterial infections and antimicrobial treatment in reptiles. *Proc N Am Vet Conf*: 771-774, 1999.

92. Jacobson ER. Use of antimicrobial drugs in reptiles. In: Fowler ME, Miller RE (eds). *Zoo & Wild Animal Medicine: Current Therapy 4*. WB Saunders Co, Philadelphia, 1999. Pp 190-200.

93. Jacobson ER, Brown MP, Chung M, et al. Serum concentration and disposition kinetics of gentamicin and amikacin in juvenile American alligators. *J Zoo Anim Med* 19:188-194, 1988.

94. Jacobson E, Kollias GV, Jr, Peters LJ. Dosages for antibiotics and parasiticides used in exotic animals. *Compend Cont Educ Pract Vet* 5:315-324, 1983.

95. Jarchow JL. Hospital care of the reptile patient. In: Jacobson ER, Kollias GV, Jr (eds). *Exotic Animals*. Churchill Livingstone, New York, 1988. Pp 19-34.

96. Jenkins JR. A formulary for reptile and amphibian medicine. *Proc Fourth Annu Avian/Exotic Anim Med Symp*, University of California, Davis, CA: 24-27, 1991.

97. Jenkins JR. Medical management of reptile patients. *Compend Cont Educ Pract Vet* 13:980-988, 1991.

98. Jenkins JR. Husbandry and diseases of Old World chameleons. *J Small Exotic Anim Med* 1:145-192, 1992.

99. Johnson JD, Mangone B, Jarchow JL. A review of mycoplasmosis infections in tortoises and options for treatment. *Proc Assoc Rept Amph Vet*: 89-92, 1998.

100. Johnson JH. Anesthesia, analgesia and euthanasia of reptiles and amphibians. *Proc Am Assoc Zoo Vet*: 132-138, 1991.

101. Johnson JH. Clinical pharmacology of reptiles. *Symp Rept Med*, Texas A&M University, College Station, TX: 90-91, 1995.

102. Johnson JH, Benson PA. Laboratory reference values for a group of captive ball pythons (*Python regius*). *Am J Vet Res* 57:1304-1307, 1996.

103. Klingenberg RJ. *Understanding Reptile Parasites*. Advanced Vivarium Systems, Lakeside, CA, 1993.

104. Klingenberg RJ. The box turtle: a practitioner's approach. *Proc Assoc Amph Rept Vet*: 37-39, 1996.

105. Klingenberg RJ. Management of the anorectic ball python. *Proc N Am Vet Conf*: 830, 1996.

106. Klingenberg RJ. New perspectives on reptile anthelmintics, insecticides and parasiticides. *Proc N Am Vet Conf*: 831-832, 1996.

107. Klingenberg RJ. Parasitology for the practitioner. *Proc N Am Vet Conf*: 826-827, 1996.

108. Klingenberg RJ. Therapeutics. In: Mader DR (ed). *Reptile Medicine and Surgery*. WB Saunders Co, Philadelphia, 1996. Pp 299-321.

109. Klingenberg RJ. Reptiles. In: Aiello SE (ed). *The Merck Veterinary Manual*. 8th ed. Merck & Co, Whitehouse Station, NJ, 1998. Pp 1402-1421.

110. Klingenberg RJ. Treating coccidia in reptiles. *Proc N Am Vet Conf*: 779, 1999.

111. Kolmstetter CM, Frazier D, Cox S, Ramsey EC. Metronidazole pharmacokinetics in yellow rat snakes (*Elaphe obsoleta quadrivittata*). *Proc Am Assoc Zoo Vet*: 26, 1997.

112. Kolmstetter CM, Frazier D, Cox S, Ramsey EC. Pharmacokinetics of metronidazole in the green iguana, *Iguana iguana*. *Bull Assoc Rept Amph Vet* 8:4-7, 1998.

113. Kopplin RP, Tarr RS, Iverson CNM. Serum profile of the iguanid lizard (*Dipsosaurus dorsalis*). *J Zoo Anim Med* 14:30-32, 1983.

114. Lawrence K, Muggleton PW, Needham JR. Preliminary study on the use of ceftazidime, a broad spectrum cephalosporin antibiotic, in snakes. *Res Vet Sci* 36:16-20, 1984.

115. Lawrence K, Needham JR, Palmer GH, et al. A preliminary study on the use of carbenicillin in snakes. *J Vet Pharmacol Ther* 7:119-124, 1984.

116. Lawrence K, Palmer GH, Needham JR. Use of carbenicillin in 2 species of tortoise (*Testudo graeca* and *T hermanni*). *Res Vet Sci* 40:413-415, 1986.

117. Lawton MPC. Anaesthesia. In: Beynon PH, Lawton MPC, Cooper JE (eds). *Manual of Reptiles*. Iowa State University Press, Ames, IA, 1992. Pp 170-183.

118. Lawton MPC. Pain management after surgery. *Proc N Am Vet Conf*: 782, 1999.

119. Lloyd ML. Reptilian dystocias review - causes, prevention, management and comments on the synthetic hormone vasotocin. *Proc Am Assoc Zoo Vet*: 290-296, 1990.

120. Lloyd ML. Crocodilian anesthesia. In: Fowler ME, Miller RE (eds). *Zoo & Wild Animal Medicine: Current Therapy 4.* WB Saunders Co, Philadelphia, 1999. Pp 205-216.

121. Lloyd ML, Reichard T, and Odum RA. Gallamine reversal in Cuban crocodiles (*Crocodilus rhombifer*) using neostigmine alone versus neostigmine with hyaluronidase. *Proc Assoc Rept Amph Vet/Am Assoc Zoo Vet:* 117-120, 1994.

122. Lock BA, Heard DJ, Dennis P. Preliminary evaluation of medetomidine/ketamine combinations for immobilization and reversal with atipamezole in three tortoise species. *Bull Assoc Rept Amph Vet* 8:6-9, 1998.

123. Mader DR. IME - Use of calcitonin in green iguanas, *Iguana iguana*, with metabolic bone disease. *Bull Assoc Rept Amph Vet* 3:5, 1993.

123a. Mader DR. Personal communication. 1999.

124. Mader DR. Gout. In: Mader DR (ed). *Reptile Medicine and Surgery.* WB Saunders Co, Philadelphia, 1996. Pp 374-379.

125. Mader DR. Reproductive surgery in the green iguana. *Semin Avian Exotic Pet Med* 5:214-221, 1996.

126. Mader DR. Specific diseases and conditions. In: Mader DR (ed). *Reptile Medicine and Surgery.* WB Saunders Co, Philadelphia, 1996. Pp 341-346.

127. Mader DR. Antibiotic therapy in reptiles. *Proc N Am Vet Conf:* 791-792, 1998.

128. Mader DR. Common bacterial disease and antibiotic therapy in reptiles. *Suppl Compend Contin Educ Pract Vet* 20:23-33, 1998.

129. Mader DR. Understanding local analgesics: practical use in the green iguana, *Iguana iguana. Proc Assoc Rept Amph Vet:* 7-10, 1998.

130. Mader DR. Understanding thermal burns in reptile patients. *Proc Assoc Rept Amph Vet:* 143-147, 1998.

131. Mader DR, Conzelman GM, Baggot JD. Effects of ambient temperature on the half-life and dosage regimen of amikacin in the gopher snake. *J Am Vet Med Assoc* 187:1134-1136, 1985.

132. Mader DR, Horvath CC, Paul-Murphy J. The hematocrit and serum profile of the gopher snake (*Pituophis melanoleucus catenifer*). *J Zoo Anim Med* 16:139-140, 1985.

133. Mader DR, Palazzolo C. Common reptile parasites not always easy to treat.*Vet Prod News* (Jan): 32-33, 1995.

134. Marks SK, Citino SB. Hematology and serum chemistry of the radiated tortoise (*Testudo radiata*). *J Zoo Wildl Med* 21:342-344, 1990.

135. Mautino M, Page CD. Biology and medicine of turtles and tortoises. *Vet Clin North Am:Small Anim Pract* 23:1251-1270, 1993.

136. Maxwell LK, Jacobson ER. Preliminary single-dose pharmacokinetics of enrofloxacin after oral and intramuscular administration in green iguanas (*Iguana iguana*). *Proc Am Assoc Zoo Vet:* 25, 1997.

137. McCracken HE. Periodontal disease in lizards. In: Fowler ME, Miller RE (eds). *Zoo & Wild Animal Medicine: Current Therapy 4.* WB Saunders Co, Philadelphia, 1999. Pp 252-257.

138. McDaniel RC, Grunow WA, Daly JJ, et al. Serum chemistry of the diamond-backed water snake (*Nerodia rhombifera rhombifera*) in Arkansas. *J Wildl Dis* 20:44-46, 1984.

139. McFarlen J. Commonly occurring reptilian intestinal parasites. *Proc Am Assoc Zoo Vet:* 120-127, 1991.

140. McKeown S. General husbandry and management. In: Mader DR (ed). *Reptile Medicine and Surgery.* WB Saunders Co, Philadelphia, 1996. Pp 9-19.

141. Messonnier SP. *Common Reptile Diseases and Treatment.* Blackwell Scientific, Cambridge, MA, 1996.

142. Messonnier S. Formulary for exotic pets. *Vet Forum* (Aug):46-49, 1996.

143. Meyer J. Gastrographin as a gastrointestinal contrast agent in the Greek tortoise (*Testudo hermanni*). *J Zoo Wildl Med* 29:183-189, 1998.

144. Miller HA, Brandt PJ, Frye FL, et al. Trichomonas associated with ocular and subcutaneous lesions in geckos. *Proc Assoc Rept Amph Vet/Am Assoc Zoo Vet*: 102-107, 1994.

145. Millichamp NJ. Surgical techniques in reptiles. In: Jacobson ER, Kollias GV, Jr (eds). *Exotic Animals*. Churchill Livingstone, New York, 1988. Pp 49-74.

146. Mitruka BM, Rawnsley HM. Clinical, Biochemical, and Hematological Reference *Values in Normal Experimental Animals and Normal Humans*, 2nd ed. Masson Publ, New York, 1981.

147. Morgan-Davies AM. Immobilization of the Nile crocodile (*Crocodilus niloticus*) with gallamine triethiodide. *J Zoo Anim Med* 11:85-87, 1980.

148. Murray MJ. Pneumonia and normal respiratory function. In: Mader DR (ed). *Reptile Medicine and Surgery*. WB Saunders Co, Philadelphia, 1996. Pp 396-405.

149. Nichols DK, Lamirande EW. Use of methohexital sodium as an anesthetic in two species of colubrid snakes. *Proc Assoc Rept Amph Vet/Am Assoc Zoo Vet*: 161-162, 1994.

150. Norton TM, Jacobson ER, Caligiuri R, et al. Medical management of a Galapagos tortoise (*Geochelone elephantopus*) with hypothyroidism. *J Zoo Wildl Med* 20:212-216, 1989.

151. Norton TM, Spratt J, Behler J, Hernandez K. Medetomidine and ketamine anesthesia with atipamezole reversal in private free-ranging gopher tortoises, *Gopherus polyphemus*. *Proc Assoc Rept Amph Vet*: 25-27, 1998.

152. Oppenheim YC, Moon PF. Sedative effects of midazolam in red-eared slider turtles (*Trachemys scripta elegans*). *J Zoo Wildl Med* 26:409-413, 1995.

153. Page CD. Current reptilian anesthesia procedures. In: Fowler ME (ed). *Zoo & Wild Animal Medicine: Current Therapy 3*. WB Saunders Co, Philadelphia, 1993. Pp 140-143.

154. Page CD, Mautino M. Clinical management of tortoises. *Compend Cont Educ Pract Vet* 12:79-85, 1990.

155. Page CD, Mautino M, Derendorf H, et al. Multiple-dose pharmacokinetics of ketoconazole administered orally to gopher tortoises (*Gopherus polyphemus*). *J Zoo Wildl Med* 22:191-198, 1991.

156. Palika L. *The Consumer's Guide to Feeding Reptiles*. Macmillan Company, New York, 1997.

157. Paré JA, Crawshaw GJ, Barta JR. Treatment of cryptosporidiosis in gila monsters (*Heloderma suspectum*) with paromycin. *Proc Assoc Rept Amph Vet*: 23, 1997.

158. Pokras MA, Sedgwick CJ, Kaufman GE. Therapeutics. In: Beynon PH, Lawton MPC, Cooper JE (eds). *Manual of Reptiles*. Iowa State University Press, Ames, IA, 1992. Pp 194-206.

159. Prezant RM, Jarchow JL. Lactated fluid use in reptiles: is there a better solution? *Proc Assoc Rept Amph Vet*: 83-87, 1997.

160. Prezant RM, Isaza R, Jacobson ER. Plasma concentrations and disposition kinetics of enrofloxacin in gopher tortoises (*Gopherus polyphemus*). *J Zoo Wildl Med* 25:82-87, 1994.

161. Pye GW, Carpenter JW. Ketamine sedation followed by propofol anesthesia in a slider, *Trachemys scripta*, to facilitate removal of an esophageal foreign body. B*ull Assoc Amph Rept Vet* 8:16-17, 1998.

162. Raiti P. Veterinary care of the common kingsnake, *Lampropeltis getula*. *Bull Assoc Rept Amph Vet* 5:11-18, 1995.

163. Raiti P. Stuck! Reproductive problems of pet snakes. *Proc N Am Vet Conf*: 795-796, 1998.

164. Ramsey EC, Dotson TK. Tissue and serum enzyme activities in the yellow rat snake (*Elaphe obsoleta quadrivittata*). *Am J Vet Res* 56:423-428, 1995.

165. Raphael B, Clark CH, Hudson R, Jr. Plasma concentrations of gentamicin in turtles. *J Zoo Anim Med* 16:136-139, 1985.

166. Raphael BL, Papich M, Cook RA. Pharmacokinetics of enrofloxacin after a single intramuscular injection in Indian star tortoises (*Geochelone elegans*). *J Zoo Wildl Med* 25:88-94, 1994.

167. Rosenthal K. Chemotherapeutic treatment of a sarcoma in a corn snake. *Proc Assoc Rept Amph Vet/Am Assoc Zoo Vet*: 46, 1994.

168. Rossi J. Practical reptile dermatology. *Proc N Am Vet Conf*: 648-649, 1995.

169. Rossi JV. Emergency medicine of reptiles. *Proc N Am Vet Conf*: 799-801, 1998.

170. Rossi JV. Practical iguana psychology. *Proc N Am Vet Conf*: 798-799, 1998.

171. Rosskopf WJ, Jr. Normal hemogram and blood chemistry values for California desert tortoises. *Vet Med:Small Anim Clin* (Jan): 85-87, 1982.

172. Rosskopf WJ, Jr, Woerpel RW, Yanoff SR. Normal hemogram and blood chemistry values for boa constrictors and pythons. *Vet Med:Small Anim Clin* (May): 822-823, 1982.

173. Samour JH, Hawkey CM, Pugsley S, et al. Clinical and pathological findings related to malnutrition and husbandry in captive giant tortoises (*Geochelone species*). *Vet Rec* (Mar 15): 299-302, 1986.

174. Schaeffer DO. Anesthesia and analgesia in nontraditional laboratory animal species. In: Kohn DF, Wixson SK, White WJ, Benson GJ (eds). *Anesthesia and Analgesia in Laboratory Animals*. Academic Press, New York, 1997. Pp 338-378.

175. Schobert E. Telazol use in wild and exotic animals. *Vet Med* 82:1080-1088, 1987.

176. Schumacher J. Reptiles and amphibians. In: Thurman JC, Tranquilli WJ, Benson GJ (eds). *Lumb and Jones' Veterinary Anesthesia*. 3rd ed. Williams & Wilkins, Baltimore, 1996. Pp 670-685.

177. Schumacher J. Respiratory diseases of reptiles. *Semin Avian Exotic Pet Med* 6:209-215, 1997.

178. Scott BW. Nutritional diseases. In: Beynon PH, Lawton MPC, Cooper JE (eds). *Manual of Reptiles*. Iowa State University Press, Ames, IA, 1992. Pp 138-152.

179. Smith DA, Barker IK, Allen OB. The effect of certain topical medications on healing of cutaneous wounds in the common garter snake (*Thamnophis sirtalis*). *Can J Vet Res* 52:129-133, 1988.

180. Smith JA, McGuire NC, Mitchell MA. Cardiopulmonary physiology and anesthesia in crocodilians. *Proc Assoc Rept Amph Vet*: 17-21, 1998.

181. Speroni JA, Giambeluca L, Errecalde EO. Farmacocinetica de cefoperazona tras su administracion intramuscular a *Tupinambis teguixin* (Sauria, Teidae). *AHA Comm Meeting*, Buenos Aires, Argentina, 1989.

182. Spiegel RA, Lane TJ, Larsen RE, et al. Diazepam and succinylcholine chloride for restraint of the American alligator. *J Am Vet Med Assoc* 185:1335-1336, 1984.

183. Spörle H, Gobel T, Schildger B. Blood-levels of some anti-infectives in the Hermann's tortoise (*Testudo hermanni*). *4th Internat Colloquium Path Med Rept Amph*, Germany, 1991.

184. Stahl SJ. Osteomyelitis in lizards and snakes. *Proc N Am Vet Conf*: 759-760, 1997.

185. Stahl SJ. Treatment and management of mites in snakes and lizards. *Proc N Am Vet Conf*: 757-758, 1997.

186. Stahl SJ. Common diseases of the green iguana. *Proc N Am Vet Conf*: 806-809, 1998.

187. Stahl SJ. Common medical problems of old world chameleons. *Proc N Am Vet Conf*: 814-817, 1998.

188. Stahl SJ. Reproductive disorders of the green iguana. *Proc N Am Vet Conf*: 810-813, 1998.

189. Stahl SJ. Medical management of bearded dragons. *Proc N Am Vet Conf*: 789-792, 1999.

190. Stahl S, Donoghue S. Pharyngostomy tube placement, management and use for nutritional support in the chelonian patient. *Proc Assoc Rept Amph Vet*: 93-97, 1997.

191. Stamper MA, Papich MG, Lewbart GA, et al. Pharmacokinetics of ceftazidime in loggerhead sea turtles (*Caretta caretta*) after single intravenous and intramuscular injections. *J Zoo Wildl Med* 30:32-35, 1999.

192. Stein G. Hematologic and blood chemistry values in reptiles. In: Mader DR (ed). *Reptile Medicine and Surgery*. WB Saunders Co, Philadelphia, 1996. Pp 473-483.

193. Stein G. Reptile and amphibian formulary. In: Mader DR (ed). *Reptile Medicine and Surgery*. WB Saunders Co, Philadelphia, 1996. Pp 465-472.

194. Stirl R, Krug P, Bonath KH. Tiletamine/zolazepam sedation in boa constrictors and its influence on respiration, circulation and metabolism. *Proc Europ Assoc Zoo Wildl Vet*: 115-119, 1996.

195. Suedmeyer WK. Iron deficiency in a group of American alligators: diagnosis and treatment. *J Small Exotic Anim Med* 1:69-72, 1991.

196. Taylor RW, Jr, Jacobson ER. Hematology and serum chemistry of the gopher tortoise, *Gopherus polyphemus. Comp Biochem Physiol* 72A:425-428, 1982.

197. Teare JA, Bush M. Toxicity and efficacy of ivermectin in chelonians. *J Am Vet Med Assoc* 183:1195-1197, 1983.

198. Whitaker BR, Krum H. Medical management of sea turtles in aquaria. In: Fowler ME, Miller RE (eds). *Zoo & Wild Animal Medicine*: Current Therapy 4. WB Saunders Co, Philadelphia, 1999. Pp 217-231.

199. Willette-Frahm M, Wright KM, Thode BC. Select protozoal diseases in amphibians and reptiles: a report for the Infectious Diseases Committee, American Association of Zoo Veterinarians. *Bull Assoc Rept Amph Vet* 5:19-29, 1995.

200. Wilson SC, Carpenter JW. Endoparasitic diseases of reptiles. *Semin Avian Exotic Pet Med* 5:64-74, 1996.

201. Wimsatt J, Johnson J, Mangone BA. Clarithromycin pharmacokinetics in the desert tortoise (*Gopherus agassizii*). *J Zoo Wildl Med* 30:36-43, 1999.

202. Wissman MA, Parsons B. Dermatophytosis of green iguanas (*Iguana iguana*). *J Small Exotic Anim Med* 2:133-136, 1993.

203. Wood FE, Critchley KH, Wood JR. Anesthesia in the green sea turtle, *Chelonia mydas. Am J Vet Res* 43:1882, 1982.

204. Wright KM, Skeba S. Hematology and plasma chemistries of captive prehensile-tailed skinks (*Corucia zebrata*). *J Zoo Wildl Med* 23:429-432, 1992.

205. Wright KM. Common medical problems of tortoises. *Proc N Am Vet Conf*: 769-771, 1997.

206. Young LA, Schumacher J, Jacobson ER, et al. Pharmacokinetics of enrofloxacin in juvenile Burmese pythons (*Python molurus bivittatus*). *Proc Assoc Rept Amph Vet/Am Assoc Zoo Vet*: 97, 1994.

Fish
Amphibians
Reptiles
Birds
Sugar Gliders
Hedgehogs
Rodents
Rabbits
Ferrets
Miniature Pigs
Primates

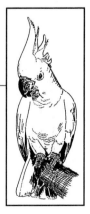

Table 18. Antimicrobial agents used in birds

Agent	Dosage	Comments
Amikacin	—	Frequently used with penicillins or cephalosporins; maintain hydration during use; least nephrotoxic of the aminoglycosides[108]
	10-15 mg/kg IM q12h[233]	Amazon parrots, cockatiels, cockatoos/PD
	10-20 mg/kg IM, IV q8-12h[133]	African grey parrots/PD
	15-20 mg/kg IM q8-12h[299]	Cockatiels/PD
	20-30 mg/kg IM q24h[371,372]	Most species/*Mycobacterium*; use in combination with other agents; see Appendix 34
	15-20 mg/kg SC, IM, IV q12h × 5 days maximum[327]	Pigeons
	20 mg/kg IM q8h[99]	Chickens/PD
	10 mg/kg SC, IM q8h × 14 days[200]	Ring-necked pheasants/PD; renal toxicosis appeared at 11 days, uric acid levels abnormal up to 7 days following cessation
	15-20 mg/kg/day divided q8-24h[34]	Red-tailed hawks/PD; use low end of dose range for smaller hawks
	15-20 mg/kg IM q24h[183]	Raptors
	7.6 mg/kg IM q8h[176]	Ostriches/PD; causes myositis; painful injection
	2 g/gal water[367]	Ratites/egg dip
	20 mg/kg IM q12h[1]	Ostrich chicks
	10 mg/kg IM q12h[50]	Cranes
Amoxicillin	100 mg/kg PO q8h[23,256]	Most species, including raptors
	200-400 mg/L drinking water[137]	Canaries/aviary use
	300-500 mg/kg soft feed[137]	Canaries/aviary use

Table 18. Antimicrobial agents used in birds (cont.)

Agent	Dosage	Comments
Amoxicillin (continued)	150-175 mg/kg PO q12h[189]	Passerines (towhee)/septic arthritis; *Pasteurella multocida* infections
	100 mg/kg IM q48h[90]	Pigeons/PD; Gram ⊕; long-acting oil suspension (not available in US)
	150 mg/kg PO, IV[346]	Pigeons/PD; *Streptococcus bovis*
	100-200 mg/kg PO, IM q4-8h[108]	Pigeons
	2-3 g/gal drinking water[139]	Pigeons
	55-110 mg/kg PO q12h[138]	Poultry/*Pasteurella*; trauma
	1 g/3 L drinking water[29]	Waterfowl
	15-22 mg/kg PO q8h[367]	Ratites
	250 mg/gal drinking water[367]	Ratites
Amoxicillin sodium	50 mg/kg IM q12-24h[90]	Pigeons/PD; only Gram ⊕
	250 mg/kg IM q12-24h[90]	Pigeons/PD; Gram ⊕ and Gram ⊖
Amoxicillin trihydrate	20 mg/kg PO q12-24h[90]	Pigeons/PD; only Gram ⊕
	100 mg/kg PO q12-24h[90]	Pigeons/PD; Gram ⊕ and Gram ⊖
Amoxicillin/ clavulanate (Clavamox, Pfizer; Augmentin, SmithKline Beecham; Synulox RTU, unavailable in US)	—	ß-lactamase inhibitor; dosage based on combined quantities of both drugs
	125 mg/kg PO q12h[256,314]	Most species, including pigeons and raptors/use with allopurinol is contraindicated
	60-120 mg/kg IM q8-12h[94]	Collared doves/PD; *Staphylococcus, E. coli*
	125-250 mg/kg PO q8-12h[94]	Collared doves/PD; *Staphylococcus, E. coli*
	500 mg/L drinking water[386]	Chickens/PD
	10-15 mg/kg PO q12h[367]	Ratites

Table 18. Antimicrobial agents used in birds (cont.)

Agent	Dosage	Comments
Amphotericin B	100 mg/kg gavage q12h × 10 days[130]	Psittacines, passerines/ megabacteriosis
	1 g/L drinking water × 10 days[130]	Psittacines, passerines/ megabacteriosis
Ampicillin	100 mg/kg IM q4h[58]	Most species
	1-2 g/L drinking water[137]	Canaries/aviary use
	2-3 g/kg soft feed[137]	Canaries/aviary use
	155 mg/kg IM q12-24h[97]	Pigeons/PD; amoxicillin preferred over ampicillin for IM use in pigeons
	55-110 mg/kg IM q8-12h[138]	Poultry/Pasteurella, trauma
	4 g/gal drinking water[313]	Galliformes/flock use
	15 mg/kg IM q12h[122]	Raptors
	15-20 mg/kg IM q12h[122,177]	Emus, cranes/PD (emus)
	11-15 mg/kg PO q8h[367]	Ratites
	4-7 mg/kg SC, IM q8h[367]	Ratites (excluding emus)
Ampicillin sodium	100 mg/kg IM q4h[100]	Amazon parrots/PD
	50 mg/kg IM q6-8h[100]	Amazon parrots/PD; localized infections
	150-200 mg/kg PO q8-12h[100]	Amazon parrots/PD; therapeutic levels not achieved in blue-naped Amazons at this dosage
	174 mg/kg/day PO[84]	Pigeons/PD; *Streptococcus bovis*
	2 g/L drinking water[84]	Pigeons/PD; *Streptococcus bovis*
	150 mg/kg IM q12-24h[90]	Pigeons/PD; only Gram ⊕
Ampicillin trihydrate	25 mg/kg PO q12-24h[90]	Pigeons/PD; only Gram ⊕
	120-175 mg/kg PO q12-24h[90]	Pigeons/PD; Gram ⊕ and Gram ⊖

111

Table 18. Antimicrobial agents used in birds (cont.)

Agent	Dosage	Comments
Apramycin (Apralan, Elanco)	0.5 g powder/L drinking water[30]	Psittacines/*Pseudomonas*; aminocyclitol; nephrotoxic; therapeutic levels not achieved in Japanese quail at 50 mg/kg IV[214]
Azithromycin (Zithromax, Pfizer)	—	*Toxoplasma, Plasmodium, Cryptosporidium, Chlamydia*
	43 mg/kg PO q24h[330]	Most species/*Mycobacterium*; used with ethambutol and rifabutin (see Appendix 34)
	50-80 mg/kg PO q24h × 3 days on, off 4 days, repeat up to 3 wk[314]	Most species/*Mycoplasma*; do not use if hepatic or renal disease; can mix with lactulose (stable refrigerated for 3-4 weeks)
mg/gal drinking disalicylate (Solutracin 200, A.L. Laboratories)	Ratites/*Clostridium perfringens*; water[367]	Bacitracin methylene 200 prepare daily
Carbenicillin (Geocillin, Roerig)	100 mg/kg IM q8h[23]	Most species
	100 mg/kg PO q12h[247]	Most species
	100 mg/kg IT q24h[58]	Most species/*Pseudomonas* respiratory infections
	127 mg (tablet)/120 ml drinking water[247]	Most species
	100-200 mg/kg IV q6-12h[314]	Most species/*Pseudomonas, Proteus*
	100 mg/kg IM q8-12h[50,140]	Pigeons, cranes
	250 mg/kg IM q12h[302]	Raptors
	11-15 mg/kg IV q8h[367]	Ratites
Cefadroxil (Cefa-Tabs, Fort Dodge)	100 mg/kg PO q12h × 7 days[139,324]	Most psittacines, pigeons/14-21 day therapy may be indicated for severe or deep pyodermas; orange flavored suspensions are preferred

112

Table 18. Antimicrobial agents used in birds (cont.)

Agent	Dosage	Comments
Cefazolin (Ancef, SmithKline Beecham)	—	Stable 10 days refrigerated; can be frozen[314]
	50-75 mg/kg IM q12h[324]	Most species
	22-110 mg/kg IM q8-12h[138]	Poultry/Pasteurella; trauma
	50-100 mg/kg PO, IM q12h[279]	Owls
	25-30 mg/kg IM, IV q8h[50]	Cranes
Cefotaxime (Claforan, Hoechst-Roussel)	—	Penetrates CSF; stable 5 days refrigerated; can be frozen[314]
	75 mg/kg IM q8h[23]	Most species
	100 mg/kg IM q8-12h[139]	Pigeons
	100 mg/kg IM q12h[183]	Raptors
	25 mg/kg IM q8h[367]	Ratites/young birds
	50-100 mg/kg IM q8-12h[50]	Cranes
Cefoxitin (Mefoxin, Merck)	50-75 mg/kg IM, IV[365]	Most species
Ceftazidime (Ceptaz, Fortaz, Glaxo Wellcome; Tazicef, SmithKline Beecham)	75-100 mg/kg IM, IV q6-8h[331]	Most species/broad spectrum; penetrates CNS
Ceftiofur (Naxcel, Pharmacia & Upjohn)	10 mg/kg IM q4h[362]	Cockatiels/PD; higher doses may be required for resistant infections
	10 mg/kg IM q8-12h[362]	Orange-winged Amazon parrots/PD
	75-100 mg IM q4-8h[107]	Most species
	0.16 mg/chick SC q24h[362]	Chickens/PD; moderately susceptible bacterial infections
	0.08-0.2 mg/chick SC q24h[362]	Chickens/susceptible *E. coli*
	0.24 mg/poult SC q24h[362]	Turkeys/PD; moderately susceptible bacterial infections

113

Table 18. Antimicrobial agents used in birds (cont.)

Agent	Dosage	Comments
Ceftiofur (continued)	0.17-0.50 mg/poult SC q24h[362]	Turkeys/susceptible *E. coli*
	10 mg/kg IM q12h[1]	Ostriches
	50 mg/kg IM q12h[1]	Ostrich chicks
Ceftriaxone (Rocephin, Roche)	—	May prolong bleeding times[314]
	75-100 mg/kg IM q4-8h[107]	Most species
	100 mg/kg IM[187] q4h	Chickens/PD; nebulization is ineffective; frequency estimated from data
Cephalexin	40-100 mg/kg PO, IM q6h[23,29]	Most species, including raptors
	100 mg/kg PO q12h[324]	Most species/14-21 day therapy may be indicated for severe or deep pyodermas
	55-110 mg/kg PO q12h[138]	Poultry/*Mycoplasma* and *Haemophilus*
	100 mg/kg PO q4-6h[44]	Pigeons, emus, cranes/PD
	100 mg/kg PO q8-12h[139]	Pigeons
	35-50 mg/kg PO,[48] IM[44] q6h	Pigeons, emus, cranes
	35-50 mg/kg IM q2-3h[44]	Quail, ducks/PD
	50 mg/kg PO q6h × 3-5 days[256]	Raptors
	15-22 mg/kg PO q8h[367]	Ratites (excluding emus)
Cephalothin (Keflin, Lilly)	100 mg/kg IM q6-8h[58]	Most species
	100 mg/kg IM q6h[44]	Pigeons, emus, cranes/PD
	100 mg/kg IM q2-3h[44]	Quail, ducks/PD
	30-40 mg/kg IM, IV q6h[367]	Ratites (excluding emus)
Cephradine (Cephradine, Biocraft)	35-50 mg/kg PO q4-6h[313]	Most species/14-21 day therapy may be indicated for severe or deep pyodermas
	100 mg/kg PO q4-6h[313]	Pigeons, emus, cranes

Table 18. Antimicrobial agents used in birds (cont.)

Agent	Dosage	Comments
Chloramphenicol	—	Bacteriostatic activity limits usefulness; palmitate not available in US, but can be compounded commercially
	50 mg/kg IM q12h[55]	Budgerigars, chickens, turkeys, ducks, geese/PD
	50-70 mg/kg PO, IM q8h[23]	Most species
	50 mg/kg IM q6h[55]	Macaws, conures/PD
	200 mg/kg IM q12h × 5 days[172]	Budgerigars/PD
	100-200 mg/L drinking water[314]	Canaries
	60-100 mg/kg IM q8h[139]	Pigeons
	250 mg/kg PO q6h[139]	Pigeons
	50 mg/kg PO q6-8h[8,313]	Galliformes (ie, turkeys)
	50 mg/kg IM q24h[55]	Peafowl, eagles/PD
	22 mg/kg IM, IV q3h[85]	Ducks/PD
	100 mg/kg SC q8h[48,50]	Cranes/PD
	35-50 mg/kg PO, SC, IM, IV q8h × 3 days[367]	Ratites
Chlorhexidine	10-30 ml/gal drinking water[315,357]	Most species, including finches/resistant Gram $\ominus$; yeast, including endoventricular mycoses;[357] topical application may be fatal to nun and parrot finches[314]
	30 ml/gal water[367]	Ratites/disinfectant egg spray at 104-108 °F (40-42 °C)
Chlorine (Na hypochlorite)	5 mg/L (5 ppm) drinking water[324]	Water disinfectant; 0.1 ml of 5.25% bleach/L approximates this concentration
Chlortetracycline	—	Most species/*Chlamydia*; doxycycline is preferred
	250 mg/16 oz drinking water[58]	Most species/limited usefulness; prepare fresh q8-12h

115

Table 18. Antimicrobial agents used in birds (cont.)

Agent	Dosage	Comments
Chlortetracycline (continued)	1,000-2,000 ppm soft mixed feed[90]	Most psittacines
	0.5% pellets × 30-45 days[23,57,58,91]	Small psittacines/reduce calcium content of diet to 0.7%
	1% pellets × 30-45 days[23,91,108,115]	Large psittacines/reduce calcium content of diet to 0.7%
	500 mg/L feed × 30-45 days[57]	Nectar feeders
	1,000-1,500 ppm drinking water[92]	Canaries
	1,500 ppm soft feed[92]	Canaries
	40-50 mg/kg PO q8h (w/grit) or q12h (w/o grit)[90]	Pigeons/PD
	1.0-1.5 g/gal drinking water[139]	Pigeons
	2,500 mg/L drinking water and 2,500 ppm feed[385]	Chickens, turkeys/PD; simultaneous medication of feed and water required to reach therapeutic level[37,388]
	250 mg/kg PO q24h[155]	Raptors
	6-10 mg/kg IM q24h[155]	Raptors
	1,000 ppm feed × 45 days[29]	Waterfowl
	15-20 mg/kg PO q8h[367]	Ratites
Ciprofloxacin (Cipro, Bayer)	20 mg/kg PO q12h[23]	Most species
	80 mg/kg PO q24h[371,372]	Most species/*Mycobacterium*; use in combination with other agents (see Appendix 34)
	5-20 mg/kg PO q12h × 5-7 days[327]	Pigeons
	250 mg/L drinking water × 5-10 days[327]	Pigeons
	5 mg/kg/day PO × 5 days[126]	Chickens/PD
	50 mg/kg PO q12h[171]	Raptors/PD

Table 18. Antimicrobial agents used in birds (cont.)

Agent	Dosage	Comments
Ciprofloxacin (continued)	3-6 mg/kg PO q12h[367]	Ratites
	10 mg/kg PO q12h × 7 days[2]	Ostrich chicks/hyperkeratosis
Citric acid	1 g/L drinking water[324]	Budgerigars, finches/ megabacteriosis; lower pH; 1 level tsp ≈ 3.85 g
Clarithromycin (Biaxin, Abbott)	85 mg/kg PO q24h[330]	Most species/*Mycobacterium;* allometrically scaled; use in combination with other agents (see Appendix 34)
Clindamycin (Antirobe, Upjohn)	25 mg/kg PO q8h[108]	Psittacines, raptors
	100 mg/kg PO q24h × 3-5 days[108,313]	Pigeons/Gram ⊕ and anaerobes
	150 mg/kg PO q24h[132]	Pigeons/osteomyelitis
	200 mg/L drinking water[71]	Pigeons
	50 mg/kg PO q12h × 7-10 days[29]	Raptors/osteomyelitis
	5.5 mg/kg PO q8h[256]	Ostrich
Clofazimine (Lamprene, Ciba Geneva)	6 mg/kg PO q12h[330,371,372]	Most species/*Mycobacterium*; use in combination with other agents (see Appendix 34)
	1.5 mg/kg PO q24h[30]	Psittacines/*Mycobacterium*
	1.5 mg/kg PO q24h × 3-12 mo[29]	Raptors/*Mycobacterium*; use in combination with other agents (see Appendix 34)
Cloxacillin (Orbenin, Beecham)	100-200 mg/kg IM q24h[256]	Most species
	250 mg/kg PO q24h[240]	Most species
	250 mg/kg PO q12h × 7-10 days[29]	Raptors
Cycloserine (Seromycin, Lilly)	5 mg/kg PO q24h × 3-12 mo[29]	Raptors/*Mycobacterium*; use in combination with other agents (see Appendix 34)
Danofloxacin	50 ppm in drinking water[249,359]	Chicken chicks/*Mycoplasma*

117

Table 18. Antimicrobial agents used in birds (cont.)

Agent	Dosage	Comments
Doxycycline (Vibramycin, Pfizer)	—	*Chlamydia, Mycoplasma*
	25-50 mg/kg PO q24h[89,108]	Most species/may cause regurgitation; use low end of dose range for macaws, cockatoos[108]
	100 mg capsule/4 oz drinking water[324]	Most species
	1 g/kg soft feed[114]	Large psittacines/10 mg/ml syrup mixed into 29% kidney beans, 29% canned corn, 29% cooked rice, 13% dry oatmeal cereal
	1,000 ppm dehulled seed PO[89]	Large psittacines/PD
	0.1% corn diet[286]	Macaws/PD
	8 mg/kg PO q12-24h[314]	Nectar feeders
	250 mg/L drinking water[92]	Canaries
	1 g/kg soft feed[92]	Canaries
	7.5 mg/kg (w/o grit), 25 mg/kg (w/grit) PO q12h[90]	Pigeons/PD
	40 mg/kg PO q24h[84]	Pigeons/PD; *Streptococcusbovis*
	500 mg/L drinking water[84]	Pigeons/PD; *Streptococcus bovis*
	100 mg/L drinking water[102]	Chickens/PD
	1-2 g/gal drinking water[138]	Poultry/*Mycoplasma, Haemophilus*; can use in combination with tylosin (2 tsp/gal drinking water)
	25 mg/kg PO q12h[183]	Raptors
	50 mg/kg PO q12h × 3-5 days[29]	Waterfowl/treat × 45 days for *Chlamydia*
	240 ppm feed × 45 days[29]	Waterfowl
	2.0-3.5 mg/kg PO q12h[89,367]	Ratites

118

Table 18. Antimicrobial agents used in birds (cont.)

Agent	Dosage	Comments
Doxycycline (Vibravenos, Pfizer)	—	Not available in US
	60-100 mg/kg SC, IM q5-7d[89,90]	Psittacines, pigeons/PD
	100 mg/kg IM q7d × 4-6 wk[23]	Psittacines/emesis may occur[25]
	75 mg/kg IM q7d × 4-6 wk[23,29]	Macaws, waterfowl
Enrofloxacin (Baytril, Bayer)	10-20 mg/kg PO q24h[90]	Psittacines, pigeons/PD
	100-200 mg/L drinking water[89]	Psittacines, pigeons/PD
	500 ppm feed[89,223]	Psittacines, including Patagonian conures/PD; mix into steamed corn diet
	15-30 mg/kg PO, IM q12h[113]	African grey parrots/PD
	0.19-0.75 mg/ml drinking water[111]	African grey parrots/PD
	1 g/kg feed[223]	Senegal parrots/PD; mix into steamed corn diet
	5 mg/kg IM, SC q12h[47]	Cockatiels/PD
	10 mg/kg PO q12h[47]	Cockatiels/PD
	250 ppm feed[89]	Budgerigars/PD
	200 mg/L drinking water[92]	Canaries
	200 mg/kg soft feed[92]	Canaries
	5-10 mg/kg SC, IM q24h[90]	Pigeons/PD
	200 mg/L drinking water × 5-7 days[327]	Pigeons
	10 mg/kg PO q12h × 4 days[12]	Chickens/PD; high efficacy for intestinal salmonellosis[335]
	50 mg/L drinking water × 5 days[192]	Chickens/PD
	5 mg/kg/day PO × 5 days[126]	Chickens/PD; accumulates in eggs

Table 18. Antimicrobial agents used in birds (cont.)

Agent	Dosage	Comments
Enrofloxacin (continued)	50 mg/L drinking water[156]	Turkeys/PD
	15 mg/kg PO, IM, IV q12h[143]	Raptors/PD; IV administration in owls results in weakness, tachycardia, vasoconstriction
	0.2 mg/ml saline, flush q24h × 10 days[29]	Raptors/nasal flush
	10-15 mg/kg PO, IM q12h × 5-7 days[29]	Waterfowl
	50 ppm × 4 hr (day 1, AM), then 25 ppm × 4 hr/day × 4 days[368]	Muscovy, Pekin ducklings/ *Riemerella (Pasteurella)*
	1.5-2.5 mg/kg PO, SC q12h[367]	Ratites
	5 mg/kg IM q12h × 2 days[367]	Ratites/may cause severe muscle necrosis
	15 mg/kg PO q12h[1]	Ostrich chicks
Erythromycin	60 mg/kg PO q12h[161]	Most species
	500 mg/gal drinking water, 10 days on, 5 days off, 10 days on[58]	Most species
	125 mg/L drinking water[92]	Canaries
	200 mg/kg soft feed[92]	Canaries
	71 mg/kg PO q24h[84]	Pigeons/PD; *Streptococcus bovis*
	125 mg/kg PO q8h[139]	Pigeons
	1 g/L drinking water[84]	Pigeons/PD; *Streptococcus bovis*
	2-3 g/gal drinking water[139]	Pigeons
	55-110 mg/kg PO q12h[138]	Poultry/*Mycoplasma*, *Haemophilus*
	5-10 mg/kg PO q8h[367]	Ratites
Ethambutol (Myambutol Lederle)	30 mg/kg PO q24h[330,371]	Most species/*Mycobacterium*; use in combination with other agents (see Appendix 34)

Table 18. Antimicrobial agents used in birds (cont.)

Agent	Dosage	Comments
Ethambutol (continued)	10 mg/kg PO q12h[23]	Most species
	20 mg/kg PO q12h × 3-12 mo[29]	Raptors/*Mycobacterium*; use in combination with other agents (see Appendix 34)
Flumequine (Flumisol)	30 mg/kg PO, IM q8-12h[90]	Pigeons/PD; quinolone; not available in US; may cause emesis
Gentamicin	—	Not generally recommended for administration in pet birds; nephrotoxic,[43] narrow margin of safety; causes polydipsia and polyuria (macaws, cockatoos, hawks);[9,32] bird should be well hydrated; amikacin is a safer alternative
	5-10 mg/kg IM q8-12h[299]	Cockatiels/PD
	5-10 mg/kg IM q4h[332]	Pigeons/PD; *Salmonella*
	5 mg/kg IM q8h[74]	Pheasants, emus, cranes/PD
	10 mg/kg IM q6h[74]	Quail/PD
	2.5 mg/kg IM q8h[31]	Raptors/PD
	5 mg/kg IM q8h[177]	Emus/PD
	1-2 mg/kg IM q8h[367]	Ratites (excluding emus)/use only as last resort
Isoniazid (Isoniazid Tablets, Duramed)	—	Most species/*Mycobacterium* (see Appendix 34)
	30 mg/kg PO q24h[226,323,371,372]	Most species
	15 mg/kg PO q12h[313]	*Mycobacterium avium* often develops resistance
Kanamycin	10-20 mg/kg IM q12h[8]	Enteric infections
Lincomycin	100 mg/kg IM q12h[30]	Psittacines
	75 mg/kg PO q12h[30]	Psittacines
	100-200 mg/L drinking water[92]	Canaries

Table 18. Antimicrobial agents used in birds (cont.)

Agent	Dosage	Comments
Lincomycin (continued)	35-50 mg/pigeon q24h × 7-14 days[244]	Pigeons
	50-75 mg/kg IM q12h × 7-10 days[29]	Raptors/pododermatitis, osteomyelitis
	100 mg/kg PO q24h[313]	Raptors
	10 g/5 L drinking water × 5-7 days[29]	Waterfowl/*Pasteurella*, mycoplasmal tenosynovitis
Lincomycin/ spectinomycin (LS-50 Water Soluble, Upjohn)	50 mg/kg PO q24h[256]	Most species
	1/8-1/4 tsp/16 oz drinking water × 10-14 days[58]	Most species
	2.5-5.0 mg/chick IM[135] once	Chicken chicks/PD; may prevent *E. coli* and *Staphylococcus aureus* infections; injectable form not available in US
	2 g/gal drinking water for first 5 days of life[136]	Turkeys/PD; *Mycoplasma* airsacculitis
Marbofloxacin (Marbocyl, Univet)	15 mg/kg PO q12h × 5-7 days[29]	Raptors/quinolone; not available in US
Metronidazole	—	Most anaerobes; see antiprotozoal dosages
	50 mg/kg PO q24h × 5 days[23,29]	Most species, including raptors
	50 mg/kg PO q12h × 30 days[324]	Amazon parrots, cockatoos/ anaerobic and hemorrhagic enteritis
Minocycline (Minocin, Lederle)	15 mg/kg PO q12h[305]	Raptors/some anaerobes
	0.5% feed[8,233]	Parakeets/PD
Neomycin	80-100 mg/L drinking water[314]	Canaries/not absorbed from gastrointestinal tract
	5-10 mg/kg IM q12h[155]	Raptors/toxic if overdosed
Nitrofurazone (NFZ 9.2, Hess & Clark)	—	Not recommended;[324] may be hepatotoxic; avoid use or reduce dosage in hot weather; do not use in finches or pigeons[327]

Table 18. Antimicrobial agents used in birds (cont.)

Agent	Dosage	Comments
Nitrofurazone (continued)	1 tsp/gal drinking water × 7-10 days[247]	Most species
	1/2 tsp/gal drinking water × 7 days[313]	Lories, mynahs/do not put in lory nectar
Norfloxacin (Noroxin, Merck; Vetriflox 20% Oral Solution, Lavet Ltd, Budapest)	10 mg/kg PO q24h[210]	Chickens, geese/PD; quinolone
	10 mg/kg PO q6-8h[210]	Turkeys/PD
	175 mg/L drinking water × 5 days[317]	Chickens
	3-5 mg/kg PO q12h[367]	Ratites
Nystatin	5,000,000 IU/L drinking water[103]	Goldfinches/megabacteriosis
Oxytetracycline (Liquamycin, LA-200, Terramycin Soluble Powder, Pfizer)	—	IM administration may cause irritation or muscle damage; may be useful in treating chlamydiosis
	50-100 mg/kg SC, IM q2-3d[112]	Cockatoos/PD
	50-75 mg/kg SC[108]	Goffin's cockatoos, blue and gold macaws/causes irritation at injection site
	58 mg/kg IM q24h[311]	Amazon parrots/PD
	200 mg/kg IM q24h[23]	Most species
	50 mg/kg PO q6-8h[139]	Pigeons
	1.0-1.5 g/gal drinking water[139]	Pigeons
	5 mg/kg SC, IM q12-24h[33]	Chicken chicks/PD; poor distribution to lung tissues; calcium affects absorption
	2.5 g/L drinking water and 2,500 ppm feed[385]	Chickens, turkeys/PD; simultaneous medication of feed and water required to reach therapeutic level
	43 mg/kg IM q24h[311]	Pheasants/PD
	16 mg/kg IM q24h[311]	Owls/PD

Table 18. Antimicrobial agents used in birds (cont.)

Agent	Dosage	Comments
Oxytetracycline (continued)	25-50 mg/kg PO q8h × 5-7 days[29]	Raptors
	200 mg/kg IM q24h × 5-7 days[29]	Waterfowl/*Pasteurella*
	10 mg/kg IM q3d[367]	Ratites/may cause severe muscle necrosis; use as last resort
Penicillin benzathine/procaine (Benza-Pen, SmithKline Beecham)	200 mg/kg IM q24h[23]	Most species
Penicillin procaine (Penicillin G Procaine, SmithKline Beecham)	100 mg/kg IM q24-48h[158]	Turkeys/PD; sulfonamide resistant *Pasteurella*
Piperacillin (Piperacil, Lederle)	150 mg/kg IM q12h[23]	Most species
	100 mg/kg IM q12h[90]	Psittacines/PD
	200 mg/kg IM q8h[233]	Budgerigars/PD
	0.02 ml (4 mg) in macaw eggs; 0.01 ml (2 mg) in small eggs[246]	Eggs/200 mg/ml solution; inject into air cell on days 14, 18, and 22
	100 mg/kg IM q8-12h[140]	Pigeons
	100 mg/kg IM q12h[50,183]	Raptors, cranes
	100 mg/kg IM q8h[304]	Raptors/pododermatitis
	25 mg/kg IM[367]	Ratite chicks (less than 6 mo)
Polymyxin B	50,000 IU/L drinking water[179]	Canaries
	50,000 IU/kg soft feed[179]	Canaries
	10-15 mg/kg IM q24h[155]	Raptors/not absorbed if given PO
Rifabutin (Mycobutin, Pharmacia)	15 mg/kg PO q24h[330,371,372]	Most species/*Mycobacterium*; use in combination with other agents (see Appendix 34)

Table 18. Antimicrobial agents used in birds (cont.)

Agent	Dosage	Comments
Rifampin (Rifadin, Marion Merrell Dow)	—	Most species/*Mycobacterium*; use in combination with other agents (see Appendix 34)
	15 mg/kg PO q12h[23]	Most species
	45 mg/kg PO q24h[226,371,372]	Most species, including Amazon parrots
	45 mg/kg PO q24h[345]	Cranes
Spectinomycin (Spectogard, Syntex; Spectam, Sanofi)	10-30 mg/kg IM q8-12h[30]	Psittacines
	200-400 mg/L drinking water[92]	Canaries
	400 mg/kg soft feed[92]	Canaries
	25-35 mg/kg IM q8-12h[140]	Pigeons
	165-275 mg/L drinking water[139]	Pigeons
Spiramycin	200-400 mg/L drinking water[92]	Canaries
	400 mg/kg soft feed[92]	Canaries
	20 mg/kg IM q24h[155]	Raptors
	250 mg/kg PO q24h[155]	Raptors/poorly absorbed
Streptomycin (Streptomycin Sulfate, Roerig)	30 mg/kg IM q12h[23]	Most species/may be nephrotoxic; consider amikacin as alternative; *Mycobacterium*; use in combination with other agents (see Appendix 34)
	25-50 mg/kg IM q24h[90]	Chickens/PD
	15 mg/kg PO q24h[155]	Raptors/highly neurotoxic
Sulfachlorpyridazine (Vetasulid, Solvay)	1/4-1/2 tsp/L drinking water × 5-10 days[8]	Most species/enteric infections
	400 mg/L drinking water × 7-10 days[326]	Pigeons
Sulfamethazine (12%)	30 mg/30 ml drinking water[314]	Small psittacines/coccidiostat with some antibacterial activity against *Pasteurella* and *Salmonella*

Table 18. Antimicrobial agents used in birds (cont.)

Agent	Dosage	Comments
Sulfamethazine (12%) (continued)	400 mg/L drinking water × 7-10 days[326]	Pigeons
Tetracycline (Tetracycline Soluble Powder, Butler; Panmycin Aquadrops, Upjohn)	200-250 mg/kg PO q12-24h[58,313]	Most species/gavage
	200 mg/gal drinking water × 5-10 days[58]	Most species
	1 Tbs powder/gal drinking water[324]	Pigeons/soluble powder (10 g/6.4 oz)
	400 mg/gal drinking water[300]	Rheas
Tiamulin (Denegard, Fermenta)	—	Mycoplasma
	25-50 mg/kg PO q24h[90]	Most species
	30 mg/kg PO q24h × 7 days[285]	Poultry adults
	60 mg/kg PO q24h × 7 days[285]	Poultry chicks
	400 mg/kg feed × 7 days (1 g powder/kg feed)[285]	Poultry
	250 mg/L drinking water × 7 days (2.2 g powder/gal)[324]	Poultry, pigeons[324]
	1 g powder/L water[285]	Poultry eggs/dip
Tiamulin/ chlortetracycline (Tetramutin, Novartis)	1.0-1.5 kg/ton feed × 7 days[352]	Chickens/*Mycoplasma*; may be used with salinomycin at 60 ppm without signs of incompatibility
Ticarcillin	200 mg/kg IM q8h[23]	Most species/*Pseudomonas*[108]
	200 mg/kg IM, IV q8-12h × 7 days[327]	Pigeons
	200 mg/kg IM q12h[183]	Raptors
Ticarcillin/ clavulanic acid (Timentin, SmithKline Beecham)	200 mg/kg IM, IV q12h[324]	Most species
Tilmicosin (Micotil 300 Injection, Elanco)	100-200 mg/L drinking water × 5 days[193]	Poultry chicks/*Mycoplasma gallisepticum*; reduction of clinical signs; macrolide

Table 18. Antimicrobial agents used in birds (cont.)

Agent	Dosage	Comments
Tilmicosin (continued)	200-300 mg/L drinking water × 5 days[193]	Poultry chicks/elimination of *M. gallisepticum*
	250-500 mg/L drinking water × 5 days[181]	Poultry chicks/*Mycoplasma synoviae* and *M. gallisepticum*; mycoplasmacidal
Tobramycin (Tobramycin, Elkins-Sinn)	5 mg/kg IM q12h[23]	Most species/aminoglycoside
	2.5-5.0 mg/kg IM q12h[313,322]	Psittacines, pheasants, cranes
	10 mg/kg IM q12h × 5-7 days[256]	Raptors
	0.25-0.50 ml intra-articular flush q24h × 7-10 days[29]	Raptors/septic arthritis
Trimethoprim (Trimethoprim, Biocraft)	15-20 mg/kg PO q8h[90]	Pigeons/PD
Trimethoprim/ sulfadiazine (Tribrissen, Schering-Plough)	12-60 mg/kg PO q12h × 5-7 days[29]	Raptors/useful for sensitive infections in neonates
	8-60 mg/kg SC, IM q12h[50]	Cranes/parenteral form not available in US; may be compounded
Trimethoprim/ sulfamethoxazole (Bactrim, Roche; Septra, Burroughs Wellcome)	75 mg/kg IM q12h[23]	Most species/reduce dose if regurgitation occurs;[108] parenteral form not available in US; may be compounded
	100 mg/kg PO q12h[23]	Most species
	48 mg/120 ml drinking water[324]	Most species
	60 mg/kg PO q24h[90]	Pigeons/PD
	360 mg/L drinking water × 10-14 days[326]	Pigeons
	48 mg/kg PO, IM q12h[183]	Raptors
	0.04% feed[289]	Geese
	960 mg/45 kg PO q12h[1]	Ostriches
	21 mg/kg PO q12h[1]	Ostriches
	60-72 mg/kg PO q12h[50]	Cranes

127

Table 18. Antimicrobial agents used in birds (cont.)

Agent	Dosage	Comments
Tylosin (Tylan, Elanco; Tylan Soluble, Elanco)	30 mg/kg IM q12h[23]	Most species
	1/2 tsp/gal drinking water[324]	Most species/approximately 4,000 mg/tsp[277]
	250-400 mg/L drinking water[92]	Canaries
	25 mg/kg IM q6h[225]	Pigeons, quail/PD
	2 tsp/gal drinking water[138,140]	Pigeons, poultry/*Mycoplasma*, *Haemophilus*
	10-40 mg/kg IM q6-8h[314]	Poultry
	500 ppm drinking water × 3 days[181,359]	Poultry chicks/ *Mycoplasma gallisepticum, M. synoviae*
	30 mg/kg IM q12h × 3 days[29]	Raptors/*Mycoplasma*
	20-30 mg/kg IM q8h × 3-7 days[29]	Waterfowl/*Mycoplasma*
	2.5 g/5 L drinking water × 3 days[29]	Waterfowl/*Mycoplasma*
	100 mg/10 ml saline nasal flush[29]	Waterfowl/*Mycoplasma*
	15 mg/kg IM q8h[225]	Cranes/PD
	25 mg/kg IM q8h[225]	Emus/PD
	17 mg/kg IM q24h × 7 days[255]	Emus/*Mycoplasma*
	2 g/gal drinking water × 4 wk[255]	Emus/*Mycoplasma*
	3-5 mg/kg IM, IV q12h[367]	Ratites
	5-10 mg/kg PO q8h[367]	Ratites

Table 19. Antifungal agents used in birds

Agent	Dosage	Comments
Acetic acid (vinegar)	15 ml/qt drinking water[179]	Most species/gastrointestinal yeast infections
Amphotericin B Fungizone, Squibb)	—	Preferred IV agent for aspergillosis; IT administration for syringeal aspergilloma may cause tracheitis
	1.5 mg/kg IV q8h × 3 days[22,105]	Most species
	1 mg/kg IT q8-12h[105,313,314]	Psittacines, raptors/aspergillosis; potentially nephrotoxic
	0.05 mg/ml sterile water[22]	Most species/nasal flush
	0.25-1.0 ml PO q24h × 4-5 days[29]	Raptors/useful in neonates; candidiasis, not absorbed from alimentary tract
	1 mg/kg IT q12h × 12 days, then q48h × 5 wk[29]	Raptors/syringeal aspergilloma
Caprylic acid (Kaprycidin A, Ecological Formulas)	271 mg/kg PO[365]	Most species/adjunctive treatment with imidazoles; seldom used
Chlorhexidine	0.05% (500 mg/L) PO[26]	Most species/ingl{uvial yeast infections
	10 ml/gal drinking water[357]	Finches/endoventricular mycoses; use with flucytosine or itraconazole
Clotrimazole (Lotrimin, Schering)	—	Psittacines/used commonly as adjunctive therapy for aspergillosis; administer via air sac, IT, nebulization, or topically
	0.2 ml (2 mg)/kg IT q24h × 5 days[324]	Psittacines/syringeal aspergilloma; apply with catheter directly into syrinx during anesthesia
	Inject 10 mg/kg into air sacs[324]	Psittacines/dilute in propylene glycol to 2.5 mg/ml; divide total dose between the 4 most accessible air sacs; toxic and may result in death in African grey parrots and other birds if injected into the muscle or viscera[324]

129

Table 19. Antifungal agents used in birds (cont.)

Agent	Dosage	Comments
Clotrimazole (continued)	10 mg/ml flush[105]	Most species/effective against *Aspergillus* at sites that can be flushed
	Nebulize 1% × 30-60 min[5,185]	Use in combination with amphotericin, flucytosine, and itraconazole
Ethyodide (Vet-A-Mix)	$^1/_4$ oz in feed q24h × 2-3 wk[5]	Ratites/air sac aspergillosis; use in combination with sodium iodine, and oral azoles
Fluconazole (Diflucan, Roerig)	—	Water soluble at pH 7; safest therapeutic index of the azoles; fungistatic; suspension available
	5-15 mg/kg PO q12h × 14-60 days or longer[324]	Most species/preferred oral azole antifungal for aspergillosis, mycelial candidiasis; use lower dose for candidiasis
	20 mg/kg PO q48h[106]	Psittacines/PD; mucosal, systemic yeast infections
	50 mg/L drinking water × 14-60 days[324]	Most species/systemic mycoses; candidiasis
	2-5 mg/kg PO q24h × 7-10 days[29,270]	Most species, including raptors/ gastrointestinal, systemic candidiasis; CNS, ocular mycoses
	4-6 mg/kg PO q12h[106]	Juvenile psittacines; candidiasis
	15 mg/kg PO q12h × 30 days following cessation of clinical signs[5]	Psittacines/chronic nasal aspergillosis
	15 mg/kg PO q12h × 4 weeks or longer[328]	Pigeons/aspergillosis
	10-20 mg/kg PO × 30 days[179]	Red-tailed hawks, gyrfalcons/ aspergillosis
	25 mg/L nectar[150]	Hummingbirds/aspergillosis

Table 19. Antifungal agents used in birds (cont.)

Agent	Dosage	Comments
Flucytosine (Ancobon, Roche)	—	Use prophylactically in raptors (especially in falcons) and waterfowl to prevent aspergillosis; may be administered as adjunctive treatment with amphotericin B; fungistatic
	60 mg/kg PO q12h (birds >500 g) or 150 mg/kg PO q12h (birds <500 g)[5]	Most species, including galliformes, swans/syringeal aspergilloma
	100-250 mg/kg PO q12h[186]	Psittacine neonates
	250 mg/kg PO q12h × 14-17 days[357]	Finches/endoventricular mycoses; can use with chlorhexidine in drinking water
	120 mg/kg PO q6h[183]	Raptors/aspergillosis
	50-75 mg/kg PO q8h[305]	Raptors/aspergillosis prophylaxis in conjunction with amphotericin B
	250 mg/kg PO q12h[183]	Raptors/candidiasis
	80-100 mg/kg PO q12h[367]	Ratites
Griseofulvin (Fulvicin U/F microsize, Schering-Plough)	30 mg/kg q24h × 21 days[2]	Ostrich chick/dermatomycoses
	35-50 mg/kg PO q24h[367]	Ratites
	10 mg/kg PO q24h × 21 days[29]	Pigeons/dermatophytoses; gavage
Iodine, sodium (20%)	50 mg/100 kg IV slowly q5d × 3 treatments[5]	Ratites/generalized air sac aspergillosis; use with ethyodide granules
Itraconazole (Sporanox, Janssen)	—	Most species/systemic mycoses; may be useful in superficial candidiasis or dermatophytosis; may be toxic if used concurrently with clotrimazole; approximately 0.35-0.39 mg/granule (approximately 285-290 granules per capsule, but number can vary considerably);[324] method of compounding with strong acid and orange juice has been reported[270]

Table 19. Antifungal agents used in birds (cont.)

Agent	Dosage	Comments
Itraconazole (continued)	10 mg/kg PO q24h × 14 days with food[270,271]	Psittacines/use in combination with other non-azoles
	2.5-5.0 mg/kg PO q24h[271]	African grey parrots/toxicity in African grey parrots (anorexia, depression)[109]
	20 mg/100 g feed up to 100 days[309]	Gouldian finches/PD; dermato-mycoses; beads from capsules are mixed with small amount of oil and seed
	5-10 mg/kg PO q12h[189]	Passerines (towhees)/aspergillosis prophylaxis
	10 mg/kg PO q12h × 21 days[357]	Finches/endoventricular mycoses; can use with chlorhexidine in drinking water
	6 mg/kg PO q12h[234]	Pigeons/PD; dosage will achieve fungicidal plasma concentrations; 26 mg/kg PO q12h is required to reach a therapeutic level of 1 µg/ml in respiratory tissues[234]
	10 mg/kg PO q12-24h[271]	Pigeons
	5 mg/kg PO q24h[5]	Galliformes, ratites, swans/air sac aspergillosis
	5-10 mg/kg PO q12-24h[183]	Raptors
	5-10 mg/kg PO q12h[313]	Waterfowl, penguins/aspergillosis, candidiasis, cryptococcosis
	6-10 mg/kg PO[177,367]	Ratites/preferred azole
Ketoconazole (Nizoral, Janssen)	—	Most species/systemic mycoses (ie, aspergillosis), candidiasis; less toxic than amphotericin B
	30 mg/kg PO q12h × 7-14 days[199]	Amazon parrots/PD

Table 19. Antifungal agents used in birds (cont.)

Agent	Dosage	Comments
Ketoconazole (continued)	10-30 mg/kg PO q12h × 30-60 days[324]	Most species/grind 200 mg tablet and mix with 5 ml simple syrup (Humco) (=40 mg/ml); dosages >20 mg/kg may cause regurgitation (if regurgitation, discontinue for 1-2 days, then restart and regurgitation usually ceases)
	20-30 mg/kg PO q8h[105]	Cockatoos
	20 mg/kg PO q12h[186]	Psittacine neonates
	200 mg/L drinking water or soft feed × 7-14 days[92]	Canaries/dissolve crushed tablet in $^1/_2$-1 tsp vinegar
	20-40 mg/kg PO q12h × 15-60 days[327]	Pigeons
	30 mg/kg PO q12h199 × 7-30 days[324]	Pigeons, raptors/prophylactic in raptors for aspergillosis
	15 mg/kg PO q12h[183]	Raptors/candidiasis
	60 mg/kg PO q12h[376]	Raptors/PD (common buzzard); aspergillosis
	50 mg/kg/day PO[67]	Toucans
	12.5 mg/kg PO q24h × 30 days[314]	Swans/candidiasis
	200 mg/L nectar[150]	Hummingbirds
	5-10 mg/kg PO q24h[367]	Ratites
	25 mg/kg PO q12h × 14 days[5]	Ratites/air sac aspergillosis
Miconazole (Daktarin, Janssen)	5 mg/kg IT q12h × 5 days[378]	Psittacines/10 mg/ml solution diluted with saline; syringeal mycoses; use with flucytosine; not available in US; Conofite (Mallinckrodt) and clotrimazole may be alternatives
Nystatin (Mycostatin, Squibb)	—	Most species/oral or gastrointestinal tract candidiasis; medication must contact the organism

Table 19. Antifungal agents used in birds (cont.)

Agent	Dosage	Comments
Nystatin (continued)	300,000 IU/kg PO q12h × 7-14 days[29,105]	Most species, including waterfowl
	100,000 IU/L drinking water[92]	Canaries
	200,000 IU/kg soft feed[92]	Canaries
	100,000 IU/kg PO q12h[140,183]	Pigeons; raptors
	250,000-500,000 IU/kg PO q12h[367]	Ratites

Table 20. Antiviral and immunomodulating agents used in birds

Agent	Dosage	Comments
Acyclovir (Zovirax, Burroughs Wellcome)	80 mg/kg PO q8h × 7 days[266]	Psittacines/PD (Quaker parakeets); psittacine herpesvirus prophylaxis or treatment
	400 mg/kg feed[70]	Psittacines (Quaker parakeets)/ psittacine herpesvirus
	1 mg/ml drinking water[70,312]	Psittacines (Quaker parakeets)/ psittacine herpesvirus; gavage
	330 mg/kg PO q12h × 4-7 days[186]	Psittacine neonates/psittacine herpes virus
	10 mg/kg IM q24h × 14 days starting 3 days post-exposure[70]	Chickens/Marek's disease
	29 mg/bird q8h × 7 days[29]	Pigeons/herpesvirus
Amantadine	10 mg/kg PO × 3 days pre- and 18 days post-exposure[70]	Turkeys/influenza viruses; must be administered before and during virus exposure
	25 mg/kg PO × 10 days following infection[70]	Chickens
	0.01% drinking water[70]	Chickens/can use simultaneously with vaccine
Interferon (Roferon-A Injection, Roche)	—	Interferon α-2a; glycoprotein which induces production of proteins, thereby inhibiting intracellular virus replication
	60-240 IU/kg SC, IM q12h[341] 300-1,200 IU/kg PO q12h[324]	Most species; stock solution: mix 1 ml (3,000,000 IU/ml) with 100 ml sterile water (30,000 IU/ml; can freeze as 2 ml vials up to 1 yr); mix 2 ml of stock into 1 L LRS (=60 IU/ml, refrigerate up to 3 mo)
	1 IU/ml or 4,000 IU/gal drinking water × 14-28 days[324,326,328]	Pigeons/may be useful against circovirus
Levamisole (Levasole, Mallinckrodt)	—	Anthelmintic with immunostimulation properties
	41 mg/gal drinking water × 3-5 wk[57]	Most species

Table 20. Antiviral and immunomodulating agents used in birds (cont.)

Agent	Dosage	Comments
Levamisole (continued)	2 mg/kg SC q14d × 3 treatments[38]	Macaws
Rimantadine (Flumadine, Forest)	0.01% drinking water[70]	Chickens/influenza viruses; must be used before and during exposure

Table 21. Antiparasitic agents used in birds

Agent	Dosage	Comments
Albendazole (11.36%) (Valbazen, SmithKline)	10 mg/kg PO once[72]	Poultry/PD; anthelmintic
	50 mg/kg PO × 3-4 days[348]	Doves, rock partridges/*Capillaria*; may be toxic in some Columbiformes at 50-100 mg/kg
	5.2 mg/kg PO q12h × 3 days, repeat in 14 days[367]	Ratites/flagellates, tapeworms
Amprolium (Corid, Merck)	—	Coccidiosis; efficacy is reduced by high doses of thiamine
	0.5 ml/L × 5 days[256]	Most species/9.6% solution
	0.25 mg/L drinking water × 7 days[378a]	Psittacines (keas)/ *Sarcocystis*; use in combination with pyramethamine and primaquine
	2 ml/gal drinking water × 5 days[242]	Parakeets, finches/9.6% solution
	25 mg/kg/day[142]	Pigeons
	8 ml/gal drinking water[139]	Pigeons/9.6% solution
	1 tsp/gal drinking water × 3-5 days[138,139]	Pigeons, poultry/20% powder
	120 g/ton (0.0175%) feed[347]	Pheasants, poultry/coccidiosis; *Sarcocystis*; interferes with thiamine absorption
	117-234 g/ton (0.0125-0.025%) feed[47, 347]	Poultry, cranes/lower dose is prophylactic; higher dose is therapeutic
	30 mg/kg PO × 5 days[155]	Raptors
	60 mg/L (0.006%) drinking water[50]	Cranes
Cambendazole (Equiben, Merck)	60-100 mg/kg PO q24h × 3-7 days[242]	Most species
	75 mg/kg PO q24h × 2 days[14]	Pigeons

Table 21. Antiparasitic agents used in birds (cont.)

Agent	Dosage	Comments
Carnidazole (Spartrix, Wildlife Pharmaceuticals)	20-30 mg/kg PO once[242]	Most species/*Trichomonas*
	30-50 mg/kg PO once, repeat in 14 days[179]	Cockatiels/*Giardia*
	0.5 mg/bird[339]	Society finches/flagellates, based on 15 g/finch
	0.25 mg/bird[339]	Society finch nestlings/flagellates; based on 7.5 g/nestling
	5 mg/bird PO[327]	Dove adults, pigeon squabs
	20 mg/kg PO139 once	Pigeons
	20 mg/kg q24h PO × 2 days[155,183]	Raptors
Chloroquine phosphate (Aralen, Sanofi)	—	*Plasmodium*; may be used with primaquine for *Haemoproteus*, *Leucocytozoon*
	25 mg/kg PO at 0 hr, then 15 mg/kg PO at 12, 24, and 48 hr[308,344]	Most species, including raptors/use with 0.75-1.0 mg/kg primaquine at 0 hr
	5 mg/kg PO q24h or in feed[347]	Game birds
	250 mg/4 oz drinking water, grape juice, or orange juice[347]	Game birds/juice covers bitter taste of drug
	10 mg/kg PO at 0 hr, then 5 mg/kg PO at 6, 24, and 48 hr[47]	Raptors/use with 0.3 mg/kg primaquine (at 24 hr following the initial chloroquine dose) q24h × 7 days
	10 mg/kg PO at 0 hr, then 5 mg/kg at 6, 18, and 24 hr[313]	Penguins
Chlorsulon (Curatrem, Merck)	20 mg/kg PO q14d × 3 treatments[63,313]	Psittacines/trematodes
	20 mg/kg PO 3 ×/wk × 2 wk[29,40]	Waterfowl, raptors/trematodes, cestodes
Clazuril (Appertex, Janssen)	7 mg/kg PO × 3 days, off 2 days, on 3 days[30]	Psittacines/coccidiostat

138

Table 21. Antiparasitic agents used in birds (cont.)

Agent	Dosage	Comments
Clazuril (continued)	2.5 mg/bird PO once[374]	Pigeons/suppresses oocyst excretion up to 2 1/2 weeks
	5-10 mg/kg PO q24h × 3 days, off 2 days, on 3 days[242]	Poultry, pigeons/coccidiostat
	5-10 mg/kg PO q72h × 3 treatments[29,40]	Waterfowl, raptors/coccidiostat
	1.1 ppm feed × 5 days[314]	Cranes
	5-10 mg/kg PO q24h × 2 days[155]	Raptors/coccidiostat
Clopidol (25%) (Coyden-25, A.L. Laboratories)	113.5-227.0 g/ton (125-250 ppm) (0.0125-0.025%) feed[347]	Game birds/coccidiosis; *Leucocytozoon; Plasmodium*
Dimetridazole (Emtryl, Jensen Salisbury)	—	*Trichomonas, Giardia, Hexamita, Spironucleus, Histomonas*; not available in US; low therapeutic index; hepatotoxic to lories, some passerines (eg, robins); not recommended for finches; 182 g/ 6.42 oz powder
	1 tsp/gal drinking water × 5 days[242,247]	Most species
	200-400 mg/L drinking water × 5 days[6]	Psittacines
	1/2 tsp/gal drinking water × 5 days[313]	Lories, mynahs
	100 mg/L drinking water[92]	Canaries
	400 mg/L drinking water × 3 days[169,170]	Pigeons/PD; bioavailability reduced with feed
	0.01875% feed[347]	Poultry, game birds
	3 g powder/L drinking water[347]	Poultry, game birds
Febantel (Vercom, Rintal, Bayer)	30 mg/kg PO once[15]	Pigeons/PD; ascarids; repeated doses required to eliminate *Capillaria obsignata*

139

Table 21. Antiparasitic agents used in birds (cont.)

Agent	Dosage	Comments
Fenbendazole (Panacur, Hoechst)	—	Most species/anthelmintic; dosages of 50 mg/kg/day may be toxic for some species, including raptors[324]
	20-100 mg/kg PO once[242]	Most species
	125 mg/L drinking water × 5 days[242]	Most species/nematodes
	25 mg/kg PO, repeat in 14 days[10]	Most species/ascarids
	50 mg/kg PO q24h × 5 days[63]	Most species/capillariasis
	50 mg/kg PO q24h × 3 days[63,327]	Most species, including pigeons/ nematodes; flukes; *Giardia* (efficacy unproven)
	50 mg/kg PO q12h × 5 days[324]	Cockatoos/use with ivermectin (0.2 mg/kg once); effective for filarid adulticide treatment
	50 mg/L drinking water × 5 days[242]	Finches
	1.5-3.9 mg/kg PO q24h × 3 days[360]	Chickens/PD; *Capillaria*
	80 ppm feed[360]	Chickens/PD; *Capillaria*
	54 g/ton feed × 5-7 days[347]	Game birds/nematodes; *capillaria*sis; gizzard worms; *Gongylonema*; cecal worms; gapeworms; flukes
	20 mg/kg PO q24h × 5 days[29]	Raptors/*Capillaria*
	20 mg/kg PO q24h × 14 days[29]	Raptors/filarial worms
	10-50 mg/kg PO, repeat in 14 days[183]	Raptors/ascarids, flukes
	20 mg/kg PO once[40]	Waterfowl/tapeworms, nematodes, acanthocephalans, gizzard worms

140

Table 21. Antiparasitic agents used in birds (cont.)

Agent	Dosage	Comments
Fenbendazole (continued)	5-15 mg/kg PO q24h × 5 days[313]	Anseriformes
	15 mg/kg PO[177]	Ostriches/wire worms; tapeworms
	100 mg/kg PO q24h × 5 days[50]	Cranes/*Capillaria*; gavage
Hydroxychloroquine sulfate (Plaquenil, Sanofi Winthrop)	100 mg/120 ml drinking water × 6 wk[179]	Pigeons/*Plasmodium*
Hygromycin B (Hygromix 8, Elanco)	12 g/ton feed × 12 wk[347]	Game birds/ascarids; cecal worms; some efficacy against capillariasis
	0.00088-0.00132% feed[347]	Game birds/ascarids
	0.0018-0.0026% feed × 2 mo[347]	Game birds/cecal worms
Ipronidazole (Ipropran, Roche)	—	*Giardia; Trichomonas; Histomonas*; not available in US; 61 g/2.65 oz
	500 mg/gal drinking water × 7days[6,13,242,278]	Most species, including pigeons
	960 mg/gal drinking water × 3-7 days[247,327]	Psittacines, pigeons
Ivermectin	—	All species/most nematodes, gapeworms, acanthocephalans, gizzard worms, leeches, most ectoparasites (including *Knemidocoptes, Dermanyssus*); can dilute with water or saline for immediate use; dilute with propylene glycol for extended use; dosages exceeding 0.2 mg/kg are probably unnecessary in birds

Table 21. Antiparasitic agents used in birds (cont.)

Agent	Dosage	Species/Comments
Ivermectin (continued)	0.2 mg/kg PO, SC, IM once[21,29,40,50,162,177,183,311,327,328,347]	Most species including psittacines, pigeons, raptors, Guinea fowl, waterfowl, ratites, cranes/ nematodes (including eye worms, gizzard worms, gapeworms), acanthocephalans; acariasis; use in combination with fenbendazole at 50 mg/kg PO q12h × 5 days for microfilaria in cockatoos
	0.2 mg/kg SC, topical on skin[95]	Canaries/quill mite acariasis; repeat in 4 days if live mites still present
	0.8-1.0 mg/L drinking water[92]	Canaries
	0.4 mg/kg SC once[189]	Passerines (towhees)/*Capillaria*
	0.4 mg/kg SC once[242]	Raptors
	0.005-0.50 mg/kg topical to eye[364]	Ocular nematodiasis
Lasalocid (Avatec, Hoffmann-La Roche)	68-113 g/ton feed continuously[347]	Game birds, chickens/coccidiosis
Levamisole (Tramisol, Mallinckrodt)	—	Many species/nematodes; immunostimulant; low therapeutic index (toxic reactions and deaths reported); IM administration may cause severe toxicity
	10-20 mg/kg SC once[242]	Most species/do not use in lories
	1.0-1.5 g (10 ml)/gal drinking water × 1-3 days[139,242]	Most species, including pigeons/ 13.65% injectable
	20 mg/kg PO once[242]	Psittacines, pigeons, raptors/ nematodes
	40 mg/kg PO once[139,242]	Psittacines, pigeons, raptors/ *Capillaria*
	80 mg/L drinking water × 3 days[314]	Finches

Table 21. Antiparasitic agents used in birds (cont.)

Agent	Dosage	Comments
Levamisole (continued)	20-25 mg/kg SC[347]	Game birds/nematodes (ie, gapeworms, capillarids, gizzard worms, eye worms)
	1-2 g/gal drinking water × 1 day, repeat in 7-14 days[347]	Game birds
	0.03-0.06% drinking water[347]	Game birds
	0.04% feed × 2 days[347]	Game birds
	20-50 mg/kg PO once[314]	Waterfowl
	30 mg/kg PO q10d[314,367]	Ratites
Mebendazole (Telmin Suspension, Telmintic Powder, Pitman-Moore)	25 mg/kg PO q12h × 5 days[314]	Psittacines/nematodes; may not be effective for proventricular and ventricular parasites
	5-6 mg/kg PO q24h × 3-5 days, repeat in 21 days[179]	Pigeons
	10-21 mg/L drinking water × 3-5 days[179]	Pigeons
	20 mg/kg PO q24h × 14 days[29]	Raptors/filarial worms
	5-15 mg/kg PO q24h × 2 days[256,314]	Waterfowl/nematodes, *Syngamus*[29]
	5-7 mg/kg PO[367]	Ostriches
	1.2 g/ton feed × 14 days[29,40]	Waterfowl/nematodes
Mefloquine HCl (Lariam, Roche)	30 mg/kg PO q12h × 1 day, then q24h × 2 days, then q7d × 6 mo[182]	Raptors/*Plasmodium*; schizonticide
Metronidazole	—	Most species/antiprotozoal, including alimentary tract protozoa (especially flagellates such as *Giardia, Histomonas, Spironucleus, Trichomonas*)
	20-35 mg/kg IM q24h × 2 days[311]	Most species
	30 mg/kg PO q12h × 10 days[262]	Psittacines

Table 21. Antiparasitic agents used in birds (cont.)

Agent	Dosage	Comments
Metronidazole (continued)	25 mg/kg PO q12h × 2-10 days[186]	Psittacine neonates
	40 mg/kg PO q24h × 7 days[297]	Budgerigars
	100 mg/L drinking water[92]	Canaries
	100 mg/kg soft feed[92]	Canaries
	10-20 mg/kg IM q24h × 2 days[242]	Pigeons
	50 mg/kg PO q12h × 5 days[327]	Pigeons
	4 g/gal drinking water[139]	Pigeons
	110 mg/kg PO q12h[138]	Poultry/*Histomonas*
	30 mg/kg PO q12h[75]	Poultry/PD
	30 mg/kg PO q12h × 5-7 days[303]	Raptors
	1.5 g/gal drinking water × 5-15 days[347]	Game birds
	20-25 mg/kg PO q12h[367]	Ratites
	1250 mg/L drinking water × 7-10 days[256]	Ratites
	40 mg/kg PO q24h[300]	Rheas
Milbemycin oxime (Interceptor, Ciba-Geigy)	2 mg/kg PO, repeat in 4 wk[154]	Galliformes/ascarids; capillarids; *Heterakis*
Monensin (Coban 45, Elanco)	90 g/ton (94 ppm) feed[52,347]	Quail, cranes/coccidiosis (including disseminated visceral coccidiosis)
	90-110 g/ton feed × 8 wk[347]	Chickens
	54-90 g/ton feed × 10 wk[347]	Turkeys
Oxfendazole (Benzelmin, Syntex)	10-40 mg/kg PO once[242]	Most species/nematodes
	20 mg/kg PO once[155]	Raptors/nematodes

Table 21. Antiparasitic agents used in birds (cont.)

Agent	Dosage	Comments
Paromomycin (Humatin, Parke-Davis)	100 mg/kg PO q12h × 7 days[59]	Macaw chicks/cryptosporidiosis; mix a 250 mg capsule with 10 ml water to facilitate dosing; macrolide; poorly absorbed; may result in overgrowth of nonsusceptible organisms, including fungi
Piperazine	—	Most species/ascarids, oxyurids; less efficacious than fenbendazole; seldom used in companion birds
	250 mg/kg PO once[242]	Psittacines, pigeons
	100 mg/kg PO, repeat in 14 days[183,242]	Raptors
	1 g/L drinking water × 3 days[29,242]	Raptors, pigeons
	50-100 mg/bird PO[347]	Chickens
	100-400 mg/bird PO[347]	Turkeys
	100-500 mg/kg PO once, repeat in 10-14 days[347]	Game birds
	0.2-0.4% feed[347]	Game birds
	1-2 g/L drinking water × 1-2 days[347]	Game birds
	45-200 mg/kg PO[313]	Waterfowl
	50-100 mg/kg PO once[256]	Emus, ostriches
Praziquantel (Droncit, Miles)	—	Most species/tapeworms, flukes
	10-20 mg/kg PO, repeat in 10-14 days[235]	Most species
	9 mg/kg IM, repeat in 10 days[30]	Psittacines/tapeworms
	12 mg (¹/₂ cat tablet) crushed and baked into 9×9×2" cake[242]	Finches/withhold regular feed
	5.75 mg (1/4 cat tablet)/bird PO, repeat in 14 days[327]	Pigeons

Table 21. Antiparasitic agents used in birds (cont.)

Agent	Dosage	Comments
Praziquantel (continued)	10 mg/kg PO[8]	Chickens
	8.5 mg/kg IM[8]	Chickens
	11 mg/kg SC once[8]	Chickens
	5-10 mg/kg PO, SC × 14 days[29]	Raptors/trematodes
	30 mg/kg PO, IM, repeat in 14 days[183]	Raptors
	10-20 mg/kg SC, IM, repeat in 10 days[40]	Waterfowl/tapeworms
	10 mg/kg PO, SC, IM q24h ×14 days[40]	Waterfowl/trematodes
	10 mg/kg IM q24h × 3 days, then PO × 11 days[127]	Toucans
	7.5 mg/kg PO[256]	Ostriches
	6 mg/kg PO, IM, repeat in 10-14 days[50]	Cranes
Primaquine (Primaquine Phosphate, Sanofi)	—	Pigeons, raptors, game birds, penguins/ hematozoa (ie, *Plasmodium, Hemoproteus, Leucocytozoon*); use with chloroquine; dosage based on amount of active base rather than total tablet weight
	0.75-1.0 mg/kg PO once[308,344]	Most species, including raptors/use with chloroquine 25 mg/kg at 0 hr then 15 mg/kg at 12, 24, and 48 hr; palliative, generally not curative
	1 mg/kg PO q24h × 45 days[378a]	Psittacines (keas)/ *Sarcocystis*; use in combination with amprolium and pyrimethamine
	0.03 mg/kg PO q24h × 3 days[58,313,347]	Game birds, penguins

Table 21. Antiparasitic agents used in birds (cont.)

Agent	Dosage	Comments
Primaquine (continued)	0.3 mg/kg PO (at 24 hr following the initial chloroquine dose) q24h × 7 days[47]	Raptors/hematozoa; use with chloroquine 10 mg/kg at 0 hr then 5 mg/kg at 6, 24, and 48 hr
Pyrantel pamoate (Nemex, Strongid, Pfizer)	—	Intestinal nematodes
	7 mg/kg PO, repeat in 14 days[63]	Most species
	560 mg/gal drinking water[324]	Psittacines, pigeons/medication floats
	20-25 mg/kg PO[140]	Pigeons
	20 mg/kg PO once[29]	Raptors
	5-7 mg/kg PO[367]	Ostriches
Pyrimethamine (Fansidar, Roche)	—	Toxoplasmosis; atoxoplasmosis; sarcocystosis; may be effective for leucocytozoonosis; supplement with folic acid or folinic acid
	0.5 mg/kg PO q12h × 14-28 days[63]	Most species
	100 mg/kg feed[63]	Most species
	0.5 mg/kg PO q12h × 45 days[378a]	Psittacines (keas)/ *Sarcocystis*; use in combination with amprolium and primaquine
	0.5-1.0 mg/kg PO q12h × 30 days[272,273]	Eclectus, Amazon parrots/ use with 30 mg/kg trimethoprim/ sulfadiazine
	1 ppm feed[347]	Game birds
	0.25-0.5 mg/kg PO q12h × 30 days[29]	Raptors, waterfowl
	0.5 mg/kg PO q12h × 30 days[40]	Waterfowl/*Sarcocystis*
Quinacrine (Atabrine, Sanofi)	—	Most species/*Plasmodium*; chloroquine and primaquine are preferred

Table 21. Antiparasitic agents used in birds (cont.)

Agent	Dosage	Comments
Quinacrine (continued)	5-10 mg/kg PO q24h × 7 days[313]	Most species
	100-300 mg/gal drinking water × 10-21 days[140]	Pigeons
Ronidazole (Ridzol 10%, Merck)	—	*Giardia; Trichomonas; Histomonas*; wide margin of safety and greater therapeutic range than other nitro imidazoles; not available in US
	6-10 mg/kg PO q24h × 6-10 days[242]	Most species
	1-2 g of 10% powder (100-200 mg)/L drinking water × 7 days[242]	Cockatiels, pigeons/higher dosage required for resistant strains in pigeons[121]
	400 mg of 10% powder (40 mg)/L drinking water × 7 days[92,242]	Passerines, including canaries
	400 mg of 10% powder (40 mg)/kg soft feed[92]	Canaries
	12.5 mg/kg/day PO × 6 days[29]	Pigeons
	400 mg/gal drinking water × 3-5 days[139]	Pigeons/treatment of choice for *Trichomonas*
Sodium chloride (10-20%)	Submerse bill × 10-15 min[209]	Waterfowl/leeches on bill
Sulfachlorpyridazine (Vetisulid, Solvay)	—	Coccidiosis
	400-500 mg/L drinking water × 5 days, off 2 days, on 5 days[242]	Most species
	200 mg/16 oz drinking water × 30 days[324]	Cockatiels, budgerigars/mixture is stable for up to 5 days if refrigerated; change daily; mix well
	150-300 mg/L drinking water[92]	Canaries
	1,200 mg/gal drinking water × 7-10 days[139]	Pigeons

Table 21. Antiparasitic agents used in birds (cont.)

Agent	Dosage	Comments
Sulfadimethoxine (12.5%) (Albon, SmithKline)	25 mg/kg PO q12h × 5 days[324]	Most species/coccidiosis
	250 mg/kg IM q24h × 3 days, off 2 days, on 3 days[41]	Pigeons/PD; close to toxic level
	1,250-1,500 mg/gal drinking water × 1 day then 750 mg/gal × 4 days[139]	Pigeons
	1/4 oz/gal drinking water × 5 days[347]	Turkeys
	1/2 oz/gal drinking water × 6 days[347]	Chickens
	25-50 mg/kg PO q24h × 3 days[183]	Raptors
Sulfadimethoxine/ ormetoprim (Rofemaid, Hoffmann-La Roche)	10 ppm feed[347]	Game birds/coccidiosis; *Leucocytozoon; Sarcosporidium*
	1,200-2,000 mg/gal drinking water[138]	Poultry
Sulfamethazine (Sulmet, Cyanamid)	—	Coccidiosis
	125 mg/L drinking water ×3 days, off 2 days, on 3 days[242]	Most species
	75 mg/kg PO q24h × 3 days, off 2 days, on 3 days[242]	Parakeets
	1,500 mg/gal drinking water × 1 day, then 750-1,000 mg/gal × 4 days[139]	Pigeons
	128-187 mg/kg PO q24h × 2 days, then 64-94 mg/kg × 4 days[179]	Chickens/coccidiosis
Sulfaquinoxaline (Sulquin 6-50, Solvay)	—	Coccidiosis
	100 mg/kg PO q24h × 3 days, off 2 days, on 3 days[242]	Lories, pigeons
	500 mg/L drinking water × 6 days, off 2 days, on 6 days[327]	Pigeons/1.8 ml/L 500 ≅ mg/L
	400 mg/L drinking water × 6 days, off 2 days, on 6 days[324]	Chickens/1.4 ml/L 400 ≅ mg/L

149

Table 21. Antiparasitic agents used in birds (cont.)

Agent	Dosage	Comments
Sulfaquinoxaline (continued)	454 g/ton feed continuously[347]	Chickens
	250 mg/L drinking water × 6 days, off 2 days, on 6 days[324]	Turkeys/0.9 ml/L ≅ 250 mg/L
	227 g/ton feed continuously[347]	Turkeys
Thiabendazole (TBZ, Omnizole, Thibenzole, Merck)	—	Most species/nematodes; generally less efficacious than fenbendazole
	40-100 mg/kg PO q24h × 7 days[242]	Most species
	100-500 mg/kg PO once[242]	Most species
	100 mg/kg PO q24h × 7-10 days[179]	Most species/tapeworms
	454 g/ton feed × 14 days[47,347]	Pheasants, cranes
	100 mg/kg PO once, repeat in 10-14 days[344]	Raptors
	50 mg/kg PO, repeat in 14 days[256]	Ostriches
Tinidazole	50 mg/kg PO once[242]	Most *species/Giardia, Trichomonas, Entamoeba*
Toltrazuril (Baycox, Bayvet)	—	Coccidiosis; efficacious for refractory coccidiosis; not available in US
	7 mg/kg PO q24h × 2-3 days[163,183]	Budgerigars, raptors
	75 mg/L drinking water × 2 days/wk × 4 wk[68]	Canaries
	20-35 mg/kg PO once[374]	Pigeons/higher dose prevents re-excretion up to 4 wk; lower dose is minimum dose required to suppress oocyst shedding
	75 mg/L drinking water × 5 days[142]	Pigeons
	25 mg/L drinking water × 2 days, repeat in 5 days[134]	Geese

150

Table 21. Antiparasitic agents used in birds (cont.)

Agent	Dosage	Comments
Trimethoprim/ sulfachlorpyridazine (1:5 ratio)	0.04% feed[179,314]	Geese
Trimethoprim/ sulfadiazine	60 mg/kg PO q12h × 3 days, off 2 days, on 3 days[29]	Raptors, waterfowl/coccidiosis
Trimethoprim/ sulfamethoxazole (Bactrim, Roche; Septra, Burroughs Wellcome)	25 mg/kg PO q24h[314] 1,200-2,000 mg/gal drinking water[138]	Toucans, mynahs/coccidiosis Poultry/coccidiosis

Table 22. Chemical restraint/anesthetic/analgesic agents used in birds

Agent	Dosage	Comments
Acepromazine	—	See ketamine for combinations
	0.25-0.50 mg/kg IM[177]	Ratites/most commonly used in combination with other anesthetics; muscle relaxation; tranquilization; seldom used in other species
	0.1-0.2 mg/kg IV[177]	
Alpha-chloralose	30 mg/kg PO once[24]	Canada geese/frequently used for immobilization of nuisance geese; prepare a suspension in corn oil, inject into individual bread baits and hand-toss to target individuals; onset approximately 60 min, duration up to 24 hr; currently available only to Wildlife Services, Dept of Agriculture
	0.37-0.43 g/cup of corn[213]	Cranes/immobilization; releasable 8-22 hr later
	0.16-0.21 g/bird[213]	Cranes/immobilization; releasable 8-22 hr later
Alphaxalone/ alphadolone (Saffan, Glaxcovet)	—	Not available in US
	5 mg/kg IV[256]	Most species
	5-10 mg/kg IV[215,216]	Psittacines, waterfowl/short duration; apnea may occur
	36 mg/kg IM, IP[215,216]	Psittacines, waterfowl/ immobilization, poor analgesia
	5-7 mg/kg IV[65]	Pigeons/duration 3-5 min; short procedures
	12-15 mg/kg IM[65]	Pigeons/duration 20-30 min; useful for radiography
	36 mg/kg IM[256]	Raptors
Atipamezole (Antisedan, Pfizer)	5x medetomidine dose IM, IV[173]	Psittacines, raptors, geese/ medetomidine reversal; righting reflex regained 3-10 min after administration

Table 22. Chemical restraint/anesthetic/analgesic agents used in birds (cont.)

Agent	Dosage	Comments
Atipamezole (continued)	250-380 µg/kg IM[30,179]	Most species, including psittacines/medetomidine and xylazine reversal
	182-281 µg/kg IV[237]	Mallard ducks/medetomidine reversal
	0.25 mg/kg IM[238]	Mallard ducks/medetomidine reversal when used with ketamine, medetomidine, midazolam combination
Atropine	0.01-0.02 mg/kg SC, IM[313]	Most species/preanesthetic; rarely indicated
	0.04-1.0 mg/kg SC, IM[57]	Preanesthetic; rarely indicated
Azaperone (Stresnil, Mallinckrodt)	0.73 mg/kg IM[367]	Ratites/sedation; butyrophenone neuroleptic
Buprenorphine (Buprenex, Reckitt & Colman)	—	Analgesia; not available in US; 0.1-0.5 mg/kg was ineffective for analgesia in African grey parrots[275]
	0.01-0.05 mg/kg IM[174]	Most species
	6.5 mg/L drinking water[363]	Most species
Butorphanol (Torbugesic, Fort Dodge)	3-4 mg/kg IM[18,184,379]	Most species, including raptors/analgesia; mild motor deficits observed; minimal cardiovascular, respiratory effects
	1-2 mg/kg IM[64,274,275]	Psittacines/analgesia; reduces isoflurane requirement for anesthesia
	1 mg/kg IM[73]	Psittacines/preanesthetic
	0.5-2.0 mg/kg IM[174]	Most species/analgesia
	0.05-0.40 mg/kg SC, IM q6-8h[327]	Pigeons/analgesia; sedation
	0.005-0.25 mg/kg IV[367]	Ratites

153

Table 22. Chemical restraint/anesthetic/analgesic agents used in birds (cont.)

Agent	Dosage	Comments
Carfentanil (Wildnil, Wildlife Pharmaceuticals)	0.03 mg/kg IM[177]	Ratites/potent narcotic; reverse with naloxone (dosage not reported)
Desflurane (Suprane, Anaquest)	—	Fluorine halogenated ether; rapid recovery, faster induction[152]
Detomidine	0.3 mg/kg IM[64]	Chickens/alpha$_2$-adrenergic agonist; marked sedation
Diazepam	—	See ketamine for combinations
	—	Used alone for sedation, tranquilization, seizures, appetite stimulation; often used with other anesthetic agents; can be used in combination with phenobarbital for seizure control; can be diluted with sterile water if used immediately
	2.5-4.0 mg/kg PO prn[314]	Most species/sedation
	0.6 mg/kg IM[19]	Most species
	1 mg/180 ml drinking water[19]	Most species
	0.5-1.0 mg/kg IM, IV prn[327]	Pigeons/sedation; seizures
	0.25-0.50 mg/kg IM, IV q24h × 2-3 days[355]	Raptors/appetite stimulant
	0.1-0.2 mg/kg IV[296]	Ratites/smooth anesthetic recovery
	0.3 mg/kg IV[177]	Ratites/tranquilization
Etorphine HCl (M-99, Wildlife Pharmaceuticals)	—	Ostriches/see ketamine for combination

Table 22. Chemical restraint/anesthetic/analgesic agents used in birds (cont.)

Agent	Dosage	Comments
Flumazenil (Romazicon, Hoffman-La Roche)	0.1 mg/kg IM[78]	Quail/PD; midazolam reversal in 1.4-1.8 min
	18.2-28.0 μg/kg IV[237]	Mallard ducks/midazolam reversal
	0.05 mg/kg intranasal[238]	Mallard ducks/midazolam reversal when used with ketamine, medetomidine, midazolam combination
Glycopyrrolate (Robinul-V, Aveco)	0.01 mg/kg IM, IV[153]	Most species/preanesthetic; rarely indicated
	0.04 mg/kg IV[367]	Ratites
Isoflurane	4-5% induction, 2.0-2.5% maintenance[324]	Most species/anesthetic of choice; butorphanol reduces isoflurane requirement in African grey parrots, cockatoos[275]
	1.115%	Emus/PD; minimum anesthetic concentration[343]
	3.5-4.0%, decrease after 30-45 min[245]	Ostriches, emus
Ketamine	—	Ketamine combinations follow
	—	Seldom used as sole agent due to prolonged violent recoveries and poor muscle relaxation;[340] can be used alone for short, non-painful procedures
	20-50 mg/kg SC, IM, IV[30,215]	Psittacines/restraint; poor analgesia; recovery up to 3 hr; smaller species require a higher dose
	25-50 mg/kg IM[66]	Pigeons/duration 30-60 min; diazepam improves muscle relaxation
	15-20 mg/kg IM, IV[153]	Raptors

Table 22. Chemical restraint/anesthetic/analgesic agents used in birds (cont.)

Agent	Dosage	Comments
Ketamine (continued)	100 mg/kg in feed[29]	Raptors/sedation to catch an escaped bird; place in a 30 g piece of meat
	20-50 mg/kg IM induction; 5 mg/kg IV q10min prn maintenance[177]	Ratites
	15-25 mg/kg IM, IV[153]	Waterfowl
Ketamine (K)/ acepromazine (A)	(K) 25-50 mg/kg/ (A) 0.5-1.0 mg/kg IM[379]	Psittacines/improved muscle relaxation over ketamine alone; thermoregulation may be affected
Ketamine (K)/ diazepam (D)	(K) 10-50 mg/kg/ (D) 0.5-2.0 mg/kg IM[379]	Psittacines/improved muscle relaxation over ketamine alone
	(K) 5-25 mg/kg/ (D) 0.5-2.0 mg/kg IV[379]	Psittacines/lower end of range is preferred
	(K) 10-25 mg/kg/ (D) 0.5-1.0 mg/kg IM, IV[327]	Pigeons/lower end of range administered IV is preferred; useful for oral procedures
	(K) 10-30 mg/kg IV/ (D) 1.0-1.5 mg/kg IM[216]	Raptors, waterfowl/induction
	(K) 8-15 mg/kg/ (D) 0.5-1.0 mg/kg IM[155]	Falcons
	(K) 3-8 mg/kg/ (D) 0.5-1.0 mg/kg IM[155]	Eagles, vultures
	(K) 5-10 mg/kg/ (D) 0.1-0.2 mg/kg IV[324]	Ratites/induction
Ketamine (K)/ etorphine (E)	(K) 200-300 mg/ (E) 6-12 mg/bird IM[177]	Ostrich adults/etorphine is inadequate when used as sole agent
Ketamine (K)/ medetomidine (M)	—	Lower (K) doses are needed when used with (M); reverse with atipamezole[215,216]
	(K) 2-5 mg/kg/ (M) 50-100 µg/kg IV[173]	Psittacines

Table 22. Chemical restraint/anesthetic/analgesic agents used in birds (cont.)

Agent	Dosage	Comments
Ketamine (K)/ medetomidine (M) (continued)	(K) 3-7 mg/kg/ (M) 75-100 g/kg IM[173]	Psittacines
	(K) 25 mg/kg/ (M) 100 g/kg IM[310]	Psittacines/anesthesia
	(K) 1.5-2.0 mg/kg/ (M) 60-85 g/kg IV[216]	Pigeons, waterfowl/sedation
	(K) 2-4 mg/kg/ (M) 25-75 g/kg IV[173]	Raptors
	(K) 3-5 mg/kg/ (M) 50-100 g/kg IM[173]	Raptors
	(K) 5-10 mg/kg/ (M) 100-200 g/kg IM, IV[173]	Geese
Ketamine (K)/ medetomidine (Me)/ midazolam (Mi)	(K) 10 mg/kg/ (Me) 0.05 g/kg/ (Mi) 2 mg/kg IV[238]	Mallard ducks/anesthesia of 30 min duration; reverse with atipamezole, flumazenil (intranasal)
Ketamine (K)/ midazolam (M)	(K) 10-25 mg/kg/ (M) 0.5-1.0 mg/kg IM[379]	Psittacines/combination needs further evaluation
Ketamine (K)/ xylazine (X)	—	(K)/ (X) combinations cause cardiac depressive effects and rough recoveries; allometrically scaled dosages for waterfowl are available[190]
	(K) 4.4 mg/kg/ (X) 2.2 mg/kg IV[215]	Psittacines/atipamezole (250-380 µg/kg IM) or yohimbine (0.1 mg/kg SC, IM) reverses xylazine
	(K) 10-30 mg/kg/ (X) 2-6 mg/kg IM[379]	Psittacines/birds <250 g require a higher dose than birds >250 g
	(K) 10 mg/kg/ (X) 0.5-1.0 mg/kg IM[245]	Ratites
	(K) 2.2-3.3 mg/kg/ (X) 2.2 mg/kg IM[177]	Ratites/(X) administered 10 min before (K)

Table 22. Chemical restraint/anesthetic/analgesic agents used in birds (cont.)

Agent	Dosage	Comments
Medetomidine (Domitor, Pfizer)	—	See ketamine for combinations; potent alpha-2 agonist; reverse with atipamezole[173]
Meperidine (Demerol, Sanofi Winthrop)	1-4 mg/kg IM[314]	Most species/sedation, analgesia; respiratory depressant
	1 mg/kg IM[367]	Ratites/analgesia postsurgery
Midazolam (Versed, Roche)	—	See ketamine for combination; short acting benzodiazepine; contraindicated with hepatic disease
	0.8 mg/kg IM, IV[153]	Most species/birds >500 g
	1.5 mg/kg IM, IV[153]	Most species/birds <500 g
	2-3 mg/kg IM[179]	Amazon parrots
	2-6 mg/kg IM[78]	Quail/PD; mild to heavy sedation depending on dose; reverse with flumazenil
	0.5-1.0 mg/kg IV, IM q8h[29]	Raptors/sedation
	0.15 mg/kg IV[177]	Ostriches/rapid sternal recumbency in adults
	0.3-0.4 mg/kg IM[245]	Ostriches, emus/premedication
	0.4 mg/kg IM[177]	Emus/sedation for adults
	4-6 mg/kg IM[179]	Waterfowl
	2.0 mg/kg IM[370]	Geese/restraint; sedation for 15-20 min
Naloxone (Narcan, DuPont)	2 mg IV[313]	Most species/narcotic antagonist; may be repeated in 14-21 hr[313] to prevent renarcotization
Phenobarbital	1-7 mg/kg PO q8-12h[129]	Most species/mild sedative effect; see psychotropic agents for other indications

Table 22. Chemical restraint/anesthetic/analgesic agents used in birds (cont.)

Agent	Dosage	Comments
Propofol (Rapinovet, Mallinckrodt)	14 mg/kg IV[104]	Pigeons/anesthesia; 2-7 min duration; may cause marked respiratory and cardiac depression, hypothermia, hypoxia;[338] too short of duration for psittacines,[30] some raptors, waterfowl;[215] limited use in birds[215,250]
	4 mg IV induction; 0.5 mg/kg/min IV maintenance[241]	Barn owls/anesthesia
	10 mg/kg IV induction; 1-4 mg boluses prn, maintenance[236,237]	Mallard ducks/anesthesia; IV catheterization, repeat boluses required for most procedures; ventilation required
Sevoflurane (Ultane, Abbott Laboratories)	Incremental increases up to 7% prn, induction[131]	Psittacines/anesthesia; similar to isoflurane; provides more rapid recovery[152,202]
Tiletamine/ zolazepam (Telazol, Fort Dodge)	—	Most species/generally not recommended for pet birds[379]
	15-20 mg/kg IM[256]	Budgerigars
	10-30 mg/kg IM[147]	Most species/restraint; anesthesia; moderate analgesia
	5-10 mg/kg IM[30,215,216]	Psittacines, waterfowl/sedation
	10 mg/kg IM[204]	Raptors (owls)/restraint
	2-8 mg/kg IV[350]	Ratite adults/induction and/or short procedures; 15 sec induction
	4-12 mg/kg IM[350]	Ratite adults/induction and/or short procedures; 10 min induction
	6.6 mg/kg IM[336]	Swans/anesthesia
Tolazoline (Priscoline, Ciba-Geigy)	15 mg/kg IV[10]	Vultures[64]/xylazine antagonist

159

Table 22. Chemical restraint/anesthetic/analgesic agents used in birds (cont.)

Agent	Dosage	Comments
Xylazine (Rompun, Miles)	—	See ketamine for combinations; seldom used in pet birds; not used as sole agent in pet birds due to cardiac depressant effects; not recommended in debilitated birds; reverse with yohimbine, tolazoline, atipamezole
	0.2-1.0 mg/kg IM[177]	Ratites/calming sedation
	1.0-2.2 mg/kg IM[177]	Ratites/pronounced sedation
	1 mg/kg IV[228]	Ducks/may cause respiratory depression
Yohimbine (Yobine, Lloyd)	—	Xylazine antagonist
	0.11-0.27 mg/kg IM once[256]	Budgerigars
	0.1 mg/kg IV[256]	Raptors
	0.125 mg/kg IV[177]	Ratites/partial reversal of xylazine effects

[a] For other analgesic recommendations, refer to Tables 23 (hormones and steroids) and 24 (nonsteroidal anti-inflammatory agents).

Table 23. Hormones and steroids used in birds

Agent	Dosage	Comments
Boldenone undecylenate (Equipoise, Solvay)	1.1 mg/kg IM q3wk[367]	Ratites/anabolic steroid
Calcitonin	4 IU/kg IM q12h × 14 days[314]	Most species/hypercalcemia (ie, secondary to rodenticide toxicity)
Chorionic gonadotropin (hCG)	500 IU/kg IM on day 1, 3, 7, 14, 21, then q14-28d[324]	Feather picking due to sexually related disorders; inhibit egg laying; dilute to 1,000 IU/ml
	500-1,000 IU/kg IM on day 1, 3, 7, then q30d prn[27,220,221]	Most species/inhibit egg laying; stable for 60 days if refrigerated after reconstitution;[220] administer on days 3 and 7 if hen lays after day 1
Dexamethasone	—	May predispose to aspergillosis and other mycoses
	2-4 mg/kg IM[19]	Most species/shock
	1 mg/kg IM once[247]	Most species/trauma
	3 mg/kg IM, IV[42]	Owls, hawks/PD; anti-inflammatory; trauma; shock; enterotoxemia
	0.5 mg/kg IM, IV q24h × 5-7 days[295]	Raptors/head trauma
	2 mg/kg IM q12h × 2 days[367]	Ratites/trauma
	4 mg/kg IM q12h × 2 days[367]	Ratites/shock
Dexamethasone Na phosphate	—	Most species/preferred steroidal anti-inflammatory agent for birds; suppresses the pituitary-adrenocortical system; may predispose to aspergillosis and other mycoses

161

Table 23. Hormones and steroids used in birds (cont.)

Agent	Dosage	Comments
Dexamethasone Na phosphate (continued)	2-4 mg/kg IM, IV q12h[182,324]	Most species, including raptors/ head trauma (until signs abate); shock (one dose); hyperthermia (until stable)
	4 mg/kg SC, IM[186]	Psittacine neonates/shock
Dinoprostone	—	See prostaglandin E2
Flumethasone (Flucort, Syntex)	1.0-1.5 mg/kg PO, SC, IM, IV[367]	Ratites/glucocorticoid; inflammation
Goserelin acetate (Zoladex, Zeneca)	3,600 µg implant[157]	Penguins/induce molt; GnRH agonist; also see leuprolide acetate
Insulin	0.002 IU/bird IM q12-48h[291]	Budgerigars/NPH insulin
	0.01-0.10 IU/bird IM q12-48h[291]	Amazon parrots/NPH insulin
	1.4 U/kg IM q12-24h[179,314]	Cockatiels, toucans (Toco)/NPH insulin
	2 IU/bird IM[261]	Toucans (Toco)/PZI or ultralente insulin; adjust dose/frequency based on glucose curves
Leuprolide acetate (Lupron, TAP)	(number of days for desired effect) $\times$ (100 µg/kg) = dosage IM once[252]	Cockatiel/GnRH depot drug to prevent ovulation; approximately 100 g/kg released daily (eg, in cockatiels, 2,800 g/kg given once will last 28 days)
	375 µg/bird IM[164,253]	Cockatiel/inhibit ovulation
	1250 µg/kg IM once[157]	Penguins/induces molt; also see goserelin acetate
Levothyroxine (L-thyroxine)	—	Hypothyroidism; obesity, lipomas; monitor weight closely

Table 23. Hormones and steroids used in birds (cont.)

Agent	Dosage	Comments
Levothyroxine (L-thyroxine) (continued)	0.02 mg/kg PO q12-24h[291]	Most species
	0.1 mg/4-12 oz drinking water[291]	Most species
Medroxy-progesterone	20 mg/kg IM[324]	Most species/aggression; inhibit egg laying; stimulate follicle resorption; some feather picking disorders; may cause polyuria, polydipsia, weight gain, immunosuppression
	0.1% feed[324]	Pigeons/inhibit ovulation
	15-30 mg/kg IM q7d × 4 treatments[157]	Penguins/induces molt
Methylprednisolone acetate	0.5-1.0 mg/kg IM[313]	Most species/allergies (Amazon foot necrosis);[314] may predispose to aspergillosis and other mycoses
	200 mg/bird IM, repeat prn[367]	Ratite adults
Mibolerone (Cheque Drops, Upjohn)	10 µg/4 oz drinking water[76]	Psittacines/potent anabolic and androgenic steroid; feather picking
Oxytocin	5 IU/kg IM, may repeat q30min[321]	Most species/egg binding; contraindicated unless uterovaginal sphincter is well dilated and uterus free of adhesions[319]
	20-30 IU/bird IM q24h × 2 treatments[367]	Ratite adults/egg binding
	3-5 IU/kg IM[29]	Waterfowl
Prednisolone	0.5-1.0 mg/kg IM, IV once[313]	Most species/may predispose to aspergillosis and other mycoses
	2 mg/kg PO q12h[30]	Psittacines/inflammation
	1.0-1.25 mg/kg PO q48h[367]	Ratites/prolonged immunosuppression

Table 23. Hormones and steroids used in birds (cont.)

Agent	Dosage	Comments
Prednisolone Na succinate (Solu-Delta-Cortef, Upjohn)	10-20 mg/kg IV, IM q15min prn[57]	Most species/shock
	0.5-1.0 mg/kg IM, IV once[324]	Most species/anti-inflammatory
	30 mg/kg IV, then 15 mg/kg IV at 2 and 6 hr, then 2.5 mg/kg/hr × 24 hr[26]	Most species/neurologic emergencies; start therapy within 4 hr of trauma
	1.5-2.0 mg/kg IM q12h[367]	Ratites/immunosuppression (see prednisolone for prolonged therapy)
	5.0-8.5 mg/kg IV q1h[367]	Ratites/shock
Prostaglandin E2 (dinoprostone) (Prepidil Gel, Upjohn)	0.1 ml intracloacal on uterine sphincter/100g[165,166,319]	Psittacines/egg binding; causes uterovaginal sphincter relaxation; may cause uterine contractions; lower dosage may be effective; freeze into aliquots
	0.02-0.10 mg/kg onto cloacal mucosa once[29]	Raptors, waterfowl/egg binding
Stanozolol (Winstrol V, Upjohn)	0.5-1.0 mg/kg IM[247]	Most species/anabolic steroid; debilitation
	2 mg/120 ml drinking water[247]	
Tamoxifen (Nolvadex, Zeneca)	40 mg/kg IM[157]	Ducks, penguins/induces molt
Testosterone	8 mg/kg IM q7d prn[8]	Most species, including canaries/anemia; libido; debilitation
	5-10 drops stock/30 ml drinking water × 5-10 days[324]	Canaries/stock solution: 100 mg parenteral suspension/30 ml drinking water
Triamcinolone	0.1-0.2 mg/kg IM once[324]	Most species/glucocorticoid; seldom used; may predispose to aspergillosis and other mycoses

Table 24. Nonsteroidal anti-inflammatory agents used in birds

Agent	Dosage	Comments
Aspirin (acetylsalicylic acid)	5 grains (325 mg)/250 ml drinking water[379]	Most species/musculoskeletal pain; antipyretic
	10 mg/kg PO q24h × 3 days[324]	
Carprofen (Rimadyl, Pfizer)	2 mg/kg IM q24h[256]	Most species/injectable form not available in US
	5-10 mg/kg PO[179]	Most species/analgesia
	5-10 mg/kg IM[216]	Raptors, anseriformes, pigeons/ post-operative analgesia
Flunixin meglumine (Banamine, Schering)	—	Analgesia; antipyretic; potentially nephrotoxic in cranes and quail[196]
	1-10 mg/kg IM[379]	Most species (including raptors)[307]
	4 mg/kg IM[73]	Psittacines/dose may not be adequate
	1.1 mg/kg IM q12h[1,3]	Ostriches/myositis[3]
Ketoprofen (Ketofen, Fort Dodge)	2 mg/kg IM[240]	Most species/analgesia; for musculoskeletal disorders
	1 mg/bird SC, IM q12-24h × 2 days[29]	Pigeons/arthritis
	1-5 mg/kg IM q12h[307]	Raptors
	1 mg/kg IM q24h × 1-10 days[29]	Waterfowl/analgesia; arthritis
Meclofenamic acid (Meclomen, Park-Davis)	2.2 mg/kg PO q24h[256]	Most species
Phenylbutazone	3.5-7.0 mg/kg PO q8-12h[313]	Psittacines
	20 mg/kg PO q8h[313]	Raptors
	10-14 mg/kg PO q12h[367]	Ratites

Table 25. Agents used in nebulizing birds

Agent	Dosage	Comments
Acetylcysteine 20% (Mucomyst, Bristol)	—	See amikacin, aminophylline, gentamicin, for combinations
	200 mg/9 ml sterile water until dissipated[324]	Most species/mucolytic; rhinitis; pneumonia; airsacculitis; syringeal aspergilloma; can mix with dexamethasone, aminoglycosides, aminophylline; tracheal irritation reported in mammals
Amikacin	50 mg/10 ml saline × 15 min q12h[329]	Most species/discontinue if polyuria develops
	50 mg/9 ml sterile water until dissipated q8h[324]	Most species/rhinitis; pneumonia; airsacculitis; tracheitis
	5 mg/ml saline[56]	Most species
	50 mg/8 ml sterile water and 1 ml acetylcysteine (20%) until dissipated q8h[324]	Most species/rhinitis; pneumonia; airsacculitis; tracheitis
Aminophylline	25 mg/9 ml sterile water or saline × 15 min[324]	Most species/bronchodilator; allergic pulmonary disease; can mix with dexamethasone, aminoglycosides, and acetylcysteine
Amphotericin B (Fungizone, Squibb)	1 mg/ml sterile water[58] or saline[329] × 15 min q12h	Most species/antifungal
	7 mg/ml saline[56]	Most species
	0.25 mg/ml saline × 15 min q12h[150]	Hummingbirds/low efficacy; may cause weight loss
Carbenicillin (Geocillin, Roerig)	200 mg/10 ml saline × 15 min q12h[329]	Psittacines/*Pseudomonas* pneumonia; use in combination with parenteral aminoglycosides
Cefotaxime	100 mg/10ml saline × 10-30 min q6-12h[329]	Most species

Table 25. Agents used in nebulizing birds (cont.)

Agent	Dosage	Comments
Ceftriaxone	—	Therapeutic blood levels were not achieved at 200 mg/ml water, with or without DMSO
	40 mg/ml water [56,187]	Poultry/PD
	40-200 mg/ml + DMSO [187]	Poultry/PD
Chloramphenicol	13 mg/ml saline [56]	Most species
Clotrimazole (Lotrimin, Schering)	10 mg/ml polyethylene glycol × 30-60 min [5,56,185]	Use in combination with systemic amphotericin B, flucytosine, and itraconazole
Doxycycline	200 mg/15ml saline [117]	Psittacines/antibiotic
Enilconazole	10 mg/ml water [30,56]	Most species/antifungal
Enrofloxacin	10 mg/ml saline [56,117]	Most species
Erythromycin (Erythro, Sanofi)	50 mg/10 ml saline × 15 min q8h [58]	Most species/airsacculitis
	20 mg/ml saline [56]	
	100 mg/10 ml saline × 15 min q8h [329]	
Gentamicin	50 mg/10ml saline × 15 min q8h [329]	Most species
	50 mg/8 ml sterile water and 1 ml acetylcysteine (20%) until dissipated q8h [324]	Most species/rhinitis; tracheitis; pneumonia; airsacculitis
	50 mg/15 ml saline and 2 ml acetylcysteine (20%) × 20 min q8h [50]	Cranes
Lincomycin	250 mg/ml water [56]	Most species
	250 mg aerosolized drug/m³ chamber × 15-30 min [54]	Chickens/PD; antibiotic; therapeutic concentrations in blood, lungs and trachea for up to 24 hr
Oxytetracycline	2 mg/ml × 60 min q4-6h [98]	Parakeets/PD
Piperacillin	100 mg/10 ml saline × 10-30 min q6-12h [329]	Most species

Table 25. Agents used in nebulizing birds (cont.)

Agent	Dosage	Comments
Polymyxin B	666,000 IU/10 ml saline[117]	Psittacines/poorly absorbed from respiratory epithelium
Spectinomycin (Spectam, Ceva)	13 mg/ml saline[56,117]	Most species
Sulfadimethoxine	13 mg/ml saline[56,117]	Most species
Tylosin (Tylan, Elanco)	1 g powder/50 ml DMSO or distilled water × 1 hr[224]	Pigeons, quail/PD; respiratory tract infections
	100 mg/10 ml saline × 10-60 min q12h[117,329]	Most species
	20 mg/ml DMSO[225]	Most species

Table 26. Chelating and related agents used in birds

Agent	Dosage	Comments
Calcium EDTA (Calcium Disodium Versenate, 3M)	—	Preferred initial chelator for lead and zinc toxicity
	35 mg/kg IM q12h × 5 days, off 3-4 days, repeat prn[206,208]	Most species
	30 mg/kg IM q12h × 3-5 days[327]	Pigeons
	35 mg/kg IM, IV q8h × 3-4 days, off 2 days, repeat prn[183]	Raptors
	25.0-52.2 mg/kg IV q12h[259]	Geese
Deferoxamine mesylate (Desferal, Ciba-Geigy)	—	Preferred chelator for iron toxicity; hemochromatosis
	20 mg/kg PO initially, then IM q4h until recovery[208]	Most species
	20 mg/kg PO q4h until recovery[208]	Most species
	100 mg/kg PO q24h up to 3 mo[256]	Most species
	40 mg/kg IM q24h × 7 days[265]	Mynahs
	100 mg/kg SC q24h × 4 mo[69]	Toucans
Diethylene triamine penta-acetic acid (DTPA)	30 mg/kg IM q12h[365]	Lead toxicity
Dimercaprol (BAL in Oil, Becton Dickinson)	2.5 mg/kg IM q4h × 2 days, then q12h × 10 days or until recovery[208]	Heavy metal toxicity; arsenic, gold; mercury, if ingestion < 2 hr;[179] rarely used
Dimercaptosuccinic acid (DMSA, Aldrich; Chemet, Bock Pharmacal)	25-35 mg/kg PO q12h × 5 days/wk × 3-5 wk[79,182,208]	Most species, including raptors/preferred oral chelator for lead toxicity; effective for zinc toxicity;[373] may be effective for mercury toxicity[182]
	40 mg/kg PO[86]	Cockatiels/lead toxicity; frequency not given; 80 mg/kg resulted in death; can use with calcium EDTA

169

Table 26. Chelating and related agents used in birds (cont.)

Agent	Dosage	Comments
Magnesium sulfate	0.5-1.0 mg/kg PO q12h × 1-3 days[29]	Waterfowl/lead toxicity; not a chelator, but increases intestinal motility
Penicillamine (Cuprimine, Merck)	—	Commercially available oral chelator; lead, zinc toxicity; preferred chelator for copper toxicity; may be used for mercury toxicity[314]
	55 mg/kg PO q12h × 1-2 wk[206,208]	Most species, including waterfowl[29]
	30-55 mg/kg PO q12h[183]	Raptors
Sodium sulfate (GoLytely, Braintree)	0.5-1.0 g/kg PO[208]	Lead toxicity; cathartic; adjunct to chelation; rarely used for lead toxicity; trials demonstrated no efficacy in cockatiels[86]

Table 27. Psychotropic agents used in birds

Agent	Dosage	Comments
Amitriptyline (Elavil, Stuart)	1-2 mg/kg PO q12-24h[365]	Most species/allergic feather picking; obsessive compulsive disorders, phobias; inhibits serotonin reuptake; antihistamine[377]
Carbamazepine (Tegretol, Basel)	3-10 mg/kg PO q24h[294] 20 mg/120 ml drinking water[324]	Most species/preferred psychotropic agent for feather picking in most psittacines;[324] convulsant, obsessive, compulsive, mutilating disorders; may cause bone marrow suppression and hepatotoxicity; combination with chlorpromazine or haloperidol recommended for initial treatment during the first 2 wk[324]
Chlorpromazine	—	Most species/feather picking; phenothiazine; dopamine antagonist;[377] correct underlying problems and discontinue within 30 days; efficacy diminishes in 14-30 days when given PO;[324] may cause ataxia, regurgitation, drowsiness[331]
	Mix 1 ml stock solution/4 oz drinking water or 0.2-1.0 ml/kg stock PO q12-24h prn[324]	Stock solution: crush five 25 mg tablets and mix with 31 ml simple syrup (Humco); start at low dose initially; mild sedation
	0.1-0.2 mg/kg IM once[324]	Cockatoos/use with carbamazepine following removal of E-collar
	0.2 mg/kg IM once prn[324]	Ringneck parakeets/mild sedation and decreases obsessive behaviors
Chorionic gonadotropin (hCG)	500 IU/kg IM on days 1, 3, 7, 14, 21, then q14-28d[324]	Most species/feather picking resulting from sexually related disorders; inhibits egg laying; dilute to 1,000 IU/ml

Table 27. Psychotropic agents used in birds (cont.)

Agent	Dosage	Comments
Clomipramine (Anafranil, Basel; Clomicalm, Novartis)	1 mg/kg/day PO q24h or divided q12h × 6 wk[298]	Most species/allergic feather picking; obsessive compulsive disorders, phobias;[377] tricyclic antidepressant; inhibits serotonin reuptake; antihistamine; may cause regurgitation, drowsiness; marginal effectiveness; crushed tablet can be suspended in a 1-2 mg/ml solution
Delmadinone (Tardak, Syntex)	1 mg/kg IM217 once	Psittacines/sexual behavior problems; not available in US
Diazepam	1.25-2.50 mg/120 ml drinking water[129]	Most species/benzodiazepine; dopamine inhibitor; GABA potentiator; stress-associated feather picking;[377] useful as sole agent or in combination with phenobarbital for seizure control; may cause sedation
	2.5-4.0 mg/kg PO q6-8h[30]	Psittacines/sedation
Diphenhydramine	2-4 mg/kg PO q12h[129,178]	Most species/allergic feather picking
	0.5 mg/240 ml drinking water[377]	Most species/allergic feather picking; antihistamine
Doxepin (Sinequan, Roerig)	0.5-1.0 mg/kg PO q12h[129,178]	Most species/allergic feather picking; tricyclic anti-depressant; antihistamine; serotonin reuptake inhibitor; may cause sedation[377]
Fluoxetine (Prozac, Dista)	2 mg/kg PO q12h[324]	Most species/adjunctive treatment for depression induced feather picking; antidepressant; serotonin reuptake inhibitor[377]
	0.4 mg/kg PO q24h[30]	Psittacines/feather picking
Haloperidol (Haldol, McNeil)	—	Most species/butyrophenone tranquilizer; inhibits dopamine; hyperexcitability and frustration induced feather picking and behavior disorders; self mutilation, obsessive compulsive disorders; may cause anorexia or depression[377]

172

Table 27. Psychotropic agents used in birds (cont.)

Agent	Dosage	Comments
Haloperidol (continued)	0.15-0.20 mg/kg PO q12h[218]	Amazon parrots, cockatoos/ birds <1 kg
	0.10-0.15 mg/kg PO q12h[218]	Amazon parrots, cockatoos/ birds >1 kg
	0.4 mg/kg PO q24h[30,217]	Psittacines/self mutilation, feather picking
	6.4 mg/L drinking water × 7 mo[168]	African grey parrots/feather picking
	1-2 mg/kg IM q21d[129]	Most species/feather picking
Hydroxyzine (Atarax, Roerig)	2.0-2.2 mg/kg PO q8h[129,205]	Most species/antihistamine; allergic feather picking
	4 mg/100-120 ml drinking water[129]	Most species/antihistamine; allergic feather picking
Medroxy-progesterone	30 mg/kg SC, repeat in 90 days prn[49,247] 20 mg/kg SC, IM, repeat in 30-60 days 1-2×[324]	Most species/progestin; potentiates GABA;[377] steroid of choice for sexually related feather picking; seasonal aggression; chronic egg laying; may cause polydipsia, polyphagia, polyuria, and weight gain
Megestrol acetate (Ovaban, Schering)	1.25-2.50 mg/120 ml drinking water × 7-10 days, then 1-2 × /wk[129]	Most species/feather picking; seldom used
	2.5 mg/kg PO q24h × 7 days then 1-2 × /wk[30,217]	Psittacines/feather picking; sexual behavior problems
Mibolerone (Cheque Drops, Upjohn)	0.1 ml (10 µg)/4 oz drinking water[76]	Psittacines/anabolic, androgenic steroid; feather picking
Naltrexone (Trexan, DuPont)	1.5 mg/kg PO q8-12h × 1-18 mo[369]	Most species/opioid antagonist; feather picking; self mutilation; contraindicated in patients with liver disease; dissolve tablet in 10 ml sterile water (preservative does not go into solution); may need to increase dosage 2-6 × to be effective

173

Table 27. Psychotropic agents used in birds (cont.)

Agent	Dosage	Comments
Nortriptyline (Pamelor, Sandoz)	2 mg/120 ml drinking water[129,178]	Most species/feather picking; seldom used
Phenobarbital	—	Most species/potentiates GABA;[377] mild sedative effect; useful as sole agent or in combination with diazepam for seizure control; sedative effects may help with feather picking
	1-7 mg/kg PO q8-12h[129]	Most species/feather picking; mild sedative effect
	5 mg/kg/day PO divided q8-12h[324]	Most species/idiopathic epilepsy
	4.5-6.0 mg/kg PO q12h to effect[26,180]	Most species, including Amazon parrots/seizures
	2.0-3.2 mg/kg PO q12h[287]	Amazon parrots/idiopathic epilepsy
	6-10 mg/120 ml drinking water[287]	Amazon parrots/idiopathic epilepsy

Table 28. Nutritional/mineral support used in birds

Agent	Dosage	Comments
Biotin (Vet-A-Min)	50 mg/kg PO q24h × 30-60 days[29]	Raptors/beak and nail regrowth
Brewers yeast	300 mg/10 birds in feed[29]	Pigeons/brittle plumage; use during molt; crush tablet and mix with feed
Calcium borogluconate (Calcibor, CBG20, Arnolds)	0.5-1.0 ml/kg IM, IV[30]	Psittacines/20% solution
	1-5 ml/kg SC, IV[29]	Raptors/hypocalcemia; dilute to 10% solution
Calcium chloride	150-200 mg/kg IV slowly, IM q8h[363]	Hypocalcemia; seldom used
Calcium glubionate (Neo-Calglucon Sandoz)	—	Most species/hypocalcemia
	25 mg/kg PO[20]	Most species
	150 mg/kg PO q12h[167]	Most species
	23 mg/kg PO q24h[186]	Psittacine neonates
	23 mg/30 ml drinking water[167]	Most species
Calcium gluconate	50-100 mg/kg IV slowly, IM (diluted)[167,313]	Most species/hypocalcemia
	50-100 mg/kg IM (diluted)[327]	Pigeons/dilute with saline or sterile water
Calcium lactate/ calcium glycerophosphate (Calphosan, Glenwood)	5-10 mg/kg IM q7d prn[20,167]	Most species/hypocalcemia
Calcium levulinate	75-100 mg/kg IM, IV[167,247]	Most species/hypocalcemia
Diatrizoate meglumine sodium (37% iodine) (Renografin-76, Solvay)	122 mg/kg IM[256,314]	Budgerigars/thyroid hyperplasia

Table 28. Nutritional/mineral support used in birds (cont.)

Agent	Dosage	Comments
Dextrose (50%)	1 ml (500 mg)/kg IV slowly[324] 2 ml (1 g)/kg IV slowly[57]	Most species/hypoglycemia; can dilute with fluids
Iodine (Lugol's iodine)	1 drop/250 ml drinking water daily[167]	Most species/thyroid hyperplasia
Iodine (sodium iodide 20%)	0.3 ml (60 mg)/kg IM[167]	Most species/thyroid hyperplasia
Iron dextran	10 mg/kg IM, repeat in 7-10 days prn[29,313]	Most species, including raptors, waterfowl/iron deficiency anemia; use cautiously in species in which iron storage disease is common (eg, toucans, mynahs, starlings, birds of paradise, other passerines)
Pancreatic enzyme powder	—	Most species/pancreatic insufficiency; maldigestion
	1/8 tsp/kg feed[8]	Most species
	1/8 tsp/2-4 oz lightly oil-coated seed[324]	Most species
	1/8 tsp/1-4 oz handfeeding formula, prn[268]	Psittacine neonates
Vitamin A (Aquasol A Parenteral, Astra)	2,000 IU/kg PO, IM[13]	Psittacines/adjunctive therapy for pox
	20,000 IU/kg IM[363]	Most species/hypovitaminosis A; maximum dose[363]
	50,000 IU/kg IM q7d[186]	Psittacine neonates
	1 ml/135 kg IM[2]	Ostriches/hypovitaminosis A
Vitamins A, D_3, E (Vital E-A+D, Schering)	10,000 IU Vit A and 1,000 IU Vit D_3 /300 g q7d[167]	Most species/hypovitaminosis A or D_3; hypervitaminosis D may occur with excessive use; alcohol in product may cause pain at injection site; product without alcohol can be compounded commercially

Table 28. Nutritional/mineral support used in birds (cont.)

Agent	Dosage	Comments
Vitamin B$_1$ (thiamine)	—	Thiamine deficiency; requirements may be higher if thiaminase present in diet
	1-3 mg/kg IM q7d[182,313]	Most species, including raptors
	1-2 mg/kg feed[276]	Vultures
	1-2 mg/kg IM q24h[276]	Vultures
Vitamin B$_{12}$ (cyanocobalamin)	250-500 g/kg q7d[314]	Most species
Vitamin B-complex	1-2 mg/kg PO q24h[314]	Raptors, penguins, cranes/ daily supplement
	2 mg thiamine/kg IM[367]	Ratites/curly toe
Vitamin C	20-40 mg/kg IM q1-7d[314]	Most species/nutritional support
	20-50 mg/kg IM q1-7d[183]	Raptors
Vitamin E (Vitamin E20, Horse Health Products)	15 mg/kg PO once[239]	Raptors/PD; administer without food; injectable vitamin E has lower efficacy
	4.4-8.8 g/kg feed[2]	Ostrich chicks/ hypo-vitaminosis E
	0.06 mg/kg IM[367]	Ratites
Vitamin E/γ - linolenic acid (2%) linoleic acid (71%) (Derm Caps, DVM Pharmaceuticals)	0.1 ml/kg PO q24h[179,256,314]	Most species/feather picking; use liquid from gel caps
	0.4% γ-linolenic acid in feed[258]	Japanese quail/PD; reduces essential fatty acid deficient hepatic lipidosis
Vitamin E/selenium (Seletoc, Schering)	0.05-0.10 mg Se/kg IM q14d[313]	Most species/neuromuscular diseases (capture myopathy white muscle disease, some cardiomyopathies); may be useful in some cockatiels with jaw, eyelid, and tongue paralysis[313]
	0.06 mg Se/kg IM q3-14d[167]	

Table 28. Nutritional/mineral support used in birds (cont.)

Agent	Dosage	Comments
Vitamin K₁	0.2-2.2 mg/kg IM q4-8h until table, then q24h × 2 wk[182,206,208]	Most species, including raptors/rodenticide toxicity
	2.5 mg/kg IM q24h until hemostasis, then q7d prn[324]	Vitamin K responsive disorders (conures); hematochezia (Amazon parrots); coagulopathies (psittacines)
	5 mg/L feed[324]	Budgerigars/vitamin K responsive bleeding disorders; mix contents of gel cap into small grain seed mix and coat seed lightly
	5 mg/kg IM[367]	Ratites/clotting disorders

Table 29. Agents used in bird emergencies

Agent	Dosage	Comments
Atropine	0.5 mg/kg IM, IV, IO, IT [324,329]	CPR
Calcium gluconate	50-100 mg/kg IV slowly,[313] IM[167]	Hypocalcemia; diluted 50 mg/ml[192]
Dexamethasone Na phosphate	2-4 mg/kg IM, IV q12h[324]	Head trauma (until signs abate); shock (one dose); hyperthermia (until stable)
	4 mg/kg SC, IM[186]	Psittacine neonates/ shock
Dextrose (50%)	1 ml/kg IV slowly[324]	Hypoglycemia; can dilute with fluids
Diazepam	0.5-1.0 mg/kg IM, IV prn[327]	Seizures
Doxapram (Dopram-V, Aveco)	20 mg/kg IM, IV, IO [324]	CPR, respiratory depression
Epinephrine (1:1,000)	0.5-1.0 ml/kg IM, IV, IO, IT [324,329]	CPR, bradycardia
Fluids	$0.025 \times$ wt (g) = ml fluids SC, IV, IO	See Appendices 27 and 28 (fluid therapy)
Prednisolone Na succinate	10-20 mg/kg IM, IV q15min prn[57]	Head trauma; CPR
Sodium bicarbonate	1 mEq/kg q15-30 min to maximum of 4 mEq/kg total dose[365]	Metabolic acidosis
	5 mEq/kg IV, IO once[324]	CPR

Table 30. Topical agents used in birds [a]

Agent	Dosage	Comments
Aloe vera	—	See heparin for combination
Ammonium solution (Penetran)	Topical prn[314]	Most species/analgesic; antipruritic; anti-inflammatory; can use on fresh wounds; avoid overusage
Amphotericin B (3% cream)	Topical to affected area q12h[179,314]	Most species/mycoses
Armor All Protectant (Armor All Protectant Corp)	Topical to affected plumage[26]	Most species/soften sticky-trap glue covered plumage; use dish soap (Dawn) to remove Armor All
Carbaryl powder (5%)	Dust plumage lightly or add to nest box litter[314]	Most species/mites, ants; remove treated litter after 24 hr
Cypermethrin (5%)	Spray with 1:100 dilution[29]	Pigeons/lice; mites
Dimethylsulfoxide (DMSO) (90%)	1 ml/kg to affected area q4-7d[314]	Most species/anti-inflammatory, analgesic; systemic absorption; use gloves during application
Detergent (Dawn, Procter & Gamble)	1-5% bath	Most species/Armor All, motor oil removal
Enilconazole (Clinafarm, Sterwin)	Topical 1:10-1:100 dilution[30]	Psittacine/mycoses
	Topical 1:10 dilution q12h × 3-4 wk[29]	Raptors/mycoses; cutaneous aspergillosis, candidiasis
Ferric subsulfate	Topical[314,324]	Most species/hemostasis of bleeding nail or beak tip; will cause necrosis if used on open skin lesions
Fipronil (Frontline, Rhone Merieux)	Spray on skin once, repeat in 30 days prn[29]	Raptors/ectoparasites; avoid plumage during application
Heparin/aloe vera	Topical to affected area[179]	Most species/anti-inflammatory; dilute 1,000 IU heparin/150 mg aloe vera
Neomycin ointment	Topical to lesions[314,324]	Most species/superficial wounds; cover with bandage; may be absorbed systemically

Table 30. Topical agents used in birds [a] (cont.)

Agent	Dosage	Comments
Permethrin	Dust plumage lightly[10]	Pigeons/lice
Povidone iodine (Betadine Surgical Scrub, Purdue Frederick)	Topical to lesions, then wash off[29]	Raptors/wound cleansing
Prostaglandin E$_2$ (dinoprostone) (Prepidil Gel, UpJohn)	0.1 ml intracloacal or on uterine sphincter/100 g[166,319]	Psittacines/egg binding; causes uterovaginal sphincter relaxation; may cause uterine contractions; lower dosage may be effective; freeze into aliquots
Pyrethrins	Topical to plumage prn[29,324]	Most species/lice; 0.15% spray
	Dust plumage moderately, prn[29,324]	Pigeons, raptors
Silver nitrate	Topical to bleeding nail tips or beak tip[324]	Most species/hemostasis control; will cause necrosis of soft tissues
Silver sulfadiazine (Silvadene Cream 1%, Marion Merrell Dow)	Topical to affected areas q12-24h[314,324]	Most species/antibacterial, antimycotic agent; burns, ulcers; Amazon foot necrosis; bandage application preferred
Skin-So-Soft (Avon)	Topical to affected plumage[26]	Most species/softens and removes sticky-trap glue from plumage; use Dawn dish detergent to remove Skin-So-Soft

[a] Many topical agents contain oils or products which can adhere to plumage. These agents should be used sparingly and generally in non-feathered regions to prevent losing the insulating properties of the plumage. Many agents may contain corticosteroids which can suppress the adrenocortical axis and cause immunosuppression.

Table 31. Ophthalmologic agents used in birds

Agent	Dosage	Comments
Atropine (0.4-0.5%)	0.6 mg/bird topical[293]	Cockatoos/PD; partial mydriasis; some birds have iridal smooth muscle; may cause ocular irritation, weakness, shallow breathing; dilute with 0.9% saline
	Topical[39]	Ratites/partial mydriasis; used in combination with curariform drugs; some ratites have iridal smooth muscle
Bacitracin/ neomycin/ polymyxin B sulfate (Neobacimyx, Schering-Plough)	Small bead topical[324]	Most species/antibiotic; corneal ulcers, conjunctivitis, excessive amounts will cause eye-wiping and soiled plumage
Chloramphenicol ophthalmic drops	1 drop topical q6-8h[179]	Pigeons/antibiotic
Gentamicin sulfate (Gentocin, Schering-Plough)	1 drop topical q4-8h[324]	Most species/antibiotic; corneal ulcers; causes irritation
Ketamine	15-20 mg/kg IM[77]	Raptors/mydriasis; will cause sedation
Neomycin/ polymyxin B/ gramicidin (Bausch & Lomb)	1 drop topical q2-8h[324]	Most species/antibiotic; corneal ulcers; conjunctivitis
Oxytetracycline/ polymyxin B (Terramycin, Pfizer)	Small bead topical[324]	Most species/antibiotic; conjunctivitis; excessive amounts will cause eye-wiping and soiled plumage
Phenylephrine	Topical[39]	Ratites/partial mydriasis; used in combination with curariform drugs; some ratites have iridal smooth muscle
Phenylephrine (4-5%)	6 mg/bird topical[293]	Cockatoos/PD; partial mydriasis; some birds have iridal smooth muscle; may cause ocular irritation, weakness, shallow breathing; dilute with 0.9% saline
Pimaricin (Natacyn, Alcon)	1 drop topical q6h, taper after 14-21 days[314]	Most species/polyene antifungal

Table 31. Ophthalmologic agents used in birds (cont.)

Agent	Dosage	Comments
d-Tubocurarine (Curarin-Asta, Asta-Werke, Bielefeld, Germany)	—	Mydriatic agent; recommended for therapeutic use only; administer into anterior chamber; high risk of intraocular injury; topical application has no effect[202]
	0.01-0.03 ml of 0.3% solution, intracameral[39,201,260]	Most species, including pigeons, raptors/dilation within 15 min, duration 4-12 hr
Vecuronium bromide (Norcuron, Organon)	—	Mydriatic agent; may cause respiratory paralysis[194] or shallow breathing, ataxia, death; neostigmine may counteract systemic effects
	0.96 mg topical[292]	Cockatoos/use caution with bilateral application
	0.096 mg/bird of 0.08% solution topical[292,293]	Cockatoos, blue-front Amazon parrots, African grey parrots/PD
	0.24-0.28 mg/kg topical[293]	Blue-front Amazon parrots
	0.18-0.22 mg/kg topical[293]	African grey parrots
	0.18-0.29 mg/kg topical[293]	Cockatoos
	2 drops of 0.4% solution topical q15min × 3 treatments[251]	Falcons/maximal effect in 65 ± 12 min
	2 drops of 0.4% solution topical q15min × 3 treatments[251]	Raptors
	0.5% solution topical[77,251]	Raptors/duration 1 hr
	1 drop of 0.4% solution topical[382]	Cormorants, loons/dilation at 30-45 min; duration >2 hr
Vecuronium (V)/ nitrous oxide (N) isoflurane (I)	(V) 0.2 mg/kg IV/1:1 ratio of O2 to 33% (N) at 0.3 L/kg/min/ (I) 1.0-2.4%[201,202]	Most species/mydriasis and anesthesia; gases are administered via air sac cannulation; vecuronium effective up to 256 min in pigeons

Table 32. Antimicrobial-impregnated polymethylmethacrylate (PMMA) agents used in birds [a]

Agent	Dosage	Comments
Bone cement (Surgical Simplex P Radiopaque Bone Cement, Howmedica)	—	Polymer powder and liquid monomer for use in making antibiotic impregnated beads[380]
Gentamicin (Gentocin, Schering)	1 ml of 50 mg/ml solution in 20 g polymer powder[380]	Raptors/pododermatitis
Gentamicin (Septopal, Merck)	Pre-made beads[285]	Commercially available in Europe; not approved in US
Itraconazole	16% intraconazole-impregnated PMMA fed as grit stones[349]	Indian peafowl/PD; antifungal agent; when used as grit, therapeutic levels achieved in 2 days and decreased over 7 days; beads from capsules mixed into PMMA uniformly before hardening; PMMA cut into 1-g size pieces (grit stone size) after hardening
Oxytetracycline (Liquamycin, Rogar/STC)	4.5 ml of 200 mg/ml solution/20 g polymer powder[380]	Raptors/pododermatitis

[a] Antimicrobial-impregnated polymethylmethacrylate is used to elute antimicrobial agents for long-term treatment of infected lesions and has been used for systemic treatment as well.[349,358,380] If antibiotic powder is available, beads can be made by mixing 1 part antimicrobial powder to 50-60 parts polymer powder. For fluid antibiotics, follow the dosages cited. A homogeneous mixture is made with the polymer powder and antibiotic, then monomer is added and mixed uniformly. The dough is placed in a catheter tip syringe and extruded, rolled into beads, and placed onto steel surgical wire. Gas sterilization is recommended and beads are aerated for at least 24 hours at room temperature. The wound is debrided and beads are placed within it until the site is no longer infected. Gentamicin-impregnated beads may elute antibiotic for up to 5 years but usually are used for weeks to months.[358,380]

Table 33. Pharmacologic treatment of oiled birds [254]

Agent	Dosage	Comments
Bismuth subsalicylate	2-5 mg/kg PO once	Adsorbent; gavage; alternatively, can use activated charcoal
Charcoal, activated (Toxiban, Vet-A-Mix)	52 mg/kg PO once	Adsorbent; gavage; alternatively, can use bismuth subsalicylate
Detergent (Dawn, Procter & Gamble)	1-5% bath	Submerse bird up to mid-neck region; rinse with water; use water at 103-105 °F (39-41 °C) and 40-60 psi
Fluid therapy	—	See Appendixes 27 and 28 for guidelines
Iron dextran	10 mg/kg IM q5-7d	If PCV <25%
Thiamine/vitamin B_1	25-30 mg/kg feed fish	Piscivores

Table 34. Agents used in avian euthanasia [a]

Agent	Dosage	Comments
Carbon dioxide (CO_2)	70%[334]	Most species/danger to person administering gas; compressed gas recommended
Carbon monoxide	Closed container[334]	Most species/danger to person administering gas; compressed gas recommended
Halothane	Saturated cotton ball in closed container or head cone[281,328,334]	Most species/very rapid induction; wing flapping and vocalizing may occur
Isoflurane	Saturated cotton ball in closed container or head cone[281,328,334]	Most species/very rapid induction; wing flapping and vocalizing may occur
Lidocaine	0.5-1.0 ml intracranially through foramen magnum[328]	Pigeons/useful for anesthetized pigeons if brain is not to be harvested for histopathology
Methoxyflurane	Saturated cotton ball in closed container or head cone[281,328,334]	Most species/induction may be slower than with halothane or isoflurane
Sodium pentobarbital	1 ml/kg IV, ICe[324]	Most species/birds react unpredictably with IV administration; ICe administration smooth and quiet

a The American Veterinary Medical Association accepts inhalant anesthetic overdose, carbon monoxide, carbon dioxide, and barbiturate overdose as humane euthanasia methods.[334] Cervical dislocation and decapitation are conditionally acceptable for research and poultry animals.[334]

Table 35. Miscellaneous agents used in birds

Agent	Dosage	Comments
Acetic acid (vinegar)	15 ml/qt drinking water[179]	Most species/gastrointestinal yeast infections
Allopurinol	10 mg/kg PO q4-12h[325]	Most species/gout; prepare 10 mg/ml suspension: crush 100 mg tablet, mix with 10 ml simple syrup (Humco); reduce dose as uricemia decreases
	30 mg/kg PO q12h[19]	Most species
	100 mg/4 oz drinking water[324]	Most species
	1 ml stock/30 ml drinking water[314]	Budgerigars/gout; stock: 100 mg tablet/10 ml water; prepare fresh
Aluminum hydroxide	30-90 mg/kg PO q12h[324]	Most species/antacid; phosphate binder
Aminopentamide (Centrine, Fort Dodge)	0.11 mg/kg SC, IM q8-12h × 1 day, then q12h × 1 day then q24h × 1 day[36]	Most species/regurgitation
	0.05 mg/kg SC, IM q12h up to 5 doses[110]	Most species/regurgitation
Aminophylline	4 mg/kg PO, IM q6-12h[324]	Most species/bronchodilator; prepare 10 mg/ml suspension: crush 100 mg tablet, mix with 10 ml simple syrup (Humco)
	10 mg/kg IV q3h, then PO after initial response[314]	Most species/diuretic, vasodilator, cardiac stimulant, lung edema
	8-10 mg/kg PO, IM, IV q8h[367]	Ratites
Anticoagulant citrate dextrose (ACD) (Formula A, Baxter; A-C-D Solution, Sanofi)	0.15 ml/1 ml whole blood[174]	Anticoagulant for transfusions; heparin can be substituted if ACD is not available[257]
Asparaginase (Elspar, Merck)	400 IU/kg IM q7d[120]	Cockatoos/lymphosarcoma; premedicate with diphenhydramine

187

Table 35. Miscellaneous agents used in birds (cont.)

Agent	Dosage	Comments
Atropine	0.2 mg/kg IM, IV q3-4h[206,207]	Most species/organophosphate toxicity
	0.5 mg/kg SC, IM, IV, IO, IT[324]	Most species/CPR
	0.5 mg/kg IM, IV[324]	Pigeons/organophosphate toxicity
	0.5 mg/kg (1/2 IV, 1/2 IM)[280]	Raptors/organophosphate toxicity
	0.03-0.05 mg/kg SC, IM, IV q8h[367]	Ratites
Barium sulfate (Barotrast, Rhone-Poulenc; Novopaque, Picker International)	25 ml/kg PO[324]	Most species/gavage; dilute 72% suspension 1:1 with water; dilute 92% suspension 1:2 with water; 60% suspension effective in Amazons;[101] more dilute concentrations (20-25%) can also be used;[333] administer 1/2 volume diluted barium and 1/2 volume air for double contrast study of crop[248]
Bismuth sulfate	1 ml/kg PO[208]	Most species/weak adsorbent, demulcent
Charcoal, activated	—	See magnesium hydroxide for combination
	2-8 g/kg PO[30,179,208]	Adsorbs toxins; use 1 g/5-10 ml water; 1 tsp =1.6 g
Cimetidine (Tagamet, Smith Kline Beecham)	5 mg/kg PO, IM q8-12h[324]	Psittacines/proventriculitis; gastric ulceration[93]
	3-5 mg/kg PO, IV q8h[367]	Ratites
	5-10 mg/kg IM q12h[367]	Ratites
Cisapride (Propulsid, Janssen)	0.5-1.5 mg/kg PO q8h[179,314]	Most species/gastrointestinal stimulant
Colchicine (Col Benemid, Merck)	0.04 mg/kg PO q12-24h[160]	Most species/gout; hepatic fibrosis/cirrhosis; dosage based on colchicine; generic agent without probenecid available

Table 35. Miscellaneous agents used in birds (cont.)

Agent	Dosage	Comments
Cyclophosphamide (Cytoxan, Squibb)	200 mg/m^2 IO q7d[120]	Cockatoos/lymphosarcoma
Digoxin	0.05 mg/kg PO q24h[383]	Quaker parakeets/PD; congestive heart failure; cardiomyopathy
	0.02 mg/kg PO q24h[8,320]	Budgerigars, mynahs, sparrows
	0.0049 mg/kg IV q12h[8]	Poultry
	0.0035 mg/kg IV q24h[8]	Turkeys
	0.019 mg/kg IV q12h[8]	Pekin ducks
Dioctyl sodium sulfosuccinate (Diocto, Barre)	1 ml/30 ml drinking water[186]	Psittacine chicks/ constipation; use only if chick is drinking
Diphenhydramine	1-4 mg/kg PO q8h[324]	Macaws, Amazon parrots/allergic rhinitis
	2-4 mg/kg IM, IV q12h[179]	Most species
	2-4 mg/100 ml drinking water[125]	Most species/hypersensitivity
	2 mg/kg IO once[120]	Cockatoos/prior to chemotherapy
Dipyrone (Novin, Vedco)	20-25 mg/kg SC, IM, IV[367]	Ratites/analgesic for intestinal disorders, antipyretic
Doxapram	—	Respiratory depression or arrest
	5-10 mg/kg IM, IV once[313]	Most species
	20 mg/kg IM, IV, IO[324]	Most species
	4-8 mg/kg IV q1h[367]	Ratites
Doxorubicin	60 mg/m2 IV q30d[88]	Blue-front Amazon parrots/ osteosarcoma; premedicate with diphenhydramine 30 min before; dilute with saline and give over 30 min (anesthesia recommended)
	30 mg/m2 IO q2d[120]	Cockatoos/lymphosarcoma; premedicate with diphen-hydramine

Table 35. Miscellaneous agents used in birds (cont.)

Agent	Dosage	Comments
Epinephrine (1:1,000)	0.5-1.0 ml/kg IM, IV, IO, IT[324]	CPR; cardiac arrest
Furosemide	0.15-2.0 mg/kg SC, IM q12-24h[313]	Most species/diuretic
	1-2 mg/kg PO q12-24h[267]	Most species/congestive heart failure; can be used with digoxin and ACE inhibitors
	5 mg/120 ml drinking water[10]	Most species; ascites
	2.5-10.0 mg/kg PO q12h × 7-14 days[324]	Cockatiels, budgerigars/ ascites
	0.15 mg/kg IM[186]	Psittacine neonates/ pulmonary congestion
	0.15 mg/kg IM q8h[191]	Mynahs/ascites, hemochromatosis
	2.2 mg/kg PO q12h[320]	Mynahs/cardiac disease
	2.2 mg/kg PO, IM, IV q12h prn[327]	Pigeons
	4-6 mg/kg PO, IM[305]	Raptors/pulmonary congestion
	0.1 ml IM q6-12h × 2 days[367]	Ratite chicks/edema
Gadopentetate dimeglumine (Magnevist, Berlex)	0.25 mmol/kg IV[318]	Contrast agent for magnetic resonance imaging
Glipizide (Glucotrol, Roerig)	1.25 mg/kg PO q24h[179]	Most species/diabetes mellitus
Glycosaminoglycan (Adequan, Luitpold)	10 mg/kg IM, IA q7d × 3 mo[356,366]	Non-infectious or traumatic joint dysfunction; 250 mg/ml for IA use; 500 mg/ml for IM use; contraindicated in septic arthritis
	500 mg IM q4d × 28 days[367]	Ratites
Heparin sodium	2 units/ml whole blood[81,83]	Cockatiels, conures/anti-coagulant for blood transfusion

Table 35. Miscellaneous agents used in birds (cont.)

Agent	Dosage	Comments
Hetastarch (Hespan, DuPont)	10-15 ml/kg IV q8h × 1-4 treatments[353]	Most species/chronic hypoproteinemia; decrease fluid treatment to $^1/_3$-$^1/_2$ maintenance fluid dose; amylopectin plasma expander colloid with a T-1/2 of 25 hr; dextrans are an alternative, but have shorter T-1/2
Hyaluronidase (Wydase, Wyeth-Ayerst)	1 ml (150 IU)/L fluids SC[182]	Most species/increases absorption rate of fluids
Hydroxyzine (Atarax, Roerig)	2.0-2.2 mg/kg PO q8h[129,205]	Amazon parrots/allergic pruritus; feather picking; self mutilation
	4 mg/100-120 ml drinking water[125,129]	Most species/respiratory allergy; feather picking
Iohexol (Omnipaque, Sarafi Winthrop)	25-30 ml/kg PO[101]	Cockatoos, Amazon parrots/ gavage; radiographic gastrointestinal contrast media; 1:1 dilution with water can also be used
Isoxsuprine (Vasodilan, Bristol Meyers)	5-10 mg/kg PO q24h × 20-40 days[29]	Raptors/peripheral vasodilator; wing tip edema
Kaolin/pectin (Kaopect, Med-Tech)	2 ml/kg PO q6-8h[19]	Psittacine neonates/intestinal protectant
Lactulose (Cephulac, Marion Merrell Dow)	0.2 ml/kg PO q12h[19] 0.3-1.0 ml/kg PO q12h[240]	Most species/hepatic encephalopathy; reduces blood ammonia levels; increases Gram $\oplus$ in the gastrointestinal tract; exerts osmotic effect in birds with caeca through fermentation to acetic and lactic acid[93]
	0.3 ml/kg PO q8-12h[186]	Psittacine neonates
Magnesium hydroxide (M)/ activated charcoal (C) (Milk of Magnesia, Roxane)	(M) 10-12 ml/ (C) 1 tsp powder[208]	Most species/cathartic; adsorbent

Table 35. Miscellaneous agents used in birds (cont.)

Agent	Dosage	Comments
Magnesium sulfate	—	See peanut butter for combination
	0.5-1.0 g/kg PO[208]	Epsom salts; cathartic; may cause lethargy; combine with dilute peanut butter as a cathartic and bulk diet[208]
	1/4 tsp/bird[367]	Ratite juveniles/obstipation
	2 Tbs/bird[367]	Ratite adults/obstipation
Mannitol	0.5 g/kg q24h IV slowly[313]	Osmotic diuretic; head trauma
	0.25-2.0 mg/kg IV[182]	Raptors/head trauma; can use with furosemide
	1,500 mg/kg IV q6h[367]	Ratites
Methocarbamol (Robaxin-V, Fort Dodge)	50 mg/kg IV slowly[314]	Swans, cranes (Demoiselle)/ capture myopathy
	50 mg/kg IV q12h[64]	Most species/muscle relaxation
	32.5 mg/kg PO q12h[314]	Swans, cranes (Demoiselle)/ capture myopathy
Metoclopramide (Reglan, Robins)	0.5 mg/kg q8-12h[314] PO, IM, IV	Most species/gastrointestinal motility disorders; regurgitation; slow crop motility
	2 mg/kg IM, IV q8h[29,307]	Raptors, waterfowl/crop stasis; ileus
	0.1 mg/kg IV[256]	Ostriches
	12.5 mg/kg PO[367]	Ratites/gastrointestinal disorders
Mineral oil	—	See peanut butter for combination
	0.3 ml/35 g or 3-5 ml/500 g[208]	Most species/cathartic
	15ml/kg PO[367]	Ratite adults/impaction
Oil	—	See mineral oil and vegetable oil

Table 35. Miscellaneous agents used in birds (cont.)

Agent	Dosage	Comments
Peanut butter	Peanut butter and mineral oil 2:1[208]	Most species/add to diet; cathartic
	Dilute peanut butter and magnesium sulfate[208]	Most species/add to diet; cathartic; dilute with water
Pralidoxime (2-PAM) (Protopam, Wyeth)	10-100 mg/kg IM q24-48h[206,208]	Organophosphate toxicity; administer within 24 hr of intoxication;[282] use lower dose in combination with atropine
	100 mg/kg IM, repeat in 6 hr[29]	Waterfowl
Probucol (Lorelco, Marion Merrell Dow)	1 drop stock/300 g PO q12h × 2-4 mo[179,314]	Most species/decreases cholesterol, lipemia, and lipomas; contains iron: use cautiously in species susceptible to hemochromatosis; may increase bile acids; use only in birds with low density lipoprotein-cholesterolemia; use with low fat diet; prepare stock: crush 250 mg tablet/7.5 ml lactulose
Propranolol (Inderal, Wyeth-Ayerst)	0.2 mg/kg IM[313]	Most species/supraventricular arrhythmia, atrial flutter, fibrillation
	0.04 mg/kg IV slowly[313]	
Psyllium (Metamucil, Procter & Gamble)	0.5 tsp/60 ml hand feeding formula[206,208]	Most species/bulk diet; can use mineral oil as alternative or in addition to psyllium
	1 Tbs in 60 ml water/bird PO, up to 120 ml/day[367]	Ratite chicks/impaction
	2 Tbs/10 kg PO[186]	Ostrich neonates/impaction
Sodium bicarbonate	1 mEq/kg q15-30min to maximum of 4 mEq/kg total dose[365]	Most species/shock; metabolic acidosis
	0.5-1.0 mEq/kg PO, SC[80]	Most species/shock; metabolic acidosis; 1 tsp = 4 g
	5 mEq/kg IV, IO once[324]	Most species/CPR
Sodium sulfate (GoLytely, Braintree)	0.5-1.0 g/kg PO[208]	Most species/cathartic

Table 35. Miscellaneous agents used in birds (cont.)

Agent	Dosage	Comments
Sucralfate (Carafate, Marion Merrell Dow)	25 mg/kg PO q8h[313]	Most species/oral, esophageal, gastric, duodenal ulcers
Terbutaline (Brethine, Novartis)	0.1 mg/kg PO q12-24h[324]	Macaws, Amazon parrots/ bronchodilator; obstructive pulmonary disease, pneumonitis
Tyrode's solution	Offer in place of drinking water[314]	Cockatiels/restores renal-medullary gradient; add 8 g NaC1, 0.13 g $CaCl_2$, 0.2 g KCl, 0.1 g $MgCl_2$, 0.05 g Na_2HPO_4, 1 g $NaHCO_3$, 1 g glucose to 1 L water
Vegetable oil	15 ml/kg PO[367]	Ratite adults/impaction
	15 ml/bird PO[367]	Ratite chicks/impaction
Vincristine sulfate (Oncovin, Lilly)	0.5 mg/m^2 IV, then 0.75 mg/m^2 q7d × 3 wk[264]	Ducks/lymphoma; lymphocytic leukemia
	0.75 mg/m^2 IO q7d × 3 wk[120]	Cockatoos/lymphosarcoma

Appendix 11. Hematologic and serum biochemical values of selected psittacines

Measurements	African grey[212,315,369a]	Amazon parrot[212,315,369a]	Blue-headed parrot[212]
Hematology			
PCV (%)	43-55	45-55	44-60
RBC (10^6/μl)	2.4-4.5	2.5-4.5	2.4-4.1
Hb (g/dl)	11.0-16.0	—	—
MCV (fl)	90-180	—	—
MCH (pg)	28-52	—	—
MCHC (g/dl)	23-33	—	—
WBC (10^3/μl)	5-11	6-11	4-11
Heterophils (%)	45-75	30-75	40-70
Lymphocytes (%)	20-50	20-65	20-50
Monocytes (%)	0-3	0-3	0-2
Eosinophils (%)	0-2	0-1	0-1
Basophils (%)	0-5	0-5	0-5
H:L ratio	—	—	0.8-3.5
Chemistries			
AP (IU/L)	20-160	15-150	—
ALT (IU/L)	—	—	—
AST (IU/L)	100-350	130-350	150-350
Bile acid (μmol/L)			
RIA	18-71	19-144	—
Colorimetric	—	—	—
Calcium (mg/dl)	8-13	8-13	10-15
Cholesterol (mg/dl)	160-425	—	—
CK (IU/L)	123-875	45-265	—
Chloride (mEq/L)	—	—	—
Creatinine (mg/dl)	0.1-0.4	0.1-0.4	0.1-0.3
GGT (IU/L)	1-10	—	—
Glucose (mg/dl)	190-350	220-350	100-300
LDH (IU/L)	150-450	160-420	200-550
Phosphorus (mg/dl)	3.2-5.4	3.1-5.5	—
Potassium (mEq/L)	2.6-4.2	3.0-4.5	3.0-4.5
Sodium (mEq/L)	134-152	136-152	130-150
Uric acid (mg/dl)	4-10	2-10	4-12
Protein, total (g/dl)	3-5	3-5	2.6-5.0
Albumin (g/dl)	1.57-3.23	1.9-3.5	—
Globulin (g/dl)	—	—	—
A:G ratio	1.6-4.3	1.9-5.9	—
Pre-albumin (g/dl)	0.03-1.35	0.35-1.05	—
α-globulin (g/dl)	$α_1$ 0.02-0.27	$α_1$ 0.05-0.32	—
	$α_2$ 0.12-0.31	$α_2$ 0.07-0.32	—
β-globulin (g/dl)	0.15-0.56	0.12-0.72	—
γ-globulin (g/dl)	0.11-0.71	0.17-0.76	—

Appendix 11. Hematologic and serum biochemical values of selected psittacines (cont.)

Measurements	Budgerigar[19,159,369a]	Cockatiel[17,46,212,369a]	Cockatoo[61,369a]
Hematology			
PCV (%)	45-57	45-57	42-52
RBC (10^6/μl)	2.3-3.9	2.5-4.7	2-4
Hb (g/dl)	13-18	11-16	12-16
MCV (fl)	90-190	90-200	120-175
MCH (pg)	27-59	28-55	35-55
MCHC (g/dl)	22-32	22-33	28-33
WBC (10^3/μl)	3-8	5-10	8-25
Heterophils (%)	40-65	40-70	15-64
Lymphocytes (%)	20-45	25-55	29-83
Monocytes (%)	0-1	0-2	0-9
Eosinophils (%)	0-1	0-2	0
Basophils (%)	0-1	0-6	0-3
H:L ratio	0.9-3.3	0.7-2.8	0-2
Chemistries			
AP (IU/L)	10-80	0-346	200-850
ALT (IU/L)	—	0-9	0-5
AST (IU/L)	55-154	100-350	120-320
Bile acid (μmol/L)			
RIA	20-65	25-85	20-70
Colorimetric	—	15-139	—
Calcium (mg/dl)	6.4-11.2	8.5-13.0	8-11
Cholesterol (mg/dl)	145-275	140-360	150-300
CK (IU/L)	54-252	30-245	140-410
Chloride (mEq/L)	—	—	110-120
Creatinine (mg/dl)	0.1-0.4	0.1-0.4	0.2-0.7
GGT (IU/L)	1-10	0-5	0-4
Glucose (mg/dl)	254-399	200-450	200-300
LDH (IU/L)	154-271	125-450	150-1000
Phosphorus (mg/dl)	3.0-5.2	3.2-4.8	3.5-6.5
Potassium (mEq/L)	2.2-3.7	2.5-4.5	3-5
Sodium (mEq/L)	139-159	132-150	145-155
Uric acid (mg/dl)	3.0-8.6	3.5-11.0	2.0-8.5
Protein, total (g/dl)	2-3	2.4-4.1	3-5
Albumin (g/dl)	—	0.7-1.8	1.0-1.6
Globulin (g/dl)	—	—	1.5-2.5
A:G ratio	—	1.5-4.3	0.6-1.0
Pre-albumin (g/dl)	—	0.8-1.6	0.3-0.6
α-globulin (g/dl)	—	$α_1$ 0.05-0.40	0.1-0.5
		$α_2$ 0.05-0.44	—
β-globulin (g/dl)	—	0.21-0.58	0.2-0.4
γ-globulin (g/dl)	—	0.11-0.43	0.5-0.5

Appendix 11. Hematologic and serum biochemical values of selected psittacines (cont.)

Measurements	Conure[212,369a]	Eclectus parrot[60]	Grey-cheek and canary-winged parakeet[212]
Hematology			
PCV (%)	42-45	45-55	46-58
RBC (10^6/μl)	2.9-4.5	2.7-3.8	—
Hb (g/dl)	12-16	13.5-16.0	—
MCV (fl)	90-190	125-175	—
MCH (pg)	28-55	40-50	—
MCHC (g/dl)	23-31	29-32	—
WBC (10^3/μl)	4-11	9-20	4.5-9.5
Heterophils (%)	40-75	35-50	40-75
Lymphocytes (%)	20-50	45-65	20-60
Monocytes (%)	0-3	1-7	0-3
Eosinophils (%)	0-3	1-1	0-1
Basophils (%)	0-5	0-3	0-5
H:L ratio	0.8-3.8	1-2	—
Chemistries			
AP (IU/L)	80-250	200-750	—
ALT (IU/L)	5-13	0-5	—
AST (IU/L)	125-350	135-230	150-750
Bile acid (μmol/L)			
RIA	20-45	—	—
Colorimetric	—	—	—
Calcium (mg/dl)	8-15	8.8-9.8	—
Cholesterol (mg/dl)	120-400	220-325	—
CK (IU/L)	35-355	200-625	—
Chloride (mEq/L)	—	112-120	—
Creatinine (mg/dl)	0.1-0.5	0.4-0.5	0.1-0.4
GGT (IU/L)	1-15	1-5	—
Glucose (mg/dl)	200-350	225-300	200-350
LDH (IU/L)	125-420	100-280	150-450
Phosphorus (mg/dl)	2-10	4.5-7.0	—
Potassium (mEq/L)	3.4-5.0	2.2-4.6	—
Sodium (mEq/L)	134-148	150-158	—
Uric acid (mg/dl)	2.5-10.5	0.7-5.0	4-12
Protein, total (g/dl)	2.5-4.5	4-5	2.5-4.5
Albumin (g/dl)	1.9-2.6	1.4-1.8	—
Globulin (g/dl)	—	1.3-2.3	—
A:G ratio	2.2-4.3	0.6-1.1	—
Pre-albumin (g/dl)	0.18-0.98	—	—
α-globulin (g/dl)	$α_1$ 0.04-0.23	0.6-1.2	—
	$α_2$ 0.08-0.26	—	
β-globulin (g/dl)	0.07-0.47	0.6-1.2	—
γ-globulin (g/dl)	0.12-0.61	0.6-1.2	—

Appendix 11. Hematologic and serum biochemical values of selected psittacines (cont.)

Measurements	Hyacinth macaw[45]	Jardine's parrot[369a]	Lovebird[369a,384]
Hematology			
PCV (%)	50-60	35-48	44-57
RBC (10^6/μl)	—	2.4-4.0	3.0-5.1
Hb (g/dl)	—	11-16	13-18
MCV (fl)	—	90-190	90-190
MCH (pg)	—	25-56	27-59
MCHC (g/dl)	—	21-33	22-32
WBC (10^3/μl)	10-16	4-10	3-8
Heterophils (%)	56-90	55-75	40-75
Lymphocytes (%)	9-44	25-45	20-55
Monocytes (%)	0-4	0-2	0-2
Eosinophils (%)	0-2	0-1	0-1
Basophils (%)	0-4	0-1	0-6
H:L ratio	1.3-10.0	1.2-3.0	0.7-3.8
Chemistries			
AP (IU/L)	—	—	10-90
ALT (IU/L)	—	—	—
AST (IU/L)	87-160	150-275	100-350
Bile acid (μmol/L)			
RIA	—	—	25-95
Colorimetric	—	—	—
Calcium (mg/dl)	7.4-12.8	7-13	9-15
Cholesterol (mg/dl)	—	—	95-335
CK (IU/L)	260-563	—	52-245
Chloride (mEq/L)	—	—	—
Creatinine (mg/dl)	0.3-0.5	—	0.1-0.4
GGT (IU/L)	—	—	2.5-18.0
Glucose (mg/dl)	255-324	200-325	200-400
LDH (IU/L)	62-89	—	100-350
Phosphorus (mg/dl)	—	—	3.2-4.9
Potassium (mEq/L)	2.3-6.2	—	2.5-3.5
Sodium (mEq/L)	144-152	—	137-150
Uric acid (mg/dl)	3.4-10.4	2.5-12.0	3-11
Protein, total (g/dl)	2.7-3.6	2.8-4.0	2.4-4.6
Albumin (g/dl)	—	—	—
Globulin (g/dl)	—	—	—
A:G ratio	—	—	—
Pre-albumin (g/dl)	—	—	—
α-globulin (g/dl)	—	—	—
β-globulin (g/dl)	—	—	—
γ-globulin (g/dl)	—	—	—

Measurements	Macaw[62]	Pionus parrot[369a]	Quaker parrot[128,369a]
Hematology			
PCV (%)	47-55	35-47	30-70
RBC ($10^6/\mu l$)	2.7-4.5	2.4-4.0	2.8-3.9
Hb (g/dl)	15-17	11-16	11-15
MCV (fl)	125-170	85-210	90-200
MCH (pg)	36-55	26-54	26-55
MCHC (g/dl)	29-35	24-31	22-32
WBC ($10^3/\mu l$)	7-22	4.0-11.5	1.2-10.7
Heterophils (%)	40-60	50-75	0-24
Lymphocytes (%)	35-60	25-45	74-90
Monocytes (%)	1-8	0-2	1-4
Eosinophils (%)	0-1	0-2	0-2
Basophils (%)	0-1	0-1	0-6
H:L ratio	0.6-1.8	1.1-3.0	—
Chemistries			
AP (IU/L)	290-750	—	—
ALT (IU/L)	0-5	—	—
AST (IU/L)	90-180	150-365	150-285
Bile acid (μmol/L)			
RIA	—	—	—
Colorimetric	—	—	—
Calcium (mg/dl)	9.5-10.5	7.0-13.5	7-12
Cholesterol (mg/dl)	100-300	130-295	—
CK (IU/L)	180-500	—	—
Chloride (mEq/L)	105-113	—	—
Creatinine (mg/dl)	0.5-0.6	0.1-0.4	—
GGT (IU/L)	0-4	—	—
Glucose (mg/dl)	280-320	125-300	200-350
LDH (IU/L)	40-250	—	—
Phosphorus (mg/dl)	4.6-6.4	2.9-6.6	—
Potassium (mEq/L)	2.2-3.9	3.5-4.6	—
Sodium (mEq/L)	148-156	145-155	—
Uric acid (mg/dl)	1-6	3.5-10.0	3.5-11.5
Protein, total (g/dl)	3.4-4.2	3.2-4.6	3.8-5.0
Albumin (g/dl)	1.3-1.7	—	—
Globulin (g/dl)	1.3-1.9	—	—
A:G ratio	0.7-1.0	—	—
Pre-albumin (g/dl)	0.3-0.6	—	—
α-globulin (g/dl)	0.1-0.4	—	—
β-globulin (g/dl)	0.2-0.6	—	—
γ-globulin (g/dl)	0.2-0.4	—	—

Appendix 11. Hematologic and serum biochemical values of selected psittacines (cont.)

Measurements	Scarlet macaw[188]	Senegal parrot[369a]
Hematology		
PCV (%)	46-53	36-48
RBC ($10^6/\mu l$)	—	2.4-4.0
Hb (g/dl)	—	11-16
MCV (fl)	—	90-200
MCH (pg)	—	27-55
MCHC (g/dl)	—	23-32
WBC ($10^3/\mu l$)	13.3-24.4	4-11
Heterophils (%)	26-72	55-75
Lymphocytes (%)	24-72	25-45
Monocytes (%)	1-10	0-2
Eosinophils (%)	0-6	0-1
Basophils (%)	0-2	0-1
H:L ratio	—	1.2-3.0
Chemistries		
AP (IU/L)	—	—
ALT (IU/L)	—	—
AST (IU/L)	86-222	100-350
Bile acid ($\mu mol/L$)		
RIA	—	20-85
Colorimetric	—	—
Calcium (mg/dl)	7.2-8.7	6.5-13.0
Cholesterol (mg/dl)	124-176	—
CK (IU/L)	98-584	100-330
Chloride (mEq/L)	100-112	—
Creatinine (mg/dl)	0.5-1.0	0.1-0.4
GGT (IU/L)	—	1-15
Glucose (mg/dl)	231-287	140-250
LDH (IU/L)	—	—
Phosphorus (mg/dl)	1.1-3.1	—
Potassium (mEq/L)	1.2-2.1	—
Sodium (mEq/L)	132-153	—
Uric acid (mg/dl)	0.4-8.2	2.3-10.0
Protein, total (g/dl)	2.3-2.7	3.0-4.5
Albumin (g/dl)	1.3-1.7	—
Globulin (g/dl)	1.1-1.6	—
A:G ratio	0.9-1.3	—
Pre-albumin (g/dl)	—	—
α-globulin (g/dl)	—	—
β-globulin (g/dl)	—	—
γ-globulin (g/dl)	—	—

Appendix 12. Hematologic and serum biochemical values for juveniles of selected psittacines

			Mean ± SD (range)		
Measurement	Cockatoos[61] (9 species) (n=152)	Umbrella cockatoo[61] (n=111)	Macaws[62] (7 species) (n=113)	Blue/gold macaw[62] (n=43)	Eclectus parrot[60] (n=111)
Hematology					
PCV (%)	39.7 ± 9.0 (25-59)	39.3	41.7 ± 8.4 (25-55)	40 ± 7.7	43.8 ± 8.4 (26-58)
RBC (10^6/µl)	2.53 ± 0.63 (1.5-4.0)	2.54	2.9 ± 0.8 (1.5-4.5)	2.7 ± 0.7	2.69 ± 0.67 (1.5-4.0)
Hgb (g/dl)	11.4 ± 2.9 (6.5-17.0)	11.6	12.3 ± 3.3 (7-17)	11.0 ± 2.9	12.5 ± 3.0 (6.5-18.0)
WBC (10^3/µl)	12.9 ± 6.3 (5.5-25.0)	16.6	19.2 ± 6.9 (7-30)	18.9 ± 5.6	13.7 ± 6.3 (5.5-25.0)
Heterophils (%)	50.8 ± 11.7 (27-74)	54.1	55.3 ± 10 (37-75)	52 ± 10	53.9 ± 11.4 (35-75)
Bands (%)	1.3 ± 2.3 (0-7)	1.31	0.6 ± 1.7 (0-5)	0.1 ± 0.7	0.5 ± 1.5 (0-5)
Lymphocytes (%)	41.2 ± 11.9 (17-65)	38.1	39 ±10 (20-60)	42 ± 10	39.5 ± 11.5 (20-65)
Monocytes (%)	5.8 ± 3.4 (0-12)	5.35	4.4 ± 2.9 (1-10)	4.3 ± 2.7	5.0 ± 2.7 (1-11)
Eosinophils (%)	0	0.02	0 ± 0.2 (0-1)	0	0.1 ± 0.3 (0-1)
Basophils (%)	0.9 ± 1.1 (0-4)	1.03	0.5 ± 1.0 (0-3)	0.9 ± 1.3	1.1 ± 1.0 (0-3)
Chemistries					
AP (IU/L)	579 ± 239 (200-1000)	440	970 ± 397 (290-1600)	1200 ± 390	489 ± 159 (200-900)
ALT (SGPT) (IU/L)	2 ± 3 (0-13)	2.1	3 ± 2 (0-9)	4 ± 3	4 ± 3 (0-10)
AST (SGOT) (IU/L)	143 ± 79 (50-400)	136	104 ± 31 (60-180)	101 ± 24	140 ± 58 (65-260)
Calcium (mg/dl)	9.6 ± 0.7 (8-11)	9.8	9.9 ± 0.5 (8.5-10.8)	10.0 ± 0.5	9.3 ± 0.4 (8.5-10.2)
Chloride (mEq/L)	110 ± 6 (97-120)	111	106 ± 6 (96-118)	104 ± 5	111 ± 5 (100-120)
Cholesterol (mg/dl)	251 ± 105 (100-500)	291	165 ± 62 (75-300)	164 ± 67	268 ± 80 (125-450)
CK (IU/L)	510 ± 235 (140-1000)	517	550 ± 312 (180-1100)	540 ± 267	616 ± 472 (200-1600)
Creatinine (mg/dl)	0.4 ± 0.1 (0.2-0.7)	0.4	0.4 ± 0.1 (0.3-0.6)	0.4 ± 0.1	0.4 ± 0.1 (0.2-0.5)

Appendix 12. Hematologic and serum biochemical values for juveniles of selected psittacines (cont.)

			Mean ± SD (range)		
Measurement	Cockatoos[61] (9 species) (n=152)	Umbrella cockatoo[61] (n=111)	Macaws[62] (7 species) (n=113)	Blue/gold macaw[62] (n=43)	Eclectus parrot[60] (n=111)
Chemistries (cont.)					
GGT (IU/L)	2.6 ± 1.7 (0-6)	2.7	1.8 ± 1.2 (0-4)	1.7 ± 1.2	4 ± 2 (0-7)
Glucose (mg/dl)	253 ± 24 (200-300)	244	281 ± 30 (225-330)	288 ± 31	258 ± 18 (220-300)
LDH (IU/L)	371 ± 285 (150-1000)	325	138 ± 84 (35-275)	144 ± 98	228 ± 101 (100-400)
Phosphorus (mg/dl)	6.1 ± 1.1 (3.5-8.0)	5.6	6.5 ± 1.0 (4.6-6.9)	6.6 ± 0.9	6.8 ± 1.2 (4.5-9.0)
Potassium (mEq/L)	3.6 ± 0.7 (2.5-5.5)	3.5	2.9 ± 0.8 (2.0-4.2)	2.7 ± 0.6	2.8 ± 0.7 (2.0-4.6)
Protein, total (g/dl)	2.8 ± 0.7 (1.5-4.0)	3.0	2.6 ± 0.6 (1.5-3.5)	2.5 ± 0.7	2.9 ± 0.5 (1.8-3.8)
Albumin (g/dl)	1.1 ± 0.3 (0.3-1.6)	1.7	1.2 ± 0.3 (0.6-1.7)	1.2 ± 0.3	1.3 ± 0.3 (0.8-1.8)
Globulin (g/dl)	1.7 ± 0.5 (0.8-2.5)	0.9	1.3 ± 0.6 (0.8-1.9)	1.3 ± 0.6	1.5 ± 0.3 (0.8-2.2)
A:G ratio	0.6 ± 0.2 (0.4-1.0)	0.6	0.8 ± 0.3 (0.5-1.0)	0.8 ± 0.2	0.9 ± 0.2 (0.6-1.1)
Sodium (mEq/L)	145 ± 6 (135-155)	145	145 ± 6 (135-156)	142 ± 6	148 ± 6 (138-158)
Urea (mg/dl)	2.0 ± 2.2 (0-6)	1.6	2.4 ± 2.3 (0-6)	1.9 ± 2.2	1.7 ± 2.4 (0-6)
Uric acid (mg/dl)	2.9 ± 2.3 (0.2-8.5)	2.7	2.3 ± 2.1 (0.2-6.0)	1.9 ± 2.5	2.0 ± 1.6 (0.2-6.5)

[a] n = number of blood samples (multiple blood samples were obtained from some individuals over time).

Appendix 13. Hematologic and serum biochemical values of selected Passeriformes

Measurements	Canary[179,369a]	Finch[212]	Mynah[212]
Hematology			
PCV (%)	37-49	45-62	44-55
RBC ($10^6/\mu l$)	2.5-3.8	2.5-4.6	2.4-4.0
Hb (g/dl)	12-16	—	—
MCV (fl)	90-210	—	—
MCH (pg)	26-55	—	—
MCHC (g/dl)	22-32	—	—
WBC ($10^3/\mu l$)	4-9	3-8	6-11
Heterophils (%)	50-80	20-65	25-65
Lymphocytes (%)	20-45	20-65	20-60
Monocytes (%)	0-1	0-1	0-3
Eosinophils (%)	0-2	0-1	0-3
Basophils (%)	0-1	0-5	0-7
H:L ratio	—	0.3-3.3	0.4-3.3
Chemistries			
AP (IU/L)	20-135	—	—
ALT (IU/L)	—	—	—
AST (IU/L)	145-345	150-350	130-350
Bile acid (μmol/L)			
RIA	23-90	—	—
Colorimetric	—	—	—
Calcium (mg/dl)	5.5-13.5	—	9-13
Cholesterol (mg/dl)	150-400	—	—
CK (IU/L)	55-350	—	—
Chloride (mEq/L)	—	—	—
Creatinine (mg/dl)	0.1-0.4	—	0.1-0.6
GGT (IU/L)	1-14	—	—
Glucose (mg/dl)	205-435	200-450	190-350
LDH (IU/L)	120-450	—	600-1000
Phosphorus (mg/dl)	2.9-4.9	—	—
Potassium (mEq/L)	2.2-4.5	—	0.3-5.1
Sodium (mEq/L)	135-165	—	136-152
Uric acid (mg/dl)	4-12	4-12	4-10
Protein, total (g/dl)	2.8-4.5	3-5	2.3-4.5
Albumin (g/dl)	—	—	—
Globulin (g/dl)	—	—	—
A:G ratio	—	—	—

Appendix 14. Hematologic and serum biochemical values of selected Galliformes

Measurements	Chicken[179]	Ringneck pheasant[387]	Turkey[179]	Quail[179]
Hematology				
PCV (%)	23-55	—	30.4-45.6	30.0-45.1
RBC ($10^6/\mu l$)	1.3-4.5	1.2-3.5	1.74-3.70	4.0-5.2
Hb (g/dl)	7.0-18.6	8.0-11.2	8.8-13.4	10.7-14.3
MCV (fl)	100-139	—	112-168	60-100
MCH (pg)	25-48	—	32.0-49.3	23-35
MCHC (g/dl)	20-34	—	23.2-35.3	28.0-38.5
WBC ($10^3/\mu l$)	9-32	18-39	16.0-25.5	12.5-24.6
Heterophil (%)	15-50	12-30	29-52	25-50
Lymphocytes (%)	29-84	63-83	35-48	50-70
Monocytes (%)	0.05-7.0	2-9	3-10	0.5-3.8
Eosinophil (%)	0-16	0	0-5	0-15
Basophils (%)	0-8	0-3	1-9	0-1.5
H:L ratio	0.2-1.7	0.14-0.48	0.6-1.5	0.4-1.0
Chemistries				
Calcium (mg/dl)	13.2-23.7	—	11.7-38.7	—
Cholesterol (mg/dl)	86-211	—	81-129	—
Creatinine (mg/dl)	0.9-1.8	—	0.8-0.9	—
GGT (IU/L)	—	—	—	—
Glucose (mg/dl)	227-300	—	275-425	—
Phosphorus (mg/dl)	6.2-7.9	—	5.4-7.1	—
Potassium (mEq/L)	3.0-7.3	—	6.0-6.4	1.4
Sodium (mEq/L)	131-171	—	149-155	180
Uric acid (mg/dl)	2.5-8.1	—	3.4-5.2	—
Protein, total (g/dl)	3.3-5.5	—	4.9-7.6	3.4-3.6
Albumin (g/dl)	1.3-2.8	—	3.0-5.9	—
Globulin (g/dl)	1.5-4.1	—	1.7-1.9	—

Appendix 15. Hematologic and serum biochemical values of selected waterfowl and Columbiformes

Measurements	Canada goose[179]	Mallard duck[387]	Pigeon[179,231,327]
Hematology			
PCV (%)	38-58	—	39.3-59.4
RBC (10⁶/μl)	1.6-2.6	2.1-3.8	2.1-4.2
Hb (g/dl)	12.7-19.1	7.4-10.9	10.7-14.9
MCV (fl)	145-174	—	118-144
MCH (pg)	53.7-70.0	—	32-48
MCHC (g/dl)	28-29	—	20-30
WBC (10³/μl)	13.0-18.5	24-40	10-30
Heterophils (%)	—	26-66	15-50
Lymphocytes (%)	—	33-63	25-70
Monocytes (%)	—	1-4	1-3
Eosinophils (%)	—	0	0-1.5
Basophils (%)	—	0-4	0-1
H:L ratio	0.5-0.9	0.4-2.0	0.21-2.00
Chemistries			
AP (IU/L)	72 ± 43	—	160-780
ALT (IU/L)	43 ± 11	—	19-48
AST (IU/L)	75 ± 17	—	45-123
Bile acid (μmol/L)			
RIA	—	—	22-60
Colorimetric	—	—	—
Calcium (mg/dl)	10.2 ± 0.7	—	7.6-10.4
Cholesterol (mg/dl)	172 ± 28	—	—
CK (IU/L)	—	—	110-480
Chloride (mEq/L)	105 ± 4	—	101-113
Creatinine (mg/dl)	0.8 ± 0.3	—	0.3-0.4
GGT (IU/L)	2 ± 3	—	0-2.9
Glucose (mg/dl)	210 ± 31	—	232-269
LDH (IU/L)	301 ± 80	—	30-205
Phosphorus (mg/dl)	2.8 ±0.9	—	1.8-4.1
Potassium (mEq/L)	3.4 ± 0.6	—	3.9-4.7
Sodium (mEq/L)	142 ± 4	—	141-149
Uric acid (mg/dl)	8.3 ± 2.3	—	2.5-12.9
Protein, total (g/dl)	4.8 ± 0.7	—	2.1-3.3
Albumin (g/dl)	2.1 ± 0.2	—	1.5-2.1
Globulin (g/dl)	2.8 ± 0.6	—	0.6-1.2
A:G ratio	0.76 ± 0.13	—	1.5-3.6

Appendix 16. Hematologic and serum biochemical values of selected Piciformes and ratites

Measurements	Toucan[212,369a]	Emu[177,179,315,369a]	Ostrich[179,369a]
Hematology			
PCV (%)	45-60	40-60	40-55
RBC ($10^6/\mu l$)	2.5-4.5	2.5-4.5	2.5-4.5
WBC ($10^3/\mu l$)	4-10	8-25	10-25
Heterophils (%)	35-65	45-75	55-90
Lymphocytes (%)	25-50	20-40	10-40
Monocytes (%)	—	0-2	0-2
Eosinophils (%)	0-4	0-1	0-1
Basophils (%)	0-5	0-1	0-1
Chemistries			
AP (IU/L)	—	—	130-220
AST (IU/L)	130-330	80-380	190-240
Bile acid (μmol/L)			
RIA	20-40	6-45	4-40
Colorimetric	—	—	—
Calcium (mg/dl)	10-15	8.8-12.5	13-20
Cholesterol (mg/dl)	—	68-170	80-170
CK (IU/L)	—	100-750	600-1200
Chloride (mEq/L)	—	—	20-60
Creatinine (mg/dl)	0.1-0.4	0.22	0-12
GGT (IU/L)	—	—	0-12
Glucose (mg/dl)	220-350	100-290	150-260
LDH (IU/L)	200-400	310-1200	225-1000
Phosphorus (mg/dl)	—	3.8-7.2	7.5-12.5
Potassium (mEq/L)	—	3.5-6.5	4.5-8.5
Sodium (mEq/L)	—	—	100-160
Uric acid (mg/dl)	4-14	4.5-14.0	6.5-14.5
Protein, total (g/dl)	3-5	3.4-5.6	2.0-5.5
Albumin (g/dl)	—	1.0-2.5	1.0-2.5

Appendix 17. Hematologic and serum biochemical values of selected raptors

Measurements	Bald eagle[9]	Golden eagle[151]	Great-horned owl[46]	Kestrel[284]
Hematology				
PCV (%)	—	35-47 (41)	30-47	—
RBC ($10^6/\mu l$)	—	1.9-2.7 (2.4)	—	—
Hb (g/dl)	—	12.1-15.2 (13.8)	—	—
WBC ($10^3/\mu l$)	—	11.7-14.7 (13.1)	14.5-32.5	14.5-57.0
Heterophils (%)	—	81-86	—	11-33
Lymphocytes (%)	—	14-22	—	24-58
Monocytes (%)	—	0	—	0.3-3.0
Eosinophils (%)	—	2-5	—	9-59
Basophils (%)	—	0-1	—	1.5-3.8
H:L ratio	—	—	—	0.2-1.4
Chemistries				
AP (IU/L)	23-30	—	21-108	—
ALT (IU/L)	—	—	0-59	—
AST (IU/L)	153-370	—	32-538	—
Calcium (mg/dl)	8.2-10.6	—	—	—
GGT (IU/L)	—	—	0-15	—
Glucose (mg/dl)	285-400	—	—	—
LDH (IU/L)	—	—	109-1320	—
Phosphorus (mg/dl)	2.4-4.3	—	—	—
Uric acid (mg/dl)	5.5-14.8	—	—	—
Protein, total (g/dl)	3.0-4.1	—	3.9-6.3	—

Appendix 17. Hematologic and serum biochemical values of selected raptors (cont.)

Measurements	Peregrine falcon[175,290]	Red-tailed hawk[9,46,179]	Sharp-shinned hawk[284]
Hematology			
PCV (%)	37-53	31-43	44-52
RBC (10^6/µl)	3-4	2.41-3.59	—
Hb (g/dl)	118-188	10.7-16.6	—
MCV (fl)	118-146	150-178	—
MCH (pg)	40.0-48.4	46.0-57.4	—
MCHC (g/dl)	319-352	297-345	—
WBC (10^3/µl)	3.3-11.0	19.1-33.4	7.7-16.8
Heterophils (%)	1-9	—	16-24
Lymphocytes (%)	1-3	—	54-75
Monocytes (%)	0.1-0.9	—	0-3
Eosinophils (%)	0-0.3	—	5-11
Basophils (%)	0-0.6	—	0-1
Chemistries			
AP (IU/L)	97-350	22-138	—
ALT (IU/L)	19-54	3-50	—
AST (IU/L)	20-52	76-492	—
Bile acid (µmol/L)			
RIA	20-118	—	—
Calcium (mg/dl)	—	10.0-12.8	—
Cholesterol (mg/dl)	175-401	—	—
CK (IU/L)	357-850	—	—
Chloride (mEq/L)	121-134	118-129	—
GGT (IU/L)	0-7	0-20	—
Glucose (mg/dl)	11-16	292-390	—
LDH (IU/L)	625-1210	0-2640	—
Phosphorus (mg/dl)	—	1.9-4.0	—
Potassium (mEq/L)	1.6-3.2	2.6-4.3	—
Sodium (mEq/L)	152-168	143-162	—
Uric acid (mg/dl)	4.4-22.0	8.1-16.8	—
Protein, total (g/dl)	2.5-4.0	3.9-6.7	2.4-3.2
Albumin (g/dl)	0.8-1.3	—	—
Globulin (g/dl)	1.6-2.8	—	—
A:G ratio	0.4-0.6	—	—

Appendix 18. Biological and physiological values of selected avian species [1,14,61,62,87,118,119,146,146,179,197,205,310,354,375]

Species	Incubation period[b] (days)	Fledgling age (days)	Weaning age (days) Parent-raised	Weaning age (days) Hand-reared	Breeding age	Longevity in captivity (years)	Body weight (g)[e]
Psittacines							
Budgerigar	16(-18)	22-26	30-40	30	6-9 mo	8-10	30
Cockatiel	18(-20)	32-38	47-52	42-49	6-12 mo	10-12	80-90
Australian parakeet	18-19	30-45	50-65	—	1-3 yr	10-12	30-110
Ring-neck parakeet	22-23	40-45	55-65	—	3 yr	—	—
Lovebirds	18(-24)	30-35	45-55	40-45	6-12 mo	—	42-48
Lories/lorikeets	21-27	42-50	62-70	50-60	2 yr	—	—
Conures	d	35-40	45-70	60	2-3 yr	—	80-100[e]
Amazon parrot	f	45-60	90-120	75-90	4-6 yr	>50	g
Small macaws	23-24(-26)	45-60	90-120	75-90	4-6 yr	50-80	h
Large macaws	26-28	70-80	120-150	95-120	5-7 yr	75	h
African grey parrot	26-28[i]	50-65	100-120	75-90	4-6 yr	50-60	554 (370-534)
Medium cockatoos	j	45-60	90-120	75-100	3-4 yr	—	k
Galah cockatoo	22-24	45-55	90-120	80-90	1 yr	—	k
Large cockatoos	j	60-80	120-150	95-120	5-6 yr	50-60	k
Eclectus parrot	26-28	72-80	120-150	100-110	4 yr	—	432 (347-512)
Passerines							
Zebra or society finch	12-16	18-20(-22)	25-28	—	9-10 mo	4-7	10-16
Canary	12-14	14	21	—	<1 yr	6-12	12-30
Mynah	14-15	30	60	—	2-3 yr	12	180-260
Columbiformes							
Pigeon	16-19	28-35	35	—	12 mo	4-8 (>20?)	240-300
Dove	12->14	18	—	—	12 mo	4-8	240-300

Appendix 18. Biological and physiological values of selected avian species (cont.)

Species	Incubation period[b] (days)	Fledgling age (days)	Weaning age (days)		Breeding age	Longevity in captivity (years)	Body weight (g)[c]
			Parent -raised	Hand-reared			
Galliformes							
Pheasant	22-24	—	Precocial	—	1 yr	10-18	—
Ratites							
Emu	50-57	—	Precocial	—	3-5 yr	30 yr	55
Ostrich	41-43	—	Precocial	—	4 yr	80 yr	150-200

a   Guidelines only. Data vary between references.

b   *Brotogeris* parakeets, 22; *Psittacula* parakeets, 23-26; Quaker parakeet, 23; Pionus parrot, 25-26; Senegal parrot, 24-25.

c   Princess of Wales parakeet, 108 (102-129); kakariki parakeet, 56 (35-43); red-rumped parakeet, 65 (62-69); Bourke's parakeet, 40 (35-43).

d   Nanday, 21-23 (-25); Patagonian, 24-25; sun, 27-28; blue-crowned, 23-24; orange-fronted, 30.

e   Queen of Bavaria, 262 (252-276).

f   Yellow-naped, yellow-fronted, yellow-crowned, double yellow-headed, 28-29; green-cheeked, blue-fronted, 26; spectacled (white-fronted), 24.

g   Blue-crowned, 740 (618-998); blue-fronted, 432 (361-485); Mexican red-headed, 360 (343-377); yellow-naped, 596 (476-795); double yellow-headed, 568 (463-694).

h   Scarlet, 1103; blue and gold, 1021; green-winged, 1179; military, 788; hyacinth, 1355 (1197-1466); red-fronted, 458.

i   Congo, 28; Timneh, 26.

j   Bare-eyed, 23-24; citron-crested, 25-26; greater sulphur-crested, 27-28; Leadbeater's, 26; lesser sulphur-crested, 24-25; Moluccan, 28-29; palm, 28-30; triton, 27-28; umbrella, 28.

k   Bare-eyed, 331; greater sulphur-crested, 806; Leadbeater's (Major Mitchell's), 423 (381-474); lesser sulphur-crested, 303; Moluccan, 808; rose-breasted, 299; triton, 559; umbrella, 552.

Appendix 19. Biological and physiological values of selected waterfowl species [118]

Species	Weight (kg) ♂	Weight (kg) ♀	Sexual maturity (yr)	Clutch size	Incubation period (days)	Longevity (yr)	Respiratory rate (BPM)	Heart rate (BPM)	Cloacal temperature °F (°C)
Common eider	2.25	2.12	1	3-6	25-30	10-15	30-95	180-230	105.8 (41)
European goldeneye	0.99-1.16	0.7-0.8	1	9-11	27-32	10-15	30-95	180-230	105.8 (41)
European wigeon	0.7	0.64	1	7-11	23-25	10-15	30-95	180-230	105.8 (41)
Mallard	1.26	1.1	1	8-12	23-29	10-15	30-95	180-230	105.8 (41)
Mandarin duck	0.44-0.55	0.44-0.55	1	9-12	28-30	10-15	30-95	180-230	105.8 (41)
Muscovy duck	2-4	1.1-1.5	1	8-15	35	10-15	30-95	180-230	105.8 (41)
Tufted duck	1.1	1.05	1	6-14	23-25	10-15	30-95	180-230	105.8 (41)
Bar-headed goose	2-3	2-3	2	4-6	27	15-20	13-40	80-150	104.9 (40.5)
Hawaiian goose	2.2	1.9	2	3-5	29	15-20	13-40	80-150	104.9 (40.5)
Pink-footed goose	2.6	2.35	2	3-5	26-27	15-20	13-40	80-150	104.9 (40.5)
Red-breasted goose	1.3-1.6	1.15	2	3-7	23-25	15-20	13-40	80-150	104.9 (40.5)
Mute swan	12.2	8.9	5	4-8	35-40	25-30	13-40	80-150	104.9 (40.5)

Appendix 20. Biological and physiological values of selected raptors [28]

Species	Minimum breeding age (yr)	Clutch size	Incubation period (days)	Interval between eggs (days)	Start of incubation
Barn owl	1	4-7	30-31	2-3	1st egg
Common kestrel	1	3-6	27-29	1-2	2nd-3rd egg
Eurasian buzzard	2-3	2-4	36-38	3	1st-2nd egg
Harris hawk	2-3	2-5	32	2-3	Penultimate or last egg
Northern eagle owl	2-3	2-4	34-36	2-3	1st-2nd egg
Northern goshawk	2-3	3-5	35-38	2-3	1st-2nd egg
Northern sparrow hawk	1-2	4-6	35	2-3	3rd-4th egg
Peregrine falcon	2	3-4	29-32	2-3	Penultimate or last egg
Snowy owl	2	3-9	30-33	2-3	1st egg

Parameter	Elevations	Decreases
PCV/RBC	Dehydration Increased oxygen demand • Chronic obstructive pulmonary disease • Obstructive airway disease • Chronic respiratory disease	Blood loss • Parasitism • Coagulopathies • Gastrointestinal bleeding Destruction • Hematozoan parasites • Bacterial septicemia • Aflatoxicosis Chronic inflammatory disease • Mycobacteriosis, chlamydiosis, aspergillosis, chronic hepatitis Neoplasia • Lymphoid leukemia
Heterophils	Inflammatory processes • Bacterial (including *Mycobacterium*) and fungal infections Excess corticosteroids • Endogenous production • Exogenous administration Birds with a high heterophil: lymphocyte ratio may mount a greater leukocytic response	Infections • Bacterial and viral (ie, PBFD) Poor sample preparation, collection, storage
Lymphocytes	Chronic antigenic stimulation • Chronic infections Lymphocytic leukemia Increased excitability	Excess corticosteroids • Endogenous release • Exogenous administration Severe viral infection Endotoxemia Septicemia Immunosuppressive drugs
Monocytes	Chlamydiosis Bacterial infections (including *Mycobacterium*) Mycotic granulomatous diseases Tissue necrosis Parasitism	Acute infection Inflammation
Eosinophils	Gastrointestinal parasitism Delayed Type IV hypersensitivity reactions	—
Basophils	Early inflammatory responses associated with histamine release	—

Appendix 21. Quick reference to abnormalities of the standard avian hematology profile (cont.)

Parameter	Elevations	Decreases
Hemostasis	—	Vitamin K deficiency
		Rodenticide toxicity
		Aflatoxicosis
		Circovirus-associated thrombocytopenia
		Conure bleeding syndrome
		Septicemia-associated DIC (as with polyomavirus and reovirus)
		Hepatic disease or failure

Appendix 22. Quick reference to abnormalities of the standard avian biochemical profile a,124,144a,184

Chemistry	Elevations		Decreases	
	Non-medical	Medical	Non-Medical	Medical
Alkaline phosphatase (IU/L)	Juveniles have higher levels	Hyperparathyroidism induced osteoclastic activity (fractures); egg laying; hepatic disease; enteritis; aflatoxicosis	—	Dietary zinc deficiency
ALT (IU/L)	Seasonal variation in raptors; sample hemolysis	—	Seasonal variation in raptors	—
Amylase (IU/L)	—	Pancreatitis; gastrointestinal disease	—	—
AST (IU/L)	Rare; severe lipemia; 300-1,000	Liver, muscle, or heart damage; vitamin E/selenium, methionine deficiency; 300-15,000	—	<50, end-stage liver disease
Bile acids (μmol/L)	Lipemia; sample hemolysis; such samples should not be analyzed	Loss of liver function, even with normal enzymes	Lipemic samples that are chemically treated	Response to therapy; liver cirrhosis; microhepatica
Calcium (mg/dl)	Lipemia (or cloudy from other causes); protein elevations; bacterial contamination	Hormonal disorders; egg production; metabolic disease; excess dietary vitamin D; dehydration; osteolytic neoplasia	EDTA; bacterial contamination; young birds have lower levels	<8; metabolic and nutritional disorders; lead poisoning; glucocorticoid administration; low albumin; African grey hypocalcemia

Appendix 22. Quick reference to abnormalities of the standard avian biochemical profile (cont.)

| Chemistry | Elevations | | Decreases | |
	Non-medical	Medical	Non-Medical	Medical
Cholesterol (mg/dl)	Postprandial;[324] high fat diet; carnivorous diet	Metabolic disease; hepatic lipidosis; bile duct obstruction; hypothyroidism; starvation	—	Liver, metabolic disease
Creatine phosphokinase (IU/L)	>300; healthy birds up to 1,000	600-25,000; muscle or heart damage; CNS disease (seizures); vitamin E/selenium deficiency; chlamydiosis; lead toxicity; IM injections	<10; bacterial contamination	Rare
Creatinine (mg/dl)	—	Not useful in birds	—	Not useful in birds
Glucose (mg/dl)	Improper dilution; postprandial; posthandling	Stress, 400-600; diabetes, 800-1500; corticosteroids	<100; unseparated blood; bacterial contamination	<100; hepatic dysfunction; septicemia; neoplasia; aspergillosis
Lactate dehydrogenase (IU/L)	Sample hemolysis	300-15,000; liver, heart, or muscle damage; hepatitis; muscle damage	<50	End-stage liver disease
Lipase (IU/L)	—	Acute pancreatitis	—	—
Phosphorus (mg/dl)	Postprandial; sample hemolysis	Severe renal disease; nutritional secondary hyperparathyroidism; hypoparathyroidism	EDTA	Hypovitaminosis D; malabsorption; chronic glucocorticoid therapy

216

Chemistry	Elevations		Decreases	
	Non-medical	Medical	Non-medical	Medical
Potassium (mEq/L)	Hemolysis; dietary supplementation	Adrenal disease; metabolic disease; severe tissue damage; renal disease; acidosis; dehydration; hemolytic anemia	—	Adrenal disease; metabolic disease; diuretic therapy; alkalosis; overhydration; dietary deficiency
Protein, total (g/dl)	Lipemia; non-temperature compensated refractometer	Inflammation; dehydration; chronic infection; gamma globulinopathy; lympho-proliferative disease; myelosis	Non-temperature compensated refractometer	Chronic hepatopathy; malabsorption; renal disease; blood loss; neoplasia; starvation/ malnutrition
Sorbitol dehydrogenase (IU/L)	—	Hepatitis	—	—
Sodium (mEq/L)	Dietary supplementation	Dehydration; salt poisoning	—	Renal disease; overhydration
Uric acid (mg/dl)	5-15; severe lipemia; dirty nail clip; carnivorous birds have higher levels	Renal disease; gout; dehydration; postprandial; ovulation; tissue damage; starvation; hypervitaminosis D	Overhydration of patient; juvenile levels are lower	End-stage liver disease

a The ranges given are not absolute and are to be used as a guide for interpretation of a wide range of avian species.

Appendix 23. Approximate resting respiratory rates of selected avian species and by weight [117,330]

Species	Respiratory rate (breaths/min)[a]
Finch	90-110
Canary	60-80
Budgerigar	60-75
Lovebird	50-60
Cockatiel	40-50
Small conure	40-50
Large conure	30-45
Toucan	15-45
Amazon parrot	15-45
Cockatoo	15-40
Macaw	20-25
Weight (g)	**Respiratory rate (breaths/min)**
100	40-52
200	35-50
300	30-45
400	25-30
500	20-30
1000	15-20

[a] Restraint can increase respiratory rate 1.5-2 × resting rate.

Appendix 24. T_4 values of selected avian species [46,179,231,369a]

Species	T_4 (µg/dl)
African grey parrot	0.3-2.1
Amazon parrot	0.1-1.1
Budgerigar	0.5-2.1
Canary	0.7-3.2
Cockatiel	0.7-2.4
Conure	0.5-2.0
Lovebird	0.2-4.3
Pigeon	0.47-2.72

Appendix 25. Applanation tonometry data for selected raptors [351]

Species (n)	Intraocular pressure (mm Hg)
Red-tailed hawk (10)	20.6 (± 3.4)
Swainson's hawk (6)	20.8 (± 2.3)
Golden eagle (7)	21.5 (± 3.0)
Bald eagle (3)	20.6 (± 2.0)
Great horned owl (6)	10.8 (± 3.6)

Appendix 26. Check list of supportive care procedures used in companion bird medicine

Because it is frequently difficult to establish an accurate diagnosis, supportive care is an essential component of companion bird medicine. Supportive care includes:

1. Minimize handling and other stressors
2. Hospitalization
   - place patient in a warm, quiet, well-ventilated environment with minimal to no disturbance
   - supplemental heat (30-32°C; 85-90°F)
     - debilitated birds are often hypothermic
3. Fluid therapy (see Appendices 27 and 28)
4. Corticosteroids (use with caution because of immunosuppressive effects, etc) in cases of:
   - shock and poor vascular perfusion
   - extreme stress
   - CNS trauma
   - selected toxemias and intoxications
5. Vitamin therapy
   - multiple vitamins (including vitamin A) as needed
   - B complex in selected cases of injury, anorexia, cachexia, CNS disorders, or blood loss
6. Antibiotics (see Table 18)
   - to control primary infections and for injured or debilitated birds where secondary infections may result
7. Iron dextran
   - iron deficiency or following hemorrhage
8. Normal photoperiod (or subdued lighting, if needed)
9. Oxygen
   - dyspnea, hypoxia, or severe pneumonia and airsacculitis
10. Maintain body weight
    - weigh daily if possible
    - offer favorite foods and avoid changing diet while ill
11. Gavage (see Appendices 27, 29-31)
    - malnourishment, anorexia, cachexia, and dehydration
    - high carbohydrate formula is initially recommended
    - high protein/high calorie formulas may be used to increase body weight during recovery

Appendix 27. Routes of administration and maximum suggested volumes of fluids to be administered to psittacines[145,301]

Bird weight (g)	Volume (ml) by route of administration[a]		
	Gavage[b]	IV bolus (initial)	Subcutaneous
10-25	0.4-0.75	0.5-0.75	1-2
25-50	0.7-3.0	0.75-1.0	2-5
50-75	3-6	1.0-1.5	5-7
75-100	6-8	1.5-2.0	7-12
100-250	8-15	2-5	12-18
250-500	15-20	5-8	18-24
500-750	20-30	8-12	24-28
750-1000	30-40	12-15	28-30

[a] Use lower dose in lighter birds.
[b] Initial volume should be much less in critically ill and anorectic patients. Adults take less proportionally than neonatal or juvenile birds.

Appendix 28. Fluid therapy recommendations for birds

Ideally, when evaluating a patient for fluid therapy, the following factors should be considered: hydration status, electrolyte balance, acid-base status, hematologic and biochemical values, and caloric balance.
- Combinations of routes (PO, SC, IO, and IV) are recommended if high fluid volumes are administered.
- When IV administration is not possible, the treatment of choice is 5% dextrose administered PO and repeated q60-90min.[140] IO administration is as effective as IV administration, but has a few complications (ie, catheter placement, osteomyelitis).[211]
- Fluids can be administered by slow IV or IO infusion, by a combination of IV bolus and SC administration, or by repeated SC administrations. A volume of 10 ml/kg/hr can be infused in healthy patients for the first 2 hr, then at 5-8 ml/kg/hr to avoid fluid overload.
- Fluid volumes using the BMR method are usually higher than other methods of fluid calculation.
- Although fluid requirements can be met in part by administering 10-15 ml/kg[283] (and up to 25 ml/kg if over a 5-7 min period) of warm lactated Ringer s solution (or 50:50 with 2-1/2-5% dextrose if the patient is hypoglycemic or caloric deficient)[257] IV as a bolus q8-12h; maintenance fluid is generally administered SC, PO, or occasionally through an intraosseous catheter. Oral administration of 5% dextrose appears to be very effective for restoring fluid deficits rapidly.
- Warming of fluids to 38-39 °C (100-102 °F) prior to administration can help prevent or correct hypothermia.
- Hetastarch at 10-15 ml/kg IV q8h up to 4 treatments may be effective for hypoproteinemia[257,283,301,361]
- Potassium chloride can be diluted in fluids to correct for potassium depletion based on electrolyte analysis (0.1-0.3 mEq/kg).
- Total parenteral nutrition is difficult in birds, but has been reported.[80,82]

Body Weight Percentage Method[324]
- Fluid replacement in ml = body weight (g) × 2.5% q8-12h as needed for dehydration
Example: A 250 g lilac-crowned Amazon parrot is dehydrated.
    (250 g) (0.025) = 6.25 ml q8-12h
    18.75 ml/day; total volume after 3 days, 56.25 ml

Maintenance and Deficit Replacement Method[257,283,288,295,301,361]
- Determine fluid deficit:
    Fluid deficit (ml) = body weight (g) x % dehydration
- Determine daily maintenance:
    Daily maintenance = 50 ml (range: 40-60 ml)/kg/day
- If possible, replace 50% of the deficit in the first 12-24 hr, the remainder over the next 24-48 hr; some clinicians recommend replacing 20-25% of the deficit in the first 4-6 hr, and the remaining volume during the next 20-28 hr.
Example: A 250 g lilac-crowned Amazon parrot is 10% dehydrated.

Weight	250 g
10% dehydration	25 ml
Maintenance at 5% body weight/day	12.5 ml

Appendix 28. Fluid therapy recommendations for birds (cont.)

1st day fluid requirements = (maintenance + 1/2 of deficit)
(12.5 + 12.5) = 25 ml/day

2nd day fluid requirements = (maintenance + 1/4 of deficit)
(12.5 + 6.0) = 18.5 ml/day

3rd day fluid requirements = (maintenance + 1/2 of deficit)
(12.5 + 6.0) = 18.5 ml/day

Total volume of fluid administered after 3 days = 62 ml

Appendix 29. Suggested initial to maximum volumes and frequency of gavage feeding in anorectic birds [288,329]

Species	Volume (ml)[a,b]	Frequency[a]
Finch	0.1-0.5	q4h
Budgerigar	0.5-3.0	q6h
Lovebird	1-3	q6h
Cockatiel	1-8	q6h
Small conure	3-12	q6h
Large conure	7-24	q6-8h
Amazon parrot	5-35	q8h
Cockatoo	10-40	q8-12h
Macaw	20-60	q8-12h

[a] Adjust volume and frequency as crop accommodates larger volumes.
[b] Generally 3-5% of body weight.[144]

Appendix 30. Suggested feeding requirements of a bird in relation to its body weight [307]

Body weight (g)	Percentage (%) of body weight required daily
100-200	18-25
201-800	11-19
801-1,200	7-11
4,000-10,000	3.5-6.0

Appendix 31. Calculation of enteral feeding requirements for birds

This appendix will aid the practitioner in calculating caloric requirements for birds. Please see Appendix 85 regarding calculation of basal metabolic rate (BMR) and maintenance energy requirement (MER). Caloric values for the three food types are:

Protein	4.29 kcal/g
Carbohydrate	4.09 kcal/g
Fat	9.29 kcal/g

Animals are unable to fully use all the calories in these nutrients, but efficiency is estimated between 80-90% depending on the type of nutrition. Commercial enteral solutions are estimated to have a digestibility of 95%. Some commercially available enteral products are listed below. Each product has varying levels of fat, carbohydrate, protein, and water. Other food sources can be used as long as nutrient levels and digestibility can be determined. Following is an example of a calculation of nutrient requirements based on BMR.

Example: A 250 g lilac-crowned Amazon parrot is debilitated and not eating because of a bacterial infection.

BMR (kcal/day) = $kW^{0.75}$
MER (kcal/day) = $(1.5 \times BMR)$
k = kcal/kg/day constant
  (non-passerines = 78, passerines = 129)

First calculate MER:
  MER = $(1.5)(78 \text{ kcal/kg/day})(0.250 \text{ kg})^{0.75}$ = 41.4 kcal/day

- An adjustment for sepsis is made by multiplying by 1.5 (see BMR appendix):
  Sepsis = $1.5 \times MER$ = $(1.5)(41.4 \text{ kcal/day})$ = 62.1 kcal/day

- Isocal HCN (2 kcal/ml) is selected as the nutrient source:
  Volume of Isocal = $(62.1 \text{ kcal/day})/(2 \text{ kcal/ml})$ = 31 ml/day

- The average Amazon parrot can be gavaged 2.5% of its body weight:
  Volume that can be gavaged = $(0.025)(250 \text{ g})$ = 6.25 ml

- Therefore, 31 ml/day of Isocal HCN can be administered via gavage feedings of 6.25 ml q5h. However, this volume may need to be reduced initially depending on the bird's degree of debilitation.

- Refer to Appendices 27, 29, and 30 for suggested volumes and frequency of gavage feeding anorectic birds.

Appendix 31. Calculation of enteral feeding requirements for birds (cont.)

• Nutrient values for selected nutritional products.[198]

Product	Protein (g)	Fat (g)	Carbohydrates (g)	Water (ml/dl)	kcal/ml
CliniCare® Feline (Pet Ag)	7.0	4.6	5.7	83	0.92
CliniCare® Canine (Pet Ag)	5.0	6.1	6.0	82	0.98
Isocal® (Mead Johnson)	3.4	4.4	13.3	84	1.0
Traumacal® (Mead Johnson)	5.5	4.5	9.5	52	1.5
Pulmocare® (Ross)	4.2	6.1	7.0	52	1.5
Isocal HCN® (Mead Johnson)	3.8	5.1	10.0	35.5	2.0
Emeraid-II® (Lafeber), 45 g + 45 ml H_2O = 100 ml	10.8	2.25	28.1	45	1.53

• Saccharide content (% of dry wt) of Emeraid-I®.

Product	Mono - (%)	Di- (%)	Tri- (%)	Tetra- (%)	kcal/ml
Emeraid-I® (Lafeber), 15 g + 30 ml H_2O = 30 ml	19.7	14.4	11.2	54.7	2.0

Appendix 32. Selected sources of formulated and medicated diets for companion and aviary birds

Harrison's Bird Diets, Inca
220 Congress Park Dr, Suite 232
Delray Beach, FL 33445, USA
(561) 279-4233
(800) 346-0269

Kaytee Products, Inc
521 Clay St
PO Box 230
Chilton, WI 53014, USA
(414) 849-2321
(800) 669-9580

LaFeber Coa
24981 N 1400 East Rd
Cornell, IL 61319, USA
(815) 358-2301
(800) 842-6445

Lakes Unlimited, Inca
639 Stryker Ave
St Paul, MN 55107, USA
(612) 290-0606
(800) 634-2473

L'Avian Pet Products
Highway 75 South
Stephen, MN 56757, USA
(800) 543-3308

Marion Zoological Scenic Birdfoods
13803 Industrial Park Blvd
Plymouth, MN 55441, USA
(612) 559-3305
(800) 327-7974

PMI Nutrition International
Mazuri Diets
1401 S Hanley Rd
St. Louis, MO 63144, USA
(314) 768-4100
(800) 227-8941

Premium Nutritional Products
ZuPreem Diets
PO Box 2094
Mission, KS 66202, USA
(913) 722-6336
(800) 345-4767

Pretty Bird International, Inca
PO Box 177
5810 Stacy Trail
Stacy, MN 55079, USA
(651) 462-1799
(800) 356-5020

Rolf C. Hagen Corp
50 Hampden Rd
Mansfield, MA 02048, USA
(508) 339-9531
(800) 225-2700

Roudybush Foodsa
3550 Watt Ave, Suite 8
Sacramento, CA 95821, USA
(888) 304-2473

Zeigler Brothers, Inca
PO Box 95
Gardners, PA 17324, USA
(717) 677-6181
(800) 841-6800

[a] Source of medicated feeds.

Appendix 33. Selected nutritional recommendations for waterfowl, raptors, and hummingbirds

Waterfowl

Geese are browsers; domestic ducks feed on mixed grains and forage. Avoid grains for goslings for the first 4 wk of life. Grit and oyster should be fed ad libitum. Piscivorous birds require higher protein and can be offered trout chow and fish.

- Starter rations (<3 wk of age): 19-22% protein[209]
- Grower rations: 12-17%,[209] reduce protein to 14% if angel wing is present in goslings[229]
- Breeder rations: 17-18% protein, 1-2 wk prior to laying[209]

Raptors (for debilitated birds)[184]

- Rehydrate - see Appendices 27 and 28 (fluid therapy)
- Oral supplementation (Ultracal, Meade Johnson) (55 ml/kg/day)
- Ground whole quail (less feet, feathers, gastrointestinal tract)
- Small amounts of quail breast meat soaked with oral electrolytes
- Whole prey after establishing normal gastrointestinal time
- Stomach capacity is approximately 40 ml/kg[306]

Hummingbird diet[381]

180 ml 24% sugar water
1 tsp (4 g) Vital High Nitrogen (Ross Laboratories)
1/8 tsp Superpreen vitamins (RHB Laboratories)
1/8 tsp Nekton Tonic-I (Nekton)

Appendix 34. Protocols used in treating mycobacteriosis in birds

Because of its zoonotic potential, controversy exists on whether to treat pet and aviary birds for *Mycobacterium avium*. Because *M. avium* isolates from birds differ from human isolates in antibiotic susceptibility, serovars, and genetic sequencing, pet birds are an unlikely source of *M. avium* in people (except immunosuppressed individuals). Nevertheless, veterinarians who treat birds with this disease do so at their own risk. The veterinarian should be aware that treatment is often lifelong for the bird, and that treatment does not necessarily prevent shedding.

There has been extensive research in humans concerning mycobacteriosis. Medications for *M. avium* complex under study in humans include macrolides (clarithromycin, azithromycin), aminoglycosides (amikacin, streptomycin, paromomycin, and the new liposomal aminoglycosides), rifamycins (rifabutin, rifapentine), a quinolone (ciprofloxacin), clofazimine, and ethambutol.[195]

All the drugs listed below, except for clofazimine, can be mixed together in the appropriate ratios in an aqueous base for short periods of time (7-10 days) for convenient dosing. Clofazimine can be diluted in vegetable oil for accurate administration.[372]

Following are antimycobacterial treatment protocols used in birds:

- Ethambutol, isoniazid, rifampin[324]
  - Ethambutol 200 mg + isoniazid 200 mg + rifampin 300 mg
  - Finely crush together, add to 10 ml of simple syrup (Humco), and administer PO q24h as follows:

Bird weight (g)	Volume (ml)
<100	0.1
100-250	0.2
250-500	0.3
500-1,000	0.4

- Ethambutol, isoniazid, rifampin[226,371]
  - Ethambutol 30 mg/kg + isoniazid 30 mg/kg + rifampin 45 mg/kg
  - Medications are mixed into a dextrose powder, mixed with a small amount of food, and administered PO q24h.

- Ethambutol, streptomycin, rifampin[23]
  - Ethambutol 10 mg/kg PO q12h + streptomycin 30 mg/kg IM q12h + rifampin 15 mg/kg PO q12h

- Ethambutol, rifabutin, enrofloxacin[371]
  - Ethambutol 30 mg/kg PO q24h
  - Rifabutin 15 mg/kg PO q24h
  - Enrofloxacin 30 mg/kg PO q24h

- Ethambutol, rifampin, enrofloxacin[371]
  - Ethambutol 30 mg/kg PO q24h
  - Rifampin 45 mg/kg PO q24h
  - Enrofloxacin 30 mg/kg PO q24h

- Ethambutol, rifampin, ciprofloxacin[371]
  - Ethambutol 30 mg/kg PO q24h
  - Rifampin 45 mg/kg PO q24h
  - Ciprofloxacin 80 mg/kg PO q24h

Appendix 34. Protocols used in treating mycobacteriosis in birds (cont.)

- •Ethambutol, rifabutin, clarithromycin[330]
  - ◦ Ethambutol 30 mg/kg PO q24h
  - ◦ Rifabutin 15 mg/kg PO q24h
  - ◦ Clarithromycin 85 mg/kg PO q24h (allometrically scaled)
  - ◦ Enrofloxacin or ciprofloxacin 15 mg/kg PO q12h or clofazimine 6 mg/kg PO q12h or amikacin 15 mg/kg IM, IV can also be added to this protocol

- •Ethambutol, rifabutin, azithromycin [330]
  - ◦ Ethambutol 30 mg/kg PO q24h
  - ◦ Rifabutin 15 mg/kg PO q24h
  - ◦ Azithromycin 43 mg/kg PO q24h
  - ◦ Enrofloxacin or ciprofloxacin 15 mg/kg PO q12h or clofazimine 6 mg/kg PO q12h or amikacin 15 mg/kg IM, IV can also be added to this protocol

- •Ethambutol, rifampin, clofazimine[372]
  - ◦ Ethambutol 30 mg/kg PO q24h
  - ◦ Rifampin 45 mg/kg PO q24h
  - ◦ Clofazimine 6 mg/kg PO 24h

- •Ethambutol, cycloserine, clofazimine, enrofloxacin (raptors)[29]
  - ◦ Ethambutol 20 mg/kg PO q12h
  - ◦ Cycloserine 5 mg/kg PO q12h
  - ◦ Clofazimine 1.5 mg/kg PO q24h
  - ◦ Enrofloxacin 10-15 mg/kg PO, IM q12h

Appendix 35. Suggested protocols for treating lymphosarcoma, lymphocytic leukemia or lymphosarcoma, and osteosarcoma in birds

C.O.P. protocol for lymphosarcoma[120]
- Prednisone 25 mg/m^2 PO q24h
- Cyclophosphamide 200/m^2 IO q7d
- Vincristine 0.75 mg/m^2 IO q7d × 3 treatments
- Doxorubicin 30 mg/m^2 IO q21d
- L-asparaginase 400 IU/kg IM q7d
- Alpha interferon 15,000 IU/m^2 SC q2d × 3 treatments
- Diphenhydramine 2 mg/kg IO before doxorubicin and L-asparaginase treatments
- Dexamethasone 1 mg/kg IM before doxorubicin and L-asparaginase treatments

Protocol for lymphocytic leukemia or lymphosarcoma[a,264]
- Vincristine sulfate 0.5 mg/m^2 IV initial dose, then 0.75 mg/m^2 q7d × 3 treatments
- Prednisone 1 mg/454 g PO q12h
- Chlorambucil 1 mg/bird PO 2×/wk

Protocol for osteosarcoma[b,88]
- Diphenhydramine 30 min before doxorubicin treatment (route not given)
- Doxorubicin 60 mg/m^2 is diluted into 6 ml sterile saline and administered IV over 30 min in an anesthetized patient via an angiocatheter in the jugular vein q30d
- Do not extravasate doxorubicin; doxorubicin may cause myelosuppression and cardiac toxicity; monitor the CBC
- Electrocardiography during treatment is recommended

[a] Dosages are for a Pekin duck (*Anas platyrhynchos domesticus*).
[b] Procedure was developed for a blue-front Amazon (*Amazona aestiva*).

Appendix 36. Vaccines used in birds (non-poultry)

Agent	Dosage	Initial	Booster	Species/Comments
Equine encephalitis (Triple-E, Solvay)	1 ml IM[342]	3 mo of age	4 mo, 5-6 mo, then biannually before and after breeding season (March/Sept)	Emus
Herpes, psittacine (Psittimune PDV, Biomune)	0.25 ml/<100 g SC[285] 0.25 ml/>100 g SC, IM[285]	Weaning	4-8 wk, then annual	Psittacines/killed vaccine; severe granuloma formation may occur at vaccination site; controversial for use in cockatoos
Paramyxovirus-1 (V.P. Vaccin Nobilis Lasota, Intervet)	Apply 1-2 drops in nostrils or eyes Add to drinking water	2-4 wk before shows/races	6-8 wk 8 wk	Pigeons, exotic doves/MLV; poor immune response Pigeons, exotic doves/1 bottle is administered to entire flock (> 100 birds), divided evenly in drinking water for 24 hr; poor immune response
Paramyxovirus-1, pigeon (Inacti/vac PMV1, Maine Biological Lab)	0.5 ml SC[285]	4 wk of age	4 wk, then annual	Pigeons, doves/killed vaccine; preferred PMV-1 vaccine
Paramyxovirus-1/Pox, pigeon (Columbovac, Solvay Duphar)	0.2 ml SC[29]	4 wk of age	?	Pigeons/killed vaccine; poor immunological response to pox

Appendix 36. Vaccines used in birds (non-poultry) (cont.)

Agent	Dosage	Initial	Booster	Species/Comments
Polyomavirus Polyomavirus (Avian Vaccine, Biomune)	0.25 ml/<200 g SC [285] 0.5 ml/>200 g SC[285]	40-50 days of age	2 wk, then annual	Psittacines/may cause discoloration, thickening, or granuloma of skin at vaccination site (usually resolves within 8 wk); birds vaccinated between 20-40 days of age during an out break should receive a second booster 4 wk after initial dose (off-label use)[324]
Pox, canary (Poximune-C, Biomune)	Wing web piercing[285]	Weaning	6-12 mo and 4 wk before breeding and vector seasons	Canaries/MLV; a "take" inflammatory reaction or scab should develop at vaccination site
Pox, pigeon (Acti/vac PP, Maine Biological Lab)	Rub into epilated follicles on thigh[285]	4 wk of age	Annual	Pigeons/MLV; annual boosters may not be necessary;[324] booster if exposure
Pox, psittacine (Maine Biological Lab)	—	—	—	Psittacines/killed vaccine; use in cockatoos is controversial; granuloma formation may occur at vaccination site and require surgical removal
Salmonella typhimurium (Sal Bac, Biomune)	0.5 ml SC[285]	2-3 wk before breeding, races, shows	3-4 wk	Pigeons/bacterin

Appendix 37. Literature cited—Birds

1. Aarons J. First aid and wound management in the ostrich. *Proc Annu Conf Assoc Avian Vet*: 201-208, 1995.

2. Aarons JE. Adverse effects of high environmental temperature on ostrich chicks. *Proc Annu Conf Assoc Avian Vet*: 153-158, 1996.

3. Aarons JE. Assessing the down bird. *Proc Annu Conf Assoc Avian Vet*: 175-179, 1997.

4. Abou-Madi N, Kollias GV. Avian fluid therapy. In: Bonagura JD, Kirk RW (eds). *Kirk's Current Veterinary Therapy XI: Small Animal Practice*. WB Saunders Co, Philadelphia, 1992. Pp 1154-1159.

5. Aguilar RF, Redig PT. Diagnosis and treatment of avian aspergillosis. In: Bonagura JD (ed). *Kirk's Current Veterinary Therapy XII: Small Animal Practice*. WB Saunders Co, Philadelphia, 1995. Pp 1294-1299.

6. Aiello SE, Mays A (eds). *The Merck Veterinary Manual*. 8th ed. Merck and Co, Whitehouse Station, NJ, 1998.

7. Alderton D. *A Birdkeeper's Guide to Pet Birds*. Tetra Press, Morris Plains, NJ, 1987.

8. Allen DG, Pringle JK, Smith DA, et al (eds). *Handbook of Veterinary Drugs*. JB Lippincott Co, Philadelphia, 1993. Pp 573-634.

9. Allen J. Avian clinical chemistries. In: Jacobson ER, Kollias GV, Jr (eds). *Exotic Animals*. Churchill Livingstone, New York, 1988. Pp 143-157.

10. Allen JL, Oosterhuis JE. Effect of tolazoline on xylazine-ketamine-induced anesthesia in turkey vultures. *J Am Vet Med Assoc* 189:1011-1012, 1986.

11. Anadón A, Bringas P, Martinez-Larrañaga MR, Diaz MJ. Bioavailability, pharmacokinetics and residues of chloramphenicol in the chicken. *J Vet Pharmacol Therap* 17:52-58, 1994.

12. Anadón A, Martinez-Larrañaga MR, Diaz MJ, et al. Pharmacokinetics and residues of enrofloxacin in chickens. *Am J Vet Res* 56:501-506, 1995.

13. Axelson RD. Avian dermatology. In: Hoefer HL (ed). *Practical Avian Medicine: The Compendium Collection*. Veterinary Learning Systems Co, Trenton, NJ,1997. Pp 186-195.

14. Axelson RD. *Caring for Your Pet Bird*. Canaviax Publ Ltd, Toronto, 1981.

15. Baert L, Van Poucke S, Vermeersch H, et al. Pharmacokinetics and anthelmintic efficacy of febantel in the racing pigeon *(Columba livia)*. *J Vet Pharmacol Therap* 16:223-231, 1993.

16. Bailey TA, Sheen RS, Samour JH, et al. Pharmacokinetics of enrofloxacin after intravenous, intramuscular and oral administration to houbara bustards *(Chlamydotis undulata macqueenii)*. *J Vet Pharmacol Therap* 20 (Suppl 1):204-205, 1997.

17. Battison AL, Buckzowski S, Archer FJ. Plasma bile acid concentration in the cockatiel. *Can Vet J* 37:233-234, 1996.

18. Bauck L. Analgesics in avian medicine. *Proc Annu Conf Assoc Avian Vet*: 239-244, 1990.

19. Bauck L. *A Practitioner's Guide to Avian Medicine*. American Animal Hospital Association, Lakewood, CO, 1993.

20. Bauck L. Nutritional problems in pet birds. *Semin Avian Exotic Pet Med* 4:3-8, 1995.

21. Bauck L, Boyer TH, Brown SA, et al. *Exotic Animal Formulary. A Supplement to AAHA's Practitioner Guides to Exotic Animal Medicine*. American Animal Hospital Association, Lakewood, CO, 1995.

22. Bauck L, Hillyer E, Hoefer H. Rhinitis: case reports. *Proc Annu Conf Assoc Avian Vet*: 134-139, 1992.

23. Bauck L, Hoefer HL. Avian antimicrobial therapy. *Semin Avian Exotic Pet Med* 2:17-22, 1993.

24. Belant JL, Seamans TW. Comparison of three formulations of alpha-chloralose for immobilization of Canada geese. *J Wildl Dis* 33:606-610, 1997.

25. Bendheim U, Lublin A. Side effects after IM Vibravenos injections. *Proc Euro Conf Avian Med Surg*: 116-119, 1993.

26. Bennett RA. Common avian emergencies. *Proc 5th Annu Internat Vet Emer Critical Care Symp*: 698-703, 1996.

27. Bennett RA. Medical and surgical management of avian reproductive disorders. *Proc Mid-Atlantic States Assoc Avian Vet Conf*: 40-44, 1997.

28. Best R. Breeding problems. In: Beynon PH, Forbes NA, Lawton MPC (eds). *BSAVA Manual of Raptors, Pigeons and Waterfowl*. Iowa State University Press, Ames, IA, 1996. Pp 202-215.

29. Beynon PH, Forbes NA, Harcourt-Brown NH. *BSAVA Manual of Raptors, Pigeons and Waterfowl*. Iowa State University Press, Ames, IA, 1996.

30. Beynon PH, Forbes NA, Lawton MPC. *BSAVA Manual of Psittacine Birds*. Iowa State University Press, Ames, IA, 1996.

31. Bird JE, Miller KW, Larson AA, et al. Pharmacokinetics of gentamicin in birds of prey. *Am J Vet Res* 44:1245-1247, 1983.

32. Bird JE, Walser MM, Duke GE. Toxicity of gentamicin in red-tailed hawks *(Buteo jamaicensis)*. *Am J Vet Res* 44:1289-1293, 1983.

33. Black WD. A study of the pharmacodynamics of oxytetracycline in the chicken. *Poult Sci* 56:1430-1434, 1977.

34. Bloomfield RB, Brooks D, Vulliet R. The pharmacokinetics of a single intramuscular dose of amikacin in red-tailed hawks *(Buteo jamaicensis)*. *J Zoo Wildl Med* 28:55-61, 1997.

35. Bonda M. Plasma glucagon, serum insulin, and serum amylase levels in normal and a hyperglycemic macaw. *Proc Annu Conf Assoc Avian Vet*: 77-88, 1996.

36. Bond MW. IME-Medication for vomiting psittacines. *J Assoc Avian Vet* 7:102, 1993.

37. Booth NH. Toxicology of drug and chemical residues. In: Booth NH, McDonald LE (eds). *Veterinary Pharmacology and Therapeutics*. 6th ed. Iowa State University Press, Ames, IA, 1988. Pp 1167-1179.

38. Breadner S. Chronic *Nocardia* infection in a hyacinth macaw. *Proc Annu Conf Assoc Avian Vet*: 283-285, 1994.

39. Brooks DE. Avian cataracts. *Semin Avian Exotic Pet Med* 6:131-137, 1997.

40. Brown MJ, Cromie RL. Weight loss and enteritis. In: Beynon PH, Forbes NA, Harcourt-Brown NH (eds). *BSAVA Manual of Raptors, Pigeons and Waterfowl*. Iowa State University Press, Ames, IA, 1996. Pp 322-328.

41. Bruch J vom, Aufinger P, Jakoby JR. Untersuchungen zur Pharmakokinetik und Wirkung von intramuskulär, oral und Über das Trinkwasser verabreichtem Sulfadimethoxine an gesunden und kokzidien-infizierten, adulten Tauben *(Columba livia* Gmel., 1789, var. dom.). (Pharmacokinetics and efficacy of sulfadimethoxine in healthy and coccidia-infected adult pigeons.) *Vet Bull* 56:7830, 1986.

42. Burns RB, Birrenkott GP. Half-life of dexamethasone and its effect on plasma corticosterone in raptors. *Proc Am Assoc Zoo Vet*: 12-13, 1988.

43. Bush M, Locke D, Neal LA, et al. Gentamicin tissue concentration in various avian species following recommended dosage therapy. *Am J Vet Res* 42:2114-2116, 1981.

233

44. Bush M, Locke D, Neal LA, et al. Pharmacokinetics of cephalothin and cephalexin in selected avian species. *Am J Vet Res* 42:1014-1017, 1981.

45. Calle PP, Stewart CA. Hematologic and serum chemistry values of captive hyacinth macaws *(Anodorhynchus hyacinthinus)*. *J Zoo Anim Med* 18:98-99, 1987.

46. Campbell TW. Biochemical evaluation of blood for the detection of hepatic disease in birds. PhD Dissertation, Kansas State University, Manhattan, KS, 1987.

47. Carpenter JW. Personal communication.

48. Carpenter JW. Cranes (Order Gruiformes). In: Fowler ME (ed). *Zoo & Wild Animal Medicine.* 2nd ed. WB Saunders Co, Philadelphia, 1986. Pp 315-326.

49. Carpenter JW. Supportive care procedures in companion bird medicine. *Kansas Vet* (Sept):10-13, 1991.

50. Carpenter JW. Infectious and parasitic diseases of cranes. In: Fowler ME (ed). *Zoo & Wild Animal Medicine: Current Therapy 3.* WB Saunders Co, Philadelphia, 1993. Pp 229-237.

51. Carpenter JW, Bossart G, Bachues K, Butine MD. Use of serum bile acids to evaluate hepatobiliary function in the cockatiel *(Nymphicus hollandicus)*. *Proc Annu Conf Assoc Avian Vet*: 73-78, 1996.

52. Carpenter JW, Novilla MN. Safety and efficacy of selected coccidiostats in cranes and implications for other avian species. *Proc Annu Conf Assoc Avian Vet*: 147-149, 1990.

53. Carpenter JW, Novilla MN, Hatfield JS. The safety and physiological effects of the anticoccidial drugs monensin and clazuril in sandhill cranes *(Grus canadensis)*. *J Zoo Wildl Med* 23:214-221, 1992.

54. Chaleva EI, Vasileva IV, Savova MD. Absorption of lincomycin through the respiratory pathways and its influence on alveolar macrophages after aerosol administration to chickens. *Res Vet Sci* 57:245-247, 1994.

55. Clark CH, Thomas JE, Milton JL, et al. Plasma concentrations of chloramphenicol in birds. *Am J Vet Res* 43:1949, 1982.

56. Clippinger TL. Diseases of the lower respiratory tract of companion birds. *Semin Avian Exotic Pet Med* 6:201-208, 1997.

57. Clubb SL. Therapeutics. In: Harrison GJ, Harrison LR (eds). *Clinical Avian Medicine and Surgery.* WB Saunders Co, Philadelphia, 1986. Pp 327-355.

58. Clubb SL. Birds. In: Johnston DE (ed). *The Bristol Veterinary Handbook of Antimicrobial Therapy.* 2nd ed. Veterinary Learning Systems Co, Trenton, NJ, 1987. Pp 188-199.

59. Clubb SL, Cray C, Greiner E, Latimer KS. Cryptosporidiosis in a psittacine nursery. *Proc Annu Conf Assoc Avian Vet*: 177-185, 1996.

60. Clubb SL, Schubot RM, Joyner K, et al. Hematologic and serum biochemical reference intervals in juvenile eclectus parrots *(Eclectus roratus)*. *J Assoc Avian Vet* 4:218-225, 1990.

61. Clubb SL, Schubot RM, Joyner K, et al. Hematologic and serum biochemical reference intervals in juvenile cockatoos. *J Assoc Avian Vet* 5:16-26, 1991.

62. Clubb SL, Schubot RM, Joyner K, et al. Hematologic and serum biochemical reference intervals in juvenile macaws *(Ara sp. [sic])*. *J Assoc Avian Vet* 5:154-162, 1991.

63. Clyde VL, Patton S. Diagnosis, treatment and control of common parasites in companion and aviary birds. *Semin Avian Exotic Pet Med* 5:75-84, 1996.

64. Clyde VL, Paul-Murphy J. Avian analgesia. In: Fowler ME, Miller RE (eds). *Zoo & Wild Animal Medicine: Current Therapy* 4. WB Saunders Co, Philadelphia, 1999. Pp 309-314.

65. Coles BH. Cage and aviary birds. In: Beynon PH, Cooper JE (eds). *Manual of Exotic Pets*. British Small Animal Veterinary Association, Worthing, UK, 1991. Pp 150-179.

66. Cooper JE. Anaesthesia of exotic animals. *Anim Technol* 35:13-20, 1984.

67. Cornelissen H. Behavior, anatomy, feeding and medical problems of toucans in captivity. *Proc Euro Conf Avian Med Surg*: 446-453, 1993.

68. Cornelissen H. IME - Treatment of common passerine conditions. *J Assoc Avian Vet* 7:103, 1993.

69. Cornelissen H, Ducatelle R, Roels S. Successful treatment of a channel-billed toucan *(Ramphastos vitellinus)* with iron storage disease by chelation therapy: Sequential monitoring of the iron content of the liver during the treatment period by quantitative chemical and image analyses. *J Avian Med Surg* 9:131-137, 1995.

70. Cross G. Antiviral therapy. *Semin Avian Exotic Pet Med* 4:96-102, 1995.

71. Crosta L, Delli Carri AP. Oral treatment with clindamycin in racing pigeons. *Proc First Conf Euro Comm Assoc Avian Vet*: 293-296, 1991.

72. Csikó GY, Banhidi GY, Semjén G, et al. Metabolism and pharmacokinetics of albendazole after oral administration to chickens. *J Vet Pharmacol Therap* 19:322-325, 1996.

73. Curro TG. Evaluation of the isoflurane-sparing effects of butorphanol and flunixin in Psittaciformes. *Proc Annu Conf Assoc Avian Vet*: 17-19, 1994.

74. Custer RS, Bush M, Carpenter JW. Pharmacokinetics of gentamicin in blood plasma of quail, pheasants, and cranes. *Am J Vet Res* 40:892-895, 1979.

75. Cybulski W, Larsson P, Tjälve H, et al. Disposition of metronidazole in hens *(Gallus gallus)* and quails *(Coturnix coturnix japonica)*: pharmacokinetics and whole-body autoradiography. *J Vet Pharmacol Therap* 19:352-358, 1996.

76. Dalhausen B. Featherpicking in pet birds. *Proc Mid-Atlantic States Assoc Avian Vet Conf*: 1-5, 1997.

77. Davidson M. Ocular consequences of trauma in raptors. *Semin Avian Exotic Pet Med* 6:121-130, 1997.

78. Day TK, Roge CK. Evaluation of sedation in quail induced by use of midazolam and reversed by use of flumazenil. *J Am Vet Med Assoc* 209:969-971, 1996.

79. Degernes LA. Toxicities in waterfowl. *Semin Avian Exotic Pet Med* 4:15-22, 1995.

80. Degernes LA. Topics in emergency medicine: fluid therapy and parenteral nutrition. *Proc Avian Specialty Advanced Prog Small Mam and Rept Med Surg (Annu Conf Assoc Avian Vet)*: 55-60, 1998.

81. Degernes LA, Crosier ML, Harrison LD, et al. Autologous, homologous and heterologous red blood cell transfusions in cockatiels *(Nymphicus hollandicus)*. *J Avian Med Surg* 13:2-9, 1999.

82. Degernes L, Davidson G, Flammer K, et al. Administration of total parenteral nutrition in pigeons. *Am J Vet Res* 55:660-665, 1994.

83. Degernes LA, Harrison LD, Smith DW, et al. Autologous, homologous and heterologous red blood cell transfusions in conures of the genus *Aratinga*. *J Avian Med Surg* 13:10-14, 1999.

84. De Herdt P, Devriese LA, De Groote B, et al. Antibiotic treatment of *Streptococcus bovis* infections in pigeons. *Proc Euro Conf Avian Med Surg*: 297-304, 1993.

85. Dein FJ, Monard DF, Kowalczyk DF. Pharmacokinetics of chloramphenicol in Chinese spot-billed ducks. *J Vet Pharmacol Therap* 3:161-168, 1980.

86. Denver MC, Tell LA, Galey FD. Comparison of oral and parenteral heavy metal chelators for the treatment of lead toxicosis in cockatiels *(Nymphicus hollandicus)*. *Proc Joint Conf Am Assoc Zoo Vet/Am Assoc Wildl Vet*: 147-148, 1998.

235

87. Dodwell GT. *The Complete Book of Canaries.* Merehurst Press, London, 1986.

88. Doolen M. Adriamycin® chemotherapy in a blue-front Amazon with osteosarcoma. *Proc Annu Conf Assoc Avian Vet*: 89-91, 1994.

89. Dorrestein G. Avian chlamydiosis therapy. *Semin Avian Exotic Pet Med* 2:23-29, 1993.

90. Dorrestein GM. Antimicrobial drug use in pet birds. In: Prescott JF, Baggot JD (eds). *Antimicrobial Therapy in Veterinary Medicine.* 2nd ed. Iowa State University Press, Ames, IA, 1993. Pp 491-506.

91. Dorrestein GM. Formulation and (bio)availability problems of drug formulations in birds. *J Vet Pharmacol Therap* 15:143-150, 1992.

92. Dorrestein GM. Infectious diseases and their therapy in Passeriformes. In: *Antimicrobial Therapy in Caged Birds and Exotic Pets.* Veterinary Learning Systems Co, Trenton, NJ, 1995. Pp 11-27.

93. Dorrestein GM. Pharmacology of the digestive tract. *Proc Avian Specialty Advanced Prog Small Mam and Rept Med Surg (Annu Conf Assoc Avian Vet)*: 43-53, 1998.

94. Dorrestein GM, Kazemi SM, Eksik N, et al. Comparative study of Synulox® and Augmentin® after intravenous, intramuscular and oral administration in collared doves *(Streptopelia decaocto).* In: Kösters J (ed). *X. Tagung der Fachgruppe "Geflügelkrankheiten."* Deutschen Veterinärmedizinischen Gesellschaft e.V., Giessen, Germany, 1996, Pp 42-54.

95. Dorrestein GM, Van Der Horst HHA, Cremers HJWM, Van Der Hage M. Quill mite *(Dermoglyphus passerinus)* infestation of canaries *(Serinus canaria)*: diagnosis and treatment. *Avian Pathol* 26:195-199, 1997.

96. Dorrestein GM, Van Gogh H, Rinzema JD. Pharmacokinetic aspects of penicillins, aminoglycosides and chloramphenicol in birds compared to mammals. A review. *Vet Quart* 6:216-224, 1984.

97. Dorrestein GM, Van Gogh H, Rinzema JD, et al. Comparative study of ampicillin and amoxicillin after intravenous, intramuscular and oral administration in homing pigeons *(Columba livia).* Res Vet Sci 42:343-348, 1987.

98. Dyer DC, Van Alstine WG. Antibiotic aerosolization: Tissue and plasma oxytetracycline concentrations in parakeets. *Avian Dis* 31:677-679, 1987.

99. El-Gammal AA, Ravis WR, Krista LM, et al. Pharmacokinetics and intramuscular bioavailability of amikacin in chickens following single and multiple dosing. *J Vet Pharmacol Therap* 15:133-142, 1992.

100. Ensley PK, Janssen DL. A preliminary study comparing the pharmacokinetics of ampicillin given orally and intramuscularly to psittacines: Amazon parrots (*Amazona* spp.) and blue-naped parrots *(Tanygnathus lucionensis). J Zoo Anim Med* 12:42-47, 1981.

101. Ernst S, Goggin JM, Biller DS, et al. Comparison of iohexol and barium sulfate as gastrointestinal contrast media in mid-sized psittacine birds. *J Avian Med Surg* 12:16-20, 1998.

102. Espigol C, Artigas C, Palmada J, Pages A. Serum levels of doxycycline during water treatment in poultry. *J Vet Pharmacol Therap* 20:192-193, 1997.

103. Filippich LJ. Megabacteria and proventricular/ventricular disease in psittacines and passerines. *Proc Annu Conf Assoc Avian Vet*: 287-293, 1990.

104. Fitzgerald G, Cooper JE. Preliminary studies on the use of propofol in the domestic pigeon *(Columba livia). Vet Sci* 49:334-338, 1990.

105. Flammer K. An overview of antifungal therapy in birds. *Proc Annu Conf Assoc Avian Vet*: 1-4, 1993.

106. Flammer K. Fluconazole in psittacine birds. *Proc Annu Conf Assoc Avian Vet*: 203-204, 1996.

107. Flammer K. A review of the pharmacology of antimicrobial drugs in birds. *Proc Avian/Exotic Anim Med Symp*, University of California, Davis, CA: 65-78, 1994.

108. Flammer K. Common bacterial infections and antibiotic use in companion birds. *Antimicrobial Therapy in Exotics: Supplement to Comp Cont Edu Pract Vet* 20(3A):34-48, 1998.

109. Flammer K. Antimicrobial therapy. *Proc Annu Conf Assoc Avian Vet*: 429-436, 1997.

110. Flammer K. Approach to the vomiting bird. *Proc 21st Annu Waltham /OSU Symp*: 19-21, 1997.

111. Flammer K, Aucoin DP, Whitt DA, et al. Plasma concentrations of enrofloxacin in African grey parrots treated with medicated water. *Avian Dis* 34:1017-1022, 1990.

112. Flammer K, Aucoin DP, Whitt DA, et al. Potential use of long-acting injectable oxytetracycline for treatment of chlamydiosis in Goffin's cockatoos. *Avian Dis* 34:228-234, 1990.

113. Flammer K, Aucoin DP, Whitt DA. Intramuscular and oral disposition of enrofloxacin in African grey parrots following single and multiple doses. *J Vet Pharmacol Therap* 41:359-366, 1991.

114. Flammer K, Aucoin DP, Whitt D. Preliminary report on the use of doxycycline-medicated feed in psittacine birds. *Proc Annu Conf Assoc Avian Vet*: 1-4, 1991.

115. Flammer K, Cassidy DR, Landgraf WW, et al. Blood concentrations of chlortetracycline in macaws fed a medicated pelleted feed. *Avian Dis* 33:199-203, 1989.

116. Flammer K, Clark CH, Drewes LA, et al. Adverse effects of gentamicin in scarlet macaws and galahs. *Am J Vet Res* 51:404-407, 1990.

117. Forbes NA. Respiratory problems. In: Beynon PH, Forbes NA, Lawton MPC (eds). *BSAVA Manual of Psittacine Birds*. Iowa State University Press, Ames, IA, 1996. Pp 147-157.

118. Forbes NA, Richardson T. Husbandry and nutrition. In: Beynon PH, Forbes NA, Harcourt-Brown NH (eds). *BSAVA Manual of Raptors, Pigeons and Waterfowl*. Iowa State University Press, Ames, IA, 1996. Pp 289-298.

119. Forshaw JM, Cooper WT. *Parrots of the World*. Doubleday & Co, Garden City, NY, 1973.

120. France M. Chemotherapy treatment of lymphosarcoma in a Moluccan cockatoo. *Proc Annu Conf Assoc Avian Vet*: 15-19, 1993.

121. Franssen FFJ, Lumeij JT. In vitro nitroimidazole resistance of *Trichomonas gallinae* and successful therapy with an increased dosage of ronidazole in racing pigeons (*Columba livia domestica*). *J Vet Pharmacol Therap* 15:409-415, 1992.

122. Frazier DL, Jones MP, Orosz SE. Pharmacokinetic considerations of the renal system in birds: Part II. Review of drugs excreted by renal pathways. *J Avian Med Surg* 9:104-121, 1995.

123. Friffin C, Snelling LR. Use of hyaluronidase in avian subcutaneous fluids. *Proc Annu Conf Assoc Avian Vet*: 239-240, 1998.

124. Fudge AM. Blood testing artifacts: interpretation and prevention. *Semin Avian Exotic Pet Med* 3:2-4, 1994.

125. Fudge AM, Reavill DR, Rosskopf WJ, Jr. Diagnosis and management of avian dyspnea: A review. *Proc Annu Conf Assoc Avian Vet*: 187-195, 1993.

126. García-Ovando H, Chiostri E, Ugnia L, et al. HPLC residues of enrofloxacin and ciprofloxacin in eggs of laying hens. *J Vet Pharmacol Therap* 20:204, 1997.

127. Giddings RF. Treatment of flukes in a toucan. *J Am Vet Med Assoc* 193:1555-1556, 1988.

128. Goodwin JS, Jacobson ER, Gaskin JM. Effects of Pacheco's parrot disease virus on hematologic and blood chemistry values of Quaker parrots (*Myopsitta monachus*). *J Zoo Anim Med* 13:127-132, 1982.

129. Gould WJ. Caring for birds' skin and feathers. *Vet Med* (Jan): 53-63, 1995.

130. Gould WJ. Common digestive tract disorders in pet birds. *Vet Med* (Jan): 40-52, 1995.

131. Greenacre CB, Quandt JE. Comparison of sevoflurane to isoflurane in psittaciformes. *Proc Annu Conf Assoc Avian Vet*: 123-124, 1997.

132. Grimm F, Serbest E. The therapy of osteomyelitis with clindamycin in patients suffering from fractures. *Proc VIII Tagung über Vogelkrankheiten,* München: 252-254, 1992.

133. Gronwall R, Brown MP, Clubb S. Pharmacokinetics of amikacin in African gray parrots. *Am J Vet Res* 50:250-252, 1989.

134. Haberkorn A, et al. The use of Bay VI 9142 (Baycox®), a new coccidiocide, in waterfowl, particularly in the goose. *Proc Conf Avian Dis*, 1988.

135. Hamdy AH, Kratzer DD, Paxton LM, et al. Effect of a single injection of lincomycin, spectinomycin, and linco-spectin on early chick mortality caused by *E. coli* and *S. aureus*. *Avian Dis* 24:164-173, 1979.

136. Hamdy AH, Saif YM, Kasson CW. Efficacy of lincomycin-spectinomycin water medication on *Mycoplasma meleagridis* air sacculitis in commercially raised turkey poults. *Avian Dis* 26: 227-233, 1981.

137. Haneveld-v Laarhoven MA, Dorrestein GM. IME - Sudden high mortality in canaries. *J Assoc Avian Vet* 4:82, 1990.

138. Harlin RW. Backyard poultry. *Proc Mid-Atlantic States Assoc Avian Vet Conf*:65-68, 1995.

139. Harlin RW. Pigeons. *Vet Clin North Am: Small Anim Pract* 24:157-173, 1994.

140. Harlin RW. Pigeons. *Proc Annu Conf Assoc Avian Vet*: 361-373, 1995.

141. Harms CA, Hoskinson JJ, Bruyette DS, et al. Development of an experimental model of hypothyroidism in cockatiels (*Nymphicus hollandicus*). *Am J Vet Res* 55:399-404, 1994.

142. Harper FDW. Poor performance and weight loss. In: Beynon PH, Forbes NA, Harcourt-Brown NH (eds). *BSAVA Manual of Raptors, Pigeons and Waterfowl.* Iowa State University Press, Ames, IA, 1996. Pp 272-278.

143. Harrenstein LA, Tell LA, Vulliet R, et al. Disposition of enrofloxacin (Baytril®) in red-tailed hawks (*Buteo jamaicensis*) and great-horned owls (*Bubo virginianus*) following a single oral, intramuscular, or intravenous dose. *Proc Joint Conf Am Assoc Zoo Vet/Am Assoc Wildl Vet*: 140-141, 1998.

144. Harris D. Therapeutic avian techniques. *Semin Avian Exotic Pet Med* 6:55-62, 1997.

144a. Harris DJ. Avian clinical pathology. *Proc Mid-Atlantic States Assoc Avian Vet Conf*: 62-67, 1996.

145. Harrison GJ. What to do until a diagnosis is made. In: Harrison GJ, Harrison LR (eds). *Clinical Avian Medicine and Surgery.* WB Saunders Co, Philadelphia, 1986. Pp 356-361.

146. Harrison GJ, Harrison LR (eds). *Clinical Avian Medicine and Surgery.* WB Saunders Co, Philadelphia, 1986. Pp 662-663.

147. Hartup BK, Miller EA. *Willowbrook Wildlife Haven Pharmaceutical Index.* Friends of the Furred and Feathered, Glen Ellyn, IL, 1992.

148. Harvey R. *Practical Incubation.* Payn Essex Printers Ltd, Sudbury, Suffolk, UK, 1990.

149. Harvey-Clark C. Clinical and research use of implantable vascular access ports in avian species. *Proc Annu Conf Assoc Avian Vet*: 191-209, 1990.

150. Harvey-Clark C, Gass CL. IME—Treating aspergillosis in hummingbirds. *J Assoc Avian Vet* 7:216, 1993.

151. Hawkey CM, Samour HJ. The value of clinical hematology in exotic birds. In: Jacobson ER, Kollias GV, Jr (eds). *Exotic Animals*. Churchill Livingstone, New York, 1988. Pp 109-141.

152. Heard DJ. Avian anesthesia: present and future trends. *Proc Annu Conf Assoc Avian Vet*: 117-122, 1997.

153. Heard DJ. IME—Overview of avian anesthesia. *AAV Today* 2:92-94, 1988.

154. Hedberg GE, Bennett RA. Preliminary studies on the use of milbemycin oxime in galliformes. *Proc Annu Conf Assoc Avian Vet*: 261-264, 1994.

155. Heidenreich M. *Birds of Prey, Medicine and Management*. Blackwell Science Ltd, Malden, MA, 1997.

156. Heinen E, DeJong A, Scheer M. Antimicrobial activity of fluoroquinolones in serum and tissues in turkeys. *J Vet Pharmacol Therap* 20 (Suppl 1):196-197, 1997.

157. Hines R, Kolattukuty PE, Sharkey P. Pharmacological induction of molt and gonadal involution in birds. *Proc Annu Conf Assoc Avian Vet*: 127-134, 1993.

158. Hirsch DC, Knox SJ, Couzelman GM, Jr, et al. Pharmacokinetics of penicillin-G in the turkey. *Am J Vet Res* 39:1219-1221, 1978.

159. Hochleithner M. Reference values for selected psittacine species using a dry chemistry system. *J Assoc Avian Vet* 3:207-209, 1989.

160. Hoefer H. IME - Hepatic fibrosis and colchicine therapy. *J Assoc Avian Vet* 5:193, 1991.

161. Hoefer HL. Antimicrobials in pet birds. In: Bonagura JD (ed). *Kirk's Current Veterinary Therapy XII: Small Animal Practice*. WB Saunders Co, Philadelphia, 1995. Pp 1278-1283.

162. Hogan HL, Joseph B, Henrickson R, et al. Efficacy and safety of ivermectin treatment for scaley leg mite infestation in parakeets. *Proc Am Assoc Zoo Vet*: 156, 1984.

163. Hooimeijer J. Coccidiosis in lorikeets infectious for budgerigar. *Proc Annu Conf Assoc Avian Vet*: 59-61, 1993.

164. Hudelson KS. A review of the mechanisms of avian reproduction and their clinical applications. *Semin Avian Exotic Pet Med* 5:189-198, 1996.

165. Hudelson KS, Hudelson P. Egg binding, hormonal control, and therapeutic considerations. *Comp Cont Edu Pract Vet* 15:427-432, 1993.

166. Hudelson KS, Hudelson P. A brief review of the female avian reproductive cycle with special emphasis on the role of prostaglandins and clinical applications. *J Avian Med Surg* 10:67-74, 1996.

167. Huff DG. Avian fluid therapy and nutritional therapeutics. *Semin Avian Exotic Pet Med* 2:13-16, 1993.

168. Iglauer F, Rasim R. Treatment of psychogenic feather picking in psittacine birds with a dopamine antagonist. *J Small Anim Pract* 34:564-566, 1993.

169. Inghelbrecht S, Vermeersch H, De Backer P, et al. Pharmacokinetics and anti-trichomonal efficacy of dimetridazole in homing pigeons (*Columba livia*). In: Kösters J (ed). *X. Tagung der Fachgruppe "Geflügelkrankheiten."* Deutschen Veterinärmedizinischen Gesellschaft e.V., Giessen, Germany, 1996. Pp 287-290.

170. Inghelbrecht S, Vermeersch H, Ronsmans S, et al. Pharmacokinetics and antitrichomonal efficacy of a dimetridazole tablet and water-soluble powder in homing pigeons (*Columba livia*). *J Vet Pharmacol Therap* 19:62-67, 1996.

171. Isaza R, Budsberg SC, Sundlof SF, et al. Disposition of ciprofloxacin in red-tailed hawks following a single oral dose. *J Zoo Wildl Med* 24:498-502, 1993.

172. Itoh N, Okada H. Pharmacokinetics and tolerability of chloramphenicol in budgerigars (*Melopsittacus undulatus*). *J Vet Med Sci* 55:439-442, 1993.

173. Jalanka HH. Medetomidine-ketamine and atipamezole: A reversible method for chemical restraint of birds. *Proc First Annu Conf Euro Comm Assoc Avian Vet*: 102-104, 1991.

174. Jenkins JR. Postoperative care of the avian patient. *Semin Avian Exotic Pet Med* 2:97-102, 1993.

175. Jennings IB. Haematology. In: Beynon PH, Forbes NA, Harcourt-Brown NH (eds). *BSAVA Manual of Raptors, Pigeons and Waterfowl.* Iowa State University Press, Ames, IA, 1996. Pp 68-78.

176. Jensen J, Westerman E. Amikacin pharmacokinetics in ostrich (*Struthio camelus*). *Proc Am Assoc Zoo Vet*: 238-242, 1990.

177. Jensen JM, Johnson JH, Weiner ST. *Husbandry & Medical Management of Ostriches, Emus & Rheas.* Wildlife and Exotic Animal TeleConsultants, College Station, TX, 1992.

178. Johnson-Delaney C. Feather picking: diagnosis and treatment. *J Assoc Avian Vet* 6:82-83, 1992.

179. Johnson-Delaney CA, Harrison LR (eds). *Exotic Companion Medicine Handbook for Veterinarians.* Wingers Publishing, Lake Worth, FL, 1996.

180. Jones MP, Orosz SE. Overview of avian neurology and neurological diseases. *Semin Avian Exotic Pet Med* 5: 150-164, 1996.

181. Jordan FTW, Horrocks BK. The minimum inhibitory concentration of tilmicosin and tylosin for *Mycoplasma gallisepticum* and *Mycoplasma synoviae* and a comparison of their efficacy in the control of *Mycoplasma gallisepticum* infection in chickens. Avian Dis 41:802-807, 1997.

182. Joseph V. Emergency care of raptors. *Vet Clin North Am: Exotic Anim Pract* 1:77-98, 1998.

183. Joseph V. Preventive health programs for falconry birds. *Proc Annu Conf Assoc Avian Vet*: 171-178, 1995.

184. Joseph V. Selected medical topics for birds of prey. *Proc Annu Conf Assoc Avian Vet*: 261-266, 1996.

185. Joseph V, Pappagianis D, Reavill DR. Clotrimazole nebulization for the treatment of respiratory aspergillosis. *Proc Annu Conf Assoc Avian Vet*: 301-306, 1994.

186. Joyner KL. Pediatric therapeutics. *Proc Annu Conf Assoc Avian Vet*: 188-199, 1991.

187. Junge RE, Naeger LL, LeBeau MA, et al. Pharmacokinetics of intramuscular and nebulized ceftriaxone in chickens. *J Zoo Wildl Med* 25:224-228, 1994.

188. Karesh WB, del Campo A, Braselton WE, et al. Health evaluation of free-ranging and hand-reared macaws (*Ara* spp.) in Peru. *J Zoo Wildl Med* 28:368-377, 1997.

189. Kasper A. Rehabilitation of California towhees. *Proc Annu Conf Assoc Avian Vet*: 83-90,1997.

190. Kaufman E, Pokras M, Sedgwick C. IME—Anesthesia in waterfowl. *AAV Today* 2:98, 1988.

191. Kaufman GE. Avian emergencies. In: Murtaugh RJ, Kaplan PM (eds). *Veterinary Emergency and Critical Care Medicine.* Mosby Year Book, Inc, St Louis, 1992. Pp 453-463.

192. Keitzmann M, Knoll U, Glünder G. Pharmacokinetics of enrofloxacin and danofloxacin in broiler chickens. *J Vet Pharmacol Therap* 20 (Suppl 1):202, 1997.

193. Kempf I, Reeve-Johnson L, Gesbert F, Guittet M. Efficacy of tilmicosin in the control of experimental *Mycoplasma gallisepticum* infection in chickens. *Avian Dis* 41:802-807, 1997.

194. Kern TJ. Avian ophthalmology. *Proc Atlantic Coast Vet Conf.* 1995.

195. Killian AD, Drusano GL, Kanyok TP. Pharmacokinetics of drugs used for the therapy of *Mycobacterium avium*-complex infection. In: Korvick JA, Benson CA (eds). *Mycobacterium avium-Complex Infection, Progress in Research and Treatment.* Marcel Dekker, New York, 1996. Pp 197-240.

196. Klein PN, Charmatz K, Langenberg J. The effect of flunixin meglumine (Banamine®) on the renal function in northern bobwhite (*Colinus virginianus*): An avian model. *Proc Annu Conf Am Assoc Zoo Vet*: 128-131, 1994.

197. Koepff C. *The New Finch Handbook.* Barron's Educational Series, Woodbury, NY, 1983.

198. Kollias GV. Nutritional support for captive wild birds. *Proc Annu Conf Am Assoc Zoo Vet*: 23-24, 1993.

199. Kollias GV, Jr, Palgut J, Rossi J, et al. The use of ketoconazole in birds: Preliminary pharmacokinetics and clinical applications. *Proc Annu Conf Assoc Avian Vet*: 103, 1986.

200. Kollias GV, Zgola MM, Weinkle TK, Schwark WS. Amikacin sulfate pharmacokinetics in ring-necked pheasants (*Phasianus colchicus*): age and route dependent effects. *Proc Am Assoc Zoo Vet*: 178-180, 1996.

201. Korbel RT. Avian ophthalmology—principles and application. *Proc Annu Conf Assoc Avian Vet*: 305-315, 1997.

202. Korbel R. Inhalation anaesthesia with isoflurane (Forene®) and sevoflurane (SEVOrane®) in domestic pigeons (*Columba livia,* Gmel., 1789, var. domestica). *Ger Vet Med Soc*: 209-217, 1998.

203. Korbel R, Spemann B, Erhardt W, Henke J. (Translated) Examinations on the systemical administration of the muscle relaxant vecuronium in ornitho-ophthalmology under the conditions of air sac perfusion anaesthesia (APA). In: Kösters J (ed). *X. Tagung der Fachgruppe "Geflügelkrankheiten."* Deutschen Veterinärmedizinischen Gesellschaft e.V., Giessen, Germany, 1996. Pp 272-276.

204. Kreeger TJ, Degernes LA, Kreeger JS, et al. Immobilization of raptors with tiletamine and zolazepam (Telazol). In: Redig PT, Cooper JE, Remple DJ, et al (eds). *Raptor Biomedicine.* University of Minnesota Press, Minneapolis, MN, 1993. Pp 141-144.

205. Krinsley M. IME - Use of DermCaps Liquid and hydroxyzine HCl for the treatment of feather picking. *J Assoc Avian Vet* 7:221, 1993.

206. LaBonde J. Household poisonings in caged birds. In: Bonagura JD (ed). *Kirk's Current Veterinary Therapy XII: Small Animal Practice.* WB Saunders Co, Philadelphia, 1995. Pp 1299-1303.

207. LaBonde J. Two clinical cases of exposure to household use of organophosphate and carbamate insecticides. *Proc Annu Conf Assoc Avian Vet*: 113-118, 1992.

208. LaBonde J. Toxicity in pet avian patients. *Semin Avian Exotic Pet Med* 4:23-31, 1995.

209. LaBonde J. Private collections of waterfowl. *Proc Annu Conf Assoc Avian Vet*: 215-224, 1996.

210. Laczay P, Semjén G, Nagy G, Lehel J. Comparative studies on the pharmacokinetics of norfloxacin in chickens, turkeys, and geese after a single oral administration. *J Vet Pharmacol Therap* 21:161-164, 1998.

211. Lamberski N, Daniel GB. Fluid dynamics of intraosseous fluid administration in birds. *J Zoo Wildl Med* 10:173-177, 1989.

212. Lane R. Basic techniques in pet avian clinical pathology. *Vet Clin North Am: Small Anim Pract* 21:1157-1179, 1991.

213. Langenberg JA, Businga NK, Nevill HE. Capture of wild sandhill cranes with alpha-chloralose: techniques and physiologic effects. *Proc Joint Conf Am Assoc Zoo Vet/Am Assoc Wildl Vet*: 50-53, 1998.

214. Lashev LD, Mihailov R. Pharmacokinetics of apramycin in Japanese quail. *J Vet Pharmacol Therap* 17:394-395, 1994.

215. Lawton MPC. Anaesthesia. In: Beynon PH, Forbes NA, Lawton MPC (eds). *BSAVA Manual of Psittacine Birds.* Iowa State University Press, Ames, IA, 1996. Pp 49-55.

216. Lawton MPC. Anaesthesia. In: Beynon PH, Forbes NA, Harcourt-Brown NH (eds). *BSAVA Manual of Raptors, Pigeons and Waterfowl.* Iowa State University Press, Ames, IA, 1996. Pp 79-88.

217. Lawton MPC. Behavioural problems. In: Beynon PH, Forbes NA, Lawton MPC (eds). *BSAVA Manual of Psittacine Birds.* Iowa State University Press, Ames, IA, 1996. Pp 106-113.

218. Lennox AM, VanDerHeyden N. Haloperidol for use in treatment of psittacine self-mutilation and feather plucking. *Proc Annu Conf Assoc Avian Vet*: 119-120, 1993.

219. Levy A, Perelman B, Waner T, et al. Reference blood chemical values in ostriches (*Struthio camelus*). *Am J Vet Res* 50:1548-1550, 1989.

220. Lightfoot TL. Clinical use and preliminary data of chorionic gonadotropin administration in psittacines. *Proc Annu Conf Assoc Avian Vet*: 303-306, 1996.

221. Lightfoot TL. How I approach chronic egg laying. *Proc North Am Vet Conf*: 757-760, 1998.

222. Limoges MJ, Semple HA, Wheler CL, Nimz EL. Plasma pharmacokinetics of an orally administered azithromycin in mealy Amazons (*Amazona farinosa*). *Proc Annu Conf Assoc Avian Vet*: 41-43,1998.

223. Lindenstruth H, Frost JW. Enrofloxacin (Baytril)- an alternative for psittacosis prevention and therapy in imported psittacines. *DTW Dtsch Tierarztl Wochenschr* 100:364-368, 1993.

224. Locke D, Bush M. Tylosin aerosol therapy in quail and pigeons. *J Zoo Anim Med* 15:67-72, 1984.

225. Locke D, Bush M, Carpenter JW. Pharmacokinetics and tissue concentrations of tylosin in selected avian species. *Am J Vet Res* 43:1807-1810, 1982.

226. Loudis BG. Soft tissue involvement of avian tuberculosis and attempted treatment—A case study. *Proc Am Assoc Zoo Vet*: 246-247, 1991.

227. Lublin Z, Mechani S, Malkinson M, et al. Efficacy of norfloxacin nicotinate treatment of broiler breeders against *Haemophilus paragallinarum. Avian Dis* 37:673-679, 1993.

228. Ludders JW, Rode J, Mitchell GS, et al. Effects of ketamine, xylazine, and a combination of ketamine and xylazine in Pekin ducks. *Am J Vet Res* 50:245, 1989.

229. Luebbert JAR. Canada goose (*Branta canadensis*) rehabilitation: a natural history guide for veterinarians. *Proc Annu Conf Assoc Avian Vet*: 245-254, 1996.

230. Lumeij JT. IME - A digest of useful clinical pathology information. *AAV Today* 2:188, 1988.

231. Lumeij JT. Appendix section: hematology and biochemistry—Columbiformes. In: Ritchie BW, Harrison GJ, Harrison LR (eds). *Avian Medicine: Principles and Application.* Wingers Publ, Lake Worth, FL, 1994.

232. Lumeij JT. Avian clinical enzymology. *Semin Avian Exotic Pet Med* 3:14-24, 1994.

233. Lumeij JT. Psittacine antimicrobial therapy. In: *Antimicrobial Therapy in Caged Birds and Exotic Pets.* Veterinary Learning Systems Co, Trenton, NJ, 1995. Pp 38-48.

234. Lumeij JT, Gorgevska D, Woestenborghs R. Plasma and tissue concentrations of itraconazole in racing pigeons (*Columba livia domestica*). *J Avian Med Surg* 9:32-35, 1995.

235. Lung NP, Romagnano A. Current approaches to feather picking. In: Bonagura JD (ed). *Kirk's Current Veterinary Therapy XII: Small Animal Practice.* WB Saunders Co, Philadelphia, 1995. Pp 1303-1307.

236. Machin KL, Caulkett NA. The cardiopulmonary effects of propofol in mallard ducks. *Proc Am Assoc Zoo Vet*: 149-154, 1996.

237. Machin KL, Caulkett NA. Cardiopulmonary effects of propofol and a medetomidine-midazolam-ketamine combination in mallard ducks. *Am J Vet Res* 59:598-602, 1998.

238. Machin KL, Caulkett NA. Investigation of injectable anesthetic agents in mallard ducks (*Anas platyrhyncus*): a descriptive study. *J Avian Med Surg* 12:255-262, 1998.

239. Mainka SA, Dierenfeld ES, Cooper RM, et al. Circulating a-tocopherol following intramuscular or oral vitamin E administration in Swainson's hawks (*Buteo swainsonii*). *J Zoo Wildl Med* 25:229-232, 1994.

240. Malley AD. Practical therapeutics for cage and aviary birds. In: Raw ME, Parkinson TJ (eds). *The Veterinary Annual.* Blackwell Scientific Publications, London, 1994. Pp 235-246.

241. Mama KR, Phillips LG, Pascoe PJ. Use of propofol for induction and maintenance of anesthesia in a barn owl (*Tyto alba*) undergoing tracheal resection. *J Zoo Wildl Med* 27:397-401, 1996.

242. Marshall R. Avian anthelmintics and antiprotozoals. *Semin Avian Exotic Pet Med* 2:33-41, 1993.

243. Martin HD, Kollias GV. Evaluation of water deprivation and fluid therapy in pigeons. *J Zoo Wildl Med* 20:173-177, 1989.

244. Marx D. Preventive health care with diagnostics. *AAV Today* 2:92-94, 1988.

245. Matthews NS. Anesthesia for big birds (ostriches and emus). *Proc North Am Vet Conf*: 705, 1993.

246. McDonald SE. IME - Injecting eggs with antibiotics. *J Assoc Avian Vet* 1:9, 1989.

247. McDonald SE. IME - Summary of medications for use in psittacine birds. *J Assoc Avian Vet* 3:120-127, 1989.

248. McMillan MC. Avian gastrointestinal radiography. In: Hoefer HL (ed). *Practical Avian Medicine: The Compendium Collection.* Veterinary Learning Systems Co, Trenton, NJ, 1997. Pp 24-29.

249. Migaki TT, Avakian AP, Barnes HJ, et al. Efficacy of danofloxacin and tylosin in the control of mycoplasmosis in chicks infected with tylosin-susceptible or tylosin-resistant field isolates of *Mycoplasma gallisepticum*. *Avian Dis* 37:508-514, 1993.

250. Mikaelian I. Intravenously administered propofol for anesthesia of the common buzzard (*Buteo buteo*), the tawny owl (*Strix aluco*), and the barn owl (*Tyto alba*). *Proc First Conf Euro Comm Assoc Avian Vet*: 97-101, 1991.

251. Mikaelian I, Paillet I, Williams D. Comparative use of various mydriatic drugs in kestrels (*Falco tinnunculus*). *Am J Vet Res* 55:270-272, 1994.

252. Millam JR. Leuprolide acetate can reversibly prevent egg laying in cockatiels. *Proc Annu Conf Assoc Avian Vet*: 46, 1993.

253. Millam JR, Finney HL. Leuprolide acetate can reversibly prevent egg laying in cockatiels (*Nymphicus hollandicus*). *Zoo Biol* 13:149-155, 1994.

254. Miller EA, Welte SC. Caring for oiled birds. In: Fowler ME, Miller RE (eds). *Zoo & Wild Animal Medicine: Current Therapy 4*. WB Saunders Co, Philadelphia, 1998. Pp 300-309.

255. Mohan R. *Mycoplasma* in ratites. *Proc Annu Conf Assoc Avian Vet*: 294-296, 1993.

256. Moore DM, Rice RL. Exotic Animal Formulary. In: Holt KM, Boothe DM, Gaumnitz J, et al. *Veterinary Values*. 5th ed. Veterinary Medicine Publishing Group, Lenexa, KS, 1998. Pp 159-245.

257. Morrisey JK. Avian emergency medicine and critical care. In: Hoefer HL (ed). *Practical Avian Medicine: The Compendium Collection*. Veterinary Learning Systems Co, Trenton, NJ, 1997. Pp 53-57.

258. Murai A, Furuse M, Okumura J-I. Involvement of (n-6) essential fatty acids and prostaglandins in liver lipid accumulation in Japanese quail. *Am J Vet Res* 57:342-345, 1996.

259. Murase T, Ikeda T, Goto I, et al. Treatment of lead poisoning in wild geese. *J Am Vet Med Assoc* 200:1726-1729, 1992.

260. Murphy CJ. Raptor ophthalmology. *Comp Contin Educ Pract Vet*: 9:241-260, 1987.

261. Murphy J. Diabetes in toucans. *Proc Annu Conf Assoc Avian Vet*: 165-170, 1992.

262. Murphy J. Psittacine trichomoniasis. *Proc Annu Conf Assoc Avian Vet*: 21-24, 1992.

263. Naether CA. *Raising Pigeons and Doves*. David McKay Co, New York, 1979.

264. Newell SM. Diagnosis and treatment of lymphocytic leukemia and malignant lymphoma in a Pekin duck (*Anas platyrhyncus domesticus*). *J Assoc Avian Vet* 5:83-86, 1991.

265. Norton TM. Bali mynah captive medical management and reintroduction program. *Proc Annu Conf Assoc Avian Vet*: 125-136, 1995.

266. Norton TM, Gaskin J, Kollias GV, et al. Efficacy of acyclovir against herpesvirus infection in Quaker parakeets. *Am J Vet Res* 52:2007-2009, 1991.

267. Oglesbee BL. Avian cardiology. *Proc North Am Vet Conf*: 730-731, 1996.

268. Oglesbee BL, McDonald S, Warthen K. Avian digestive system disorders. In: Birchard SJ, Sherding RG (eds). *Saunders Manual of Small Animal Practice*. WB Saunders Co, Philadelphia, 1994. Pp 1290-1301.

269. Olsen GH, Carpenter JW. Andean condor medicine, reproduction and husbandry. *Proc Annu Conf Assoc Avian Vet*: 147-152, 1995.

270. Orosz SE, Frazier DL. Antifungal agents: A review of their pharmacology and therapeutic indications. *J Avian Med Surg* 9:8-18, 1995.

271. Orosz SE, Schroeder EC, Frazier DL. Itraconazole: A new antifungal drug for birds. *Proc Annu Conf Assoc Avian Vet*: 13-19, 1994.

272. Page DC. A clinical review of apicomplexan parasites in non-domestic birds. *Proc Annu Conf Am Coll Vet Internal Med Forum*: 1072, 1995.

273. Page DC, Schmidt RE, English JH, et al. Antemortem diagnosis and treatment of sarcocystosis in two species of psittacines. *J Zoo Wildl Med* 23:77-85, 1992.

274. Paul-Murphy J. Advances in avian analgesia. *Proc Am Assoc Zoo Vet*: 131-133, 1997.

275. Paul-Murphy J. Evaluation of analgesic properties of butorphanol and buprenorphine for the psittacine bird. *Proc Annu Conf Assoc Avian Vet*: 125-127, 1997.

276. PÇricard JM, Andral B. Thiamine deficiency as a possible cause for the "staggers" syndrome of the Griffon vulture (*Gyps fulvus*). *Proc Euro Conf Avian Med Surg*: 191-198, 1993.

277. Plumb DC. *Veterinary Drug Handbook*. 3rd ed. Pharma Vet Pub, White Bear Lake, MN, 1999.

278. Pokras MA. Trichomoniasis. *Proc N Am Vet Conf*: 778-779, 1998.

279. Porter SL. Vehicular trauma in owls. *Proc Annu Conf Assoc Avian Vet*: 164-170, 1990.

280. Porter SL. Organophosphate/carbamate poisoning in birds of prey. *Proc Am Assoc Zoo Vet/Am Assoc Wildl Vet*: 176, 1992.

281. Porter SL. Euthanasia techniques for wildlife. *Proc Atlantic Coast Vet Conf.*, 1995.

282. Porter SL. The toxicity of cholinesterase inhibitors to birds. *Proc N Am Vet Conf*: 880-881, 1996.

283. Powers L. Fluid therapy in birds. *Proc Annu Conf Assoc Avian Vet*: 259-262, 1997.

283a. Powers LV. Interpretation of avian hematologic abnormalities. *Proc Mid-Atlantic States Assoc Avian Vet Conf*: 36-39, 1997.

284. Powers LV, Pokras M, Rio K, et al. Hematology and occurrence of hemoparasites in migrating sharp-shinned hawks (*Accipiter striatus*) during Fall migration. *J Raptor Res* 28:178-185, 1994.

285. Product insert.

286. Prus SE, Clubb SL, Flammer K. Doxycycline plasma concentrations in macaws fed a medicated corn diet. *Avian Dis* 36:480-483, 1992.

287. Quesenberry K. Avian neurologic disorders. In: Birchard SJ, Sherding RG (eds). *Saunders Manual of Small Animal Practice*. WB Saunders Co, Philadelphia, 1994. Pp 1312-1316.

288. Quesenberry KE, Hillyer EV. Supportive care and emergency therapy. In: Ritchie BW, Harrison GJ, Harrison LR (eds). *Avian Medicine: Principles and Application*. Wingers Publ, Lake Worth, FL, 1994. Pp 382-416.

289. Quesenberry KE. Avian antimicrobial therapeutics. In: Jacobson ER, Kollias GV, Jr (eds). *Exotic Animals*. Churchill Livingstone, New York, 1988. Pp 177-207.

290. Quintavalla F, Zucca P. Birds of prey: blood chemistry profile for peregrine falcons (*Falco peregrinus*) and eagle owls (*Bubo bubo*) in a raptor centre in north Italy. *Proc Euro Conf Assoc Avian Vet*: 544-551, 1993.

291. Rae M. Endocrine disease in pet birds. *Semin Avian Exotic Pet Med* 4:32-38, 1995.

292. Ramer JC, Paul-Murphy J, Brunson D, Murphy CJ. Induction of mydriasis in three psittacine species. *Proc Am Assoc Zoo Vet*: 288-289, 1994.

293. Ramer JC, Paul-Murphy J, Brunson D, Murphy CJ. Effects of mydriatic agents in cockatoos, African gray parrots, and blue-fronted Amazon parrots. *J Am Vet Med Assoc* 208:227-230, 1996.

294. Ramsay E. Personal communication.

295. Ramsay E. Emergency medicine and critical care of raptors. *Proc Avian/Exotic Anim Med Symp*, University of California, Davis, CA: 75-79, 1990.

296. Ramsay E. Ratite restraint, immobilization and anesthesia. *Proc Avian/Exotic Anim Med Symp*, University of California, Davis, CA: 176-179, 1991.

297. Ramsay EC, Drew ML, Johnson B. Trichomoniasis in a flock of budgerigars. *Proc Annu Conf Assoc Avian Vet*: 309-311, 1990.

298. Ramsay EC, Grindlinger H. Use of clomipramine in the treatment of obsessive behavior in psittacine birds. *J Assoc Avian Vet* 8:9, 1994.

299. Ramsay EC, Vulliet R. Pharmacokinetic properties of gentamicin and amikacin in the cockatiel. *Avian Dis* 37:628-634, 1993.

300. Randolph K. Equine encephalitis virus in ratites. *Proc Annu Conf Assoc Avian Vet*: 249-252, 1995.

301. Redig PT. Fluid therapy and acid-base balance in the critically ill avian patient. *Proc Annu Conf Assoc Avian Vet*: 59-73, 1984.

302. Redig PT. Treatment protocol for bumblefoot types 1 and 2. *AAV Today* 1:207-208, 1987.

303. Redig PT. Health management of raptors trained for falconry. *Proc Annu Conf Assoc Avian Vet*: 258-264, 1992.

304. Redig PT. Bumblefoot treatment in raptors. In: Fowler ME (ed). *Zoo & Wild Animal Medicine: Current Therapy 3*. WB Saunders Co, Philadelphia, 1993. Pp 181-188.

305. Redig P. *Medical Management of Birds of Prey: A Collection of Notes on Selected Topics.* The Raptor Center, St. Paul, MN, 1993.

306. Redig PT. Avian emergency. In: Beynon PH, Forbes NA, Harcourt-Brown NH (eds). *BSAVA Manual of Raptors, Pigeons and Waterfowl.* Iowa State University Press, Ames, IA, 1996. Pp 40-41.

307. Redig PT. Nursing avian patients. In: Beynon PH, Forbes NA, Harcourt-Brown NH (eds). *BSAVA Manual of Raptors, Pigeons and Waterfowl.* Iowa State University Press, Ames, IA, 1996. Pp 42-46.

308. Redig PT, Talbot B, Guarnera T. Avian malaria. *Proc Annu Conf Assoc Avian Vet*: 173-181, 1993.

309. Reiss AE, Badcock NR. Itraconazole levels in serum, skin and feathers of Gouldian finches (*Chloebia gouldiae*) following in-seed medication. *Proc Joint Conf Am Assoc Zoo Vet/Am Assoc Wildl Vet*: 142-143, 1998.

310. Reither NP. Medetomidine and atipamezole in avian practice. *Proc Euro Conf Avian Med Surg*: 43-48, 1993.

311. Ritchie BW. Avian therapeutics. *Proc Annu Conf Assoc Avian Vet*: 415-431, 1990.

312. Ritchie BW. Diagnosing and preventing common viral infections in companion birds. *Proc 21st Annu Waltham/OSU Symp*: 7-13, 1997.

313. Ritchie BW, Harrison GJ. Formulary. In: Ritchie BW, Harrison GJ, Harrison LR (eds). *Avian Medicine: Principles and Application.* Wingers Publ, Lake Worth, FL, 1994. Pp 457-478.

314. Ritchie BW, Harrison GJ. Formulary. In: Ritchie BW, Harrison GJ, Harrison LR (eds). *Avian Medicine: Principles and Application, Abridged edition.* Wingers Publ, Lake Worth, FL, 1997. Pp 227-253.

315. Ritchie BW, Harrison GJ, Harrison LR (eds). *Avian Medicine: Principles and Application.* Wingers Publ, Lake Worth, FL, 1994. Pp 1331-1347.

316. Roberts MF. *Pigeons.* TFH Publ, Jersey City, NJ, 1962.

317. Rolinski Z, Kowalski C, Wlaz P. Distribution and elimination of norfloxacin from broiler chicken tissues and eggs. *J Vet Pharmacol Ther* 20:200-201, 1997.

318. Romagnano A. Magnetic resonance imaging of the avian brain and abdominal cavity. *Proc Annu Conf Assoc Avian Vet*: 307-309, 1995.

319. Romagnano A. Avian obstetrics. *Semin Avian Exotic Pet Med* 5:180-188, 1996.

320. Rosenthal K, Stamoulis M. Diagnosis of congestive heart failure in an Indian Hill mynah bird (*Gracula religiosa*). *J Assoc Avian Vet* 7:27-30, 1993.

321. Rosskopf WJ, Jr, Woerpel RW. Avian obstetrical medicine. *Proc Annu Conf Assoc Avian Vet*: 323-336, 1993.

322. Rosskopf WJ, Woerpel RW. Practical avian therapeutics with dosages of commonly used medications. *Proc Basics Avian Med* (Sydney, Australia): 75-81, 1996.

323. Rosskopf WJ, Jr, Woerpel RW, Asterino R. Successful treatment of avian tuberculosis in pet psittacines. *Proc Annu Conf Assoc Avian Vet*: 238-251, 1991.

324. Rupiper DJ. Personal communication.

325. Rupiper DJ. IME—Allopurinol in simple syrup for gout. *J Assoc Avian Vet* 7:219, 1993.

326. Rupiper DJ. Diseases that affect race performance of homing pigeons. Part 1: husbandry, diagnostic strategies, and viral diseases. *J Avian Med Surg* 12:70-77, 1998.

327. Rupiper DJ, Ehrenberg M. Introduction to pigeon practice. *Proc Annu Conf Assoc Avian Vet*: 203-211, 1994.

328. Rupiper DJ, Ehrenberg M. Practical pigeon medicine. *Proc Annu Conf Assoc Avian Vet*: 479-497, 1997.

329. Rupley AE. Emergency procedures; recovering from disaster. *Proc Annu Conf Assoc Avian Vet*: 249-257, 1997.

330. Rupley AE. Respiratory bacterial, fungal and parasitic diseases. *Proc Avian Specialty Advanced Prog Small Mam and Rept Med Surg* (Annu Conf Assoc Avian Vet): 23-44, 1997.

331. Rupley AE. Critical care of pet birds; procedures, therapeutics, and patient support. *Vet Clin North Am: Exotic Anim Pract* 1:11-41, 1998.

332. Sabrautzki S. The course of gentamicin concentrations in serum and tissues of pigeons. Inaugural dissertation. Tierarztliche Fakultat der Ludwig-Maximilians-Universitat München. *Vet Bull* 54:5915, 1983.

333. Sander JE. Using contrast radiography to diagnose gastrointestinal diseases in birds. *Vet Med* (July): 652-655, 1996.

334. Schaeffer DO. Avian euthanasia. *Proc Annu Conf Assoc Avian Vet*: 287-288, 1996.

335. Scheer M, DeJong A, Froyman R, Heinen E. Antimicrobial activity in the digestive tract of broiler chickens treated orally with enrofloxacin. *J Vet Pharmacol Ther* 20:201-202, 1997.

336. Schobert E. Telazol® use in wild and exotic animals. *Vet Med* (Oct): 1080-1088, 1987.

337. Schöpf A, Vasicek L. Blood chemistry in canary finches (*Serinus canaria*). *Proc Euro Assoc Avian Vet*: 437-439, 1991.

338. Schumacker J, Bennett RA, Citino SB. Propofol: applications and limitations in exotic species. *Proc Euro Assoc Zoo Wildl Vet*: 427-430, 1998.

339. Scott JR. Passerine aviary diseases: diagnosis and treatment. *Proc Annu Conf Assoc Avian Vet*: 39-48, 1996.

340. Sedgwick CJ. Anesthesia of caged birds. In: Kirk RW (ed). *Current Veterinary Therapy VII: Small Animal Practice*. WB Saunders, Philadelphia, 1980. Pp 653-656.

341. Sellers C. Personal communication.

342. Shane SM, Tully TN. Equine encephalitis in emus—cause, diagnosis and prevention. *Emu Today and Tomorrow* (Feb): 38-39, 1993.

343. Smith JA, Tully TN, Cornick JL. Determination of isoflurane minimum anesthetic concentration in emus. *Proc Annu Conf Assoc Avian Vet*: 181-182, 1997.

344. Smith SA. Parasites of birds of prey: their diagnosis and treatment. *Semin Avian Exotic Pet Med* 5:97-105, 1996.

345. Snyder SB, Richard MJ. Treatment of avian tuberculosis in a whooping crane (*Grus americana*). Proc Am Assoc Zoo Vet: 167-170, 1994.

346. Soenens J, Vermeersch H, Baert K, et al. Pharmacokinetics and efficacy of amoxycillin in the treatment of an experimental *Streptococcus bovis* infection in racing pigeons (*Columba livia*). *J Vet Pharmacol Ther* 20:182-183, 1997.

347. Stadler C, Carpenter JW. Parasites of backyard game birds. *Semin Avian Exotic Pet Med* 5:85-96, 1996.

348. Stalis IH, Rideout BA, Allen JL, et al. Possible albendazole toxicity in birds. *Proc Am Assoc Zoo Vet*: 216-217, 1995.

349. Stetter MD, Sheppard C, Cook RA. Itraconazole-impregnated synthetic grit for sustained release dosing in avian species. *Proc Am Assoc Zoo Vet*: 181-185, 1996.

350. Stewart JS. IME—Restraint and anesthesia of ratites. *J Assoc Avian Vet* 4:90, 1990.

351. Stiles J, Buyukmihci NC, Farver TB. Tonometry of normal eyes in raptors. *Am J Vet Res* 55:477-479, 1994.

352. Stipkovits L, Burch DGS, Salyi G, Glavits R. Study to test the compatibility of Tetramutin® given in feed at different levels with salinomycin (60 ppm) in chickens. *J Vet Pharmacol Ther* 20:191-192, 1997.

353. Stone EG. Preliminary evaluation of hetastarch for the management of hypoproteinemia and hypovolemia. *Proc Annu Conf Assoc Avian Vet*: 197-199, 1994.

354. Stunkard JA. *Diagnostics, Treatment and Husbandry of Pet Birds.* Stunkard Publ Co, Edgewater, MD, 1984.

355. Suarez DL. Appetite stimulation in raptors. In: Redig PT, Cooper JE, Remple DJ, et al (eds). *Raptor Biomedicine.* University of Minnesota Press, Minneapolis, MN, 1993. Pp 225-228.

356. Suedmeyer WK. IME—Use of Adequan in articular diseases of avian species. *J Assoc Avian Vet* 7:105, 1993.

357. Suedmeyer WK, Haynes N, Roberts D. Clinical management of endoventricular mycoses in a group of African finches. *Proc Annu Conf Assoc Avian Vet*: 225-227, 1997.

358. Swalec-Tobias K, Schneider RK, Besser TE. Use of antimicrobial-impregnated polymethylmethacrylate. *J Am Vet Med Assoc* 208:841-845, 1996.

359. Tanner AC, Avakian AP, Barnes HJ, et al. A comparison of danofloxacin and tylosin in the control of induced *Mycoplasma gallisepticum* infection in broiler chicks. *Avian Dis* 37:515-522, 1993.

360. Taylor SM, Kenny J, Houston A, et al. Efficacy, pharmacokinetics and effect on egg-laying and hatchability of two dose rates of in-feed fenbendazole for the treatment of *Capillaria* species infections in chickens. *Vet Rec* 133:519-521, 1993.

361. Tell LA. Fluid therapy in raptors. *Proc N Am Vet Conf*: 572-573, 1995.

362. Tell L, Harrenstien L, Wetzlich S, et al. Pharmacokinetics of ceftiofur sodium in exotic and domestic avian species. *J Vet Pharmacol Ther* 21:85-91, 1998.

363. Tennant B. *Small Animal Formulary.* Stephens & George Ltd, Mid Glamorgan, Wales, UK, 1994.

364. Thomas-Baker B, Dew RD, Patton S. Ivermectin treatment of ocular nematodiasis in birds. *J Am Vet Med Assoc* 189:1113, 1986.

365. Tully TN. Personal communication.

366. Tully TN. A treatment protocol for non-responsive arthritis in companion birds. *Proc Annu Conf Assoc Avian Vet*: 45-49, 1994.

367. Tully TN, Shane SM. Ratite formulary. In: Tully TN, Shane SM (eds). *Ratite Management, Medicine and Surgery.* Krieger Publishing, Malabar, FL, 1996. Pp 158-163.

368. Turbahn A, De Jäckel S, Greuel E, et al. Dose response study of enrofloxacin against *Riemerella anatipestifer* septicaemia in Muscovy and Pekin ducklings. *Avian Pathol* 26:791-802, 1997.

369. Turner R. Trexan (naltrexone hydrochloride) use in feather picking in avian species. *Proc Annu Conf Assoc Avian Vet*: 116-118, 1993.

369a. University of Miami School of Medicine, Comparative Pathology Laboratory, Miami, FL.

370. Valverde A, Honeyman VL, Dyson DH, et al. Determination of a sedative dose and influence of midazolam on cardiopulmonary function in Canada geese. *Am J Vet Res* 51:1071-1074, 1990.

371. VanDerHeyden N. Update on avian mycobacteriosis. *Proc Annu Conf Assoc Avian Vet*: 53-62, 1994.

372. VanDerHeyden N. New strategies in the treatment of avian mycobacteriosis. *Semin Avian Exotic Pet Med* 6:25-33, 1997.

373. Van Sant F. Zinc and clinical disease in parrots. *Proc Annu Conf Assoc Avian Vet*: 387-391, 1997.

374. Vercruysse J. Efficacy of toltrazuril and clazuril against experimental infections with *Eimeria labbeana* and *E. columbarum* in racing pigeons. *Avian Dis* 34:73-79, 1990.

375. Vriends MM. *Simon & Schuster's Guide to Pet Birds.* Simon & Schuster, New York, 1984.

376. Wagner CH, Hochleitner M, Rausch W-D. Ketoconazole plasma levels in buzzards. *Proc First Conf Euro Comm Assoc Avian Vet*: 333-340, 1991.

377. Welle KR. A review of psychotropic drug therapy. *Proc Annu Conf Assoc Avian Vet*: 121-124, 1998.

378. Westerhof I. Treatment of tracheal obstruction in psittacine birds using a suction technique: A retrospective study of 19 birds. *J Avian Med Surg* 9:45-49, 1995.

378a. Weston HS. The successful treatment of sarcocystosis in two keas (*Nestor nobilis*) at the Franklin Park Zoo. *Proc Am Assoc Zoo Vet*: 186-191, 1996.

379. Wheler C. Avian anesthetics, analgesics and tranquilizers. *Semin Avian Exotic Pet Med* 2:7-12, 1993.

380. Wheler CL, Machin KL, Lew LJ. Use of antibiotic-impregnated polymethyl-methacrylate beads in the treatment of chronic osteomyelitis and cellulitis in a juvenile bald eagle (*Haliaeetus leucocephalus*). *Proc Annu Conf Assoc Avian Vet*: 187-194, 1996.

381. White J. Neotropical songbirds and veterinary medicine: are we giving them the attention they deserve? *Proc Annu Conf Assoc Avian Vet*: 77-82, 1997.

382. Williams M, Smith PJ, Loerzel SM, Dunn JL. Evaluation of the efficacy of vecuronium bromide as a mydriatic in several different species of aquatic birds. *Proc Annu Conf Assoc Avian Vet*: 113-117, 1996.

383. Wilson RC, Zenoble RD, Horton CR, et al. Single dose digoxin pharmacokinetics in the Quaker conure (*Myopsitta monachus*). *J Zoo Wildl Med* 20:432-434, 1989.

384. Woerpel RW, Rosskopf WJ, Jr. Clinical experience with avian laboratory diagnostics. *Vet Clin North Am: Small Anim Pract* 14:249-286, 1984.

385. Ziv G, Shem-Tov M, Glickman A, et al. Serum oxytetracycline and chlortetracycline concentrations in broilers and turkeys treated with high doses of the drugs via the feed and water. *J Vet Pharmacol Ther* 20:190-191, 1997.

386. Ziv G, Shem-Tov M, Glickman A, Saran A. Concentrations of amoxycillin and clavulanic acid in the serum of broilers during continuous and pulse-dosing of the drinking water. *J Vet Pharmacol Therap* 20:183-184, 1997.

387. Zuchowska E. Some blood parameters in zoo birds. *Proc Euro Conf Avian Med Surg*: 493-506, 1993.

388. Zwijnenberg RJG, Vulto AG, Van Miert ASJPAM, Lumeij JT. Evaluation of antibiotics for racing pigeons (*Columba livia* var. *domestica*) available in the Netherlands. *J Vet Pharmacol Therap* 15:364-378, 1992.

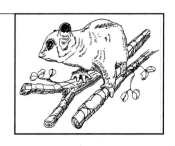

Table 36. Antimicrobial agents used in sugar gliders [a]

Agent	Dosage	Comments
Amoxicillin	30 mg/kg IM q24h[7]	
Amoxicillin/clavulanic acid (Clavamox, Pfizer)	12.5 mg/kg SC q24h[16]	Injectable form not available in US
Cephalexin	30 mg/kg SC q24h[16]	Injectable form not available in US
Enrofloxacin	5 mg/kg PO, IM q12h[16]	Tissue necrosis may occur when administered parenterally
Lincomycin	30 mg/kg IM q24h[7]	
Metronidazole	80 mg/kg PO q24h[7]	
Trimethoprim/ sulfamethoxazole	15 mg/kg PO q12h[13] 50-57 mg/kg PO q24h[9]	

[a] Dosages of select drugs may also be based on the low end of ranges for cats, ferrets, or hedgehogs.[10]

Table 37. Antiparasitic agents used in sugar gliders [a]

Agent	Dosage	Comments
Carbaryl powder (5%)	Topical[2]	Ectoparasites; use sparingly; can be used in nest boxes
Fenbendazole	20-50 mg/kg PO q24h × 3 days[2]	Roundworms, hookworms, whipworms; cestodes
Ivermectin	0.2 mg/kg PO, SC, repeat in 14 days[2]	Roundworms, hookworms, whipworms; ascariasis
Oxfendazole	5 mg/kg PO single dose[2]	Roundworms; cestodes (adult)
Pyrethrin powder	Topical[14]	Ectoparasites; use products safe for kittens

[a] Dosages of select antiparasitic agents may also be based on the low end of ranges for cats, ferrets, or hedgehogs.[10]

Table 38. Chemical restraint/anesthetic/analgesic agents used in sugar gliders [a,b]

Agent	Dosage	Comments
Acepromazine	—	See butorphanol, ketamine for combinations
Butorphanol	—	Butorphanol combination follows [3]
	0.5 mg/kg IM[13]	Analgesia
Butorphanol (B)/ acepromazine (A)	(B) 1.7 mg/kg/ (A) 1.7 mg/kg PO[9]	Post-operative sedation and analgesia to prevent self-trauma to incision site; dilute with normal saline to administer
Flunixin meglumine	0.1 mg/kg IM[13]	Analgesia; non-steroidal anti-inflammatory
Isoflurane	5% induction;[1] 2-3% maintenance[16]	Anesthetic of choice
Ketamine	—	Ketamine combination follows
	20 mg/kg IM[7]	Followed with isoflurane
Ketamine (K)/ acepromazine (A)	(K) 10 mg/kg/ (A) 1mg/kg SC[9]	Post-operative sedation and analgesia to prevent self-trauma to incision site

[a] Dosages of select drugs may also be based on the low end of ranges for cats, ferrets, or hedgehogs.[10]

[b] Do not use tiletamine/zolazepam because it has caused neurologic syndromes and death in squirrel gliders at doses of 10 mg/kg.[6]

Appendix 38. Biological and physiologic values of the sugar glider [4,5,8,12,15,17-19]

Parameter	Normal values
Average life span (wild) Male Female	 4-5 yr 5-7 yr
Maximum reported life span (captivity)	15 yr
Adult weight[a]	♂, 115-160 g (av 140 g) ♀, 95-135 g (av 115 g)
Body length	16-21 cm (av 17 cm)
Tail length	16.5-21.0 cm (av 19 cm)
Heart rate	200-300 beats/min
Respiratory rate	16-40 breaths/min
Rectal temperature	$36.2 \pm 0.4\ °C\ (97.2 \pm 0.7\ °F)$
Basal metabolic rate	$2.54\ W^{0.75}$
Estrus cycle • Type • Length	 Seasonally polyestrus 29 days
Gestation period	15-17 days
Litter size	1-2 (usually 2)
Birth weight	0.19 g
Pouch emergence	60-70 days
Weaning age	110-120 days
Sexual maturity	♂, 12-14 mo; ♀, 8-12 mon

a Weights are for adult sugar gliders (*Petaurus breviceps breviceps*). Many sugar gliders in
  the US are the New Guinean spp which are smaller. Weights of ≤ 100 g are more
  typical.[11,13]

Appendix 39. Hematologic values of the sugar glider [a]

Measurement	International Species Information System values[8]	Currumbin Sanctuary Queensland Australia values [b,2]
PCV (%)	43.7 ± 4.0 (18)	47.6 [40-51] (7)
RBC ($10^6/\mu l$)	7.9 ± 0.9 (17)	7.5 [6.5-8.3] (7)
Hemoglobin (g/dl)	15.5 ± 1.6 (18)	15.1 [12.8-16.2] (7)
WBC ($10^3/\mu l$)	5.3 ± 3.2 (17)	16.3 [9.1-22.8] (7)
Segmented neutrophils ($10^3/\mu l$)	1.3 ± 1.1 (17)	1.0 [0.5-1.8] (7)
Band neutrophils ($10^3/\mu l$)	0.12 ± 0.05 (2)	—
Lymphocytes ($10^3/\mu l$)	3.8 ± 2.2 (17)	15.0 [8.3-21.2] (7)
Monocytes ($10^3/\mu l$)	0.17 ± 0.18 (15)	0.05 [0.0-0.23] (7)
Eosinophils ($10^3/\mu l$)	0.10 ± 0.06 (13)	0.23 [0.0-0.99] (7)
Basophils ($10^3/\mu l$)	—	0 (7)
NRBC/100 WBC	2 ± 1 (6)	0 (7)
Platelets ($10^3/\mu l$)	728 ±176 (3)	—

[a] Sample size is presented in ( ); range is in [ ].
[b] Reference ranges for *Petaurus breviceps breviceps*; blood collected from the medial tibial artery.

Appendix 40. Serum biochemical values of the sugar glider [a]

Measurement	International Species Information System values[8]	Currumbin Sanctuary Queensland Australia values [b,2]
AP (IU/L)	182 ± 30 (3)	188 (1)
ALT (IU/L)	78 ± 41 (11)	36 [28-44] (3)
AST (IU/L)	79 ± 72 (13)	49.7 [20-70] (3)
Bilirubin, total (mg/dl)	0.3 ± 0.2 (10)	—
Calcium (mg/dl)	8.9 ± 0.2 (3)	9.6 (1)
Chloride (mEq/L)	106 ± 1 (3)	105 [101-109] (5)
Cholesterol (mg/dl)	161 ± 2 (3)	200 [128-248] (3)
CPK (IU/L)	503 ± 48 (3)	224 (1)
Creatinine (mg/dl)	0.7 ± 0.1 (3)	0.8 [0.2-1.5] (7)
Glucose (mg/dl)	154 ± 78 (12)	50 [5-124] (3)[c]
LDH (IU/L)	246 ± 33 (3)	—
Phosphorus (mg/dl)	5.5 ± 0.5 (3)	8.1 (1)
Potassium (mEq/L)	3.2 ± 0.4 (3)	5.4 [4.4-6.3] (3)
Protein, total (g/dl)	6.0 ± 0.6 (11)	5.9 [4.0-6.9] (7)
Albumin (g/dl)	4.6 ± 0.2 (3)	3.3 [3.0-3.5] (7)
Globulin (g/dl)	1.7 ± 0.2 (3)	2.6 [0.6-3.0] (7)
Sodium (mEq/L)	145 ± 2 (3)	144 [138-158] (4)
Urea nitrogen (mg/dl)	33 ± 56 (12)	18 [10-27] (7)

[a] Sample size is presented in ( ); range is in [ ].
[b] Reference ranges for *Petaurus breviceps breviceps*; blood collected from the medial tibial artery.
[c] Glucose test was performed on whole blood up to 24 hr post-collection; therefore, values may be invalid.

Appendix 41. Dietary components for sugar gliders in captivity [1]

Fruit	Oranges, watermelon, paw paw, pears, kiwifruit, apricots, berries, bananas, apples, mangos, grapes, melons, figs
Invertebrates	Mealworms, grasshoppers, moths, fly pupae, crickets
Blossoms and branches	*Eucalyptus, Banksia, Leptospermum, Grevillea, Acacia, Melaleuca, Callistemum, Hakea*
Supplements	Puppy chow,[a] nectar mix,[b] vitamins, minerals

[a]   Pelleted diets for sugar gliders are being developed and may be preferable.
[b]   Gliderade, Avico; Nekton-Lori, Nekton USA.

Appendix 42. Suggested sugar glider diets [a,5]

Diet 1[a,3]		
Items (mixed into a slurry)	% of diet by weight	Amount (g) per adult animal
• Chopped, mixed fruit[b]	40	12.0
• Cooked, chopped vegetables[c]	8	2.5
• Peach or apricot nectar	34	10.0
• Ground, dry, low-iron bird diet[d]	18	5.5
Total	**100**	**30.0**

Diet 2[e,11]

50% Leadbeater's mixture (150 ml warm water; 150 ml honey; 1 shelled, hard-boiled egg; 25 g high protein baby cereal; 1 tsp vitamin/mineral supplement)
- Mix warm water and honey
- In separate container, blend egg until homogenized
- Gradually add honey/water, then vitamin powder, then baby cereal, and blend after each addition until smooth
- Keep refrigerated until served

50% Insectivore/carnivore diet (ie, Mazuri Brand, Purina Mills, St. Louis, MO; Reliable Protein Products, Palm Desert, CA; ZuPreem, Mission, KS)

[a]   Insects can be added to this diet to help prevent dental problems.
[b]   Any fruit, but less than 10% citrus.
[c]   Steamed or microwaved; 50:50 starchy:nonstarchy vegetables (eg, 50% sweet potato, 50% carrot).
[d]   Zeigler Lo-iron Bird of Paradise pellets (Zeigler Brothers, Inc., Gardners, PA) or Marion Zoological Red Apple Jungle Scenic Birdfood (Marion Zoological Scenic Birdfoods, Plymouth, MN).
[e]   Feed fresh portions in evening; chop items together to reduce only favorite foods being selected. Can offer treats (meats, diced fruits with multiple vitamin/mineral powder, bee pollen, worms, and crickets and other gut-loaded insects) at ≈ 5% of daily intake.

Appendix 43. Growth and development of sugar gliders [2]

Age (days)	Weight (g)	Feed[a] (ml/day)	Development
1	0.2	—	Mouth and forelimbs most developed feature
20	0.8	—	Ears free from head; papillae of mystacial vibrissae (whiskers) visible
35	2	1	Mystacial vibrissae erupt; ears pigmented
40	3	1.5	Start to pigment on shoulders; eyeslits present
60	12	3	Detaching from teat; fur emerging; dorsal stripe developing
70	20	4	Eyes open; fully furred; left in nest
80	35	6	Fur lengthens
90	44	7	—
100	54	8	Emerging from nest; start eating solids
130	78	—	Weaned

[a] Based on a low-lactose milk replacer.

Appendix 44. Literature cited - Sugar gliders

1. Booth RJ. Medicine and husbandry: dasyurids, possums, and bats. *Proc 233 Wildl Post Grad Comm Vet Sci*: 423-441, 1994.

2. Booth RJ. General husbandry and medical care of sugar gliders. In: Bonagura JD (ed). *Kirk's Current Veterinary Therapy XIII: Small Animal Practice*. WB Saunders Co, Philadelphia, 2000. Pp 1157-1163.

3. Dempsey J. Personal communication. 1997.

4. Grzimek B, Ganslosser U. Ringtails and gliders. In: Grzimek B (ed). *Grzimek's Encyclopedia of Mammals*. Vol 1. McGraw-Hill Publishing Co, New York, 1990. Pp 318-324.

5. Henry SR, Suckling GC. A review of the ecology of the sugar glider. In: Smith PA, Hume ID (eds). *Possums and Gliders*. Australian Mammal Society, Sydney, 1984. Pp 355-358.

6. Holz P. Immobilization of marsupials with tiletamine and zolazepam. *J Zoo Wildl Med* 23:426-428, 1992.

7. Hough I, Reuter RE, Rahaley RS, et al. Cutaneous lymphosarcoma in a sugar glider. *Aust Vet J* 69:93-94, 1992.

8. *International Species Information System (ISIS)*, 12101 Johnny Cake Rd, Apple Valley, MN.

9. Johnson SD. Orchiectomy of the mature sugar glider (*Petaurus breviceps*). *Exotic Pet Pract* 2:71, 1997.

10. Johnson-Delaney CA. *Exotic Companion Medicine Handbook for Veterinarians* (Supplement). Wingers Publishing, Lake Worth, FL, 1996. Pp 17-23.

11. Johnson-Delaney CA. The marsupial pet: sugar gliders, exotic possums, and wallabies. *Proc Assoc Avian Vet*: 329-339, 1998.

12. MacPherson C. *Sugar Gliders (A Complete Pet Owner's Manual)*. Barron's Educational Series, Inc., Hong Kong, 1997.

13. MacPherson C. Personal communication. 1998.

14. Ness RD. Introduction to sugar gliders. *N Am Vet Conf Proc*: 864-865, 1998.

15. Nowak RM. *Walker's Mammals of the World*. 5th ed. Vol 1. Johns Hopkins University Press, Baltimore, MD, 1991. Pp 74-76.

16. Pye GW, Carpenter JW. A guide to medicine and surgery in sugar gliders. *Vet Med* (Oct): 891-905, 1999.

17. Strahan R. *The Mammals of the World*. Reed Books, Chatswood, Australia. 1995.

18. Tyndale-Biscoe CH. Reproductive physiology of possums and gliders. In: Smith PA, Hume ID (eds). *Possums and Gliders*. Australian Mammal Society, Sydney, 1984. Pp 79-87.

19. Tyndale-Biscoe CH, Renfree M. *Reproductive Physiology of Marsupials*. Cambridge University Press, Cambridge, UK, 1987.

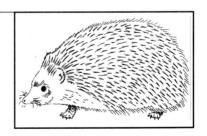

Table 39. Antimicrobial and antifungal agents used in hedgehogs

Agent	Dosage	Comments
Ampicillin	10 mg/kg IM q12h[6,7]	
Amoxicillin	15 mg/kg IM q12h[6]	
Amoxicillin/ clavulanate (Clavamox, Pfizer)	12.5 mg/kg PO[14] q12h	
Chloramphenicol	30 mg/kg IM q12h[6,7] 50 mg/kg PO, SC, IM, q12h[5-7]	Acute salmonellosis
Clindamycin (Antirobe, Upjohn)	5.5 mg/kg PO q12h[14]	Anaerobes; dental disease
Enilconazole (Imaverol, Janssen)	Topical q24h[14]	Dermatophytosis; dilute 1:50
Enrofloxacin	2.5-5.0 mg/kg PO, IM[10] q12h 5-10 mg/kg PO, SC, IM q12h[5]	
Erythromycin	10 mg/kg PO, IM q12h[6,7]	Penicillin-resistant gram + cocci; *Mycoplasma; Pasteurella; Bordetella*
Gentamicin	2 mg/kg SC, IM q8h[5]	Rarely indicated
Griseofulvin (microsize)	— 25 mg/kg PO q12h[6] 50 mg/kg PO q24h[6]	Skin and deep mycoses; long-term therapy
Ketoconazole	10 mg/kg PO q24h[6] × 6-8 wk	Mycoses; use long-term
Lime sulfur	Topical[4]	Dermatophytosis
Oxytetracycline	50 mg/kg PO q24h[3]	*Bordetella*; may be administered in food
Penicillin G	40,000 IU/kg IM q24h[6]	
Spiramycin	15 mg/kg PO × 8 days[6]	Gingivitis
Sulfadimethoxine	2-20 mg/kg PO, SC, IM q24h[5,6]	
Trimethoprim/sulfa	30 mg/kg PO, SC, IM q12h[5,10]	Respiratory infections
Tylosin (Tylan, Elanco)	10 mg/kg PO[6] q12h[7]	*Mycoplasma; Clostridium;* do not administer IM (causes muscle necrosis)

Table 40. Antiparasitic agents used in hedgehogs

Agent	Dosage	Comments
Amitraz (Mitaban, Upjohn)	0.3% topical q7d × 2-3 wk[8]	Mites (*Chorioptes*, sarcoptic, *Demodex*, etc.); may dilute; use with caution
Fenbendazole	5 mg/kg PO q24h × 5 days[14]	Nematodes
	10-30 mg/kg PO × 5 days[7]	Nematodes (ie, *Crenosoma, Capillaria*)
	20-30 mg/kg PO q10d[5]	Nematodes
Flea products (feline)	Topical[4]	Use sparingly
Ivermectin	0.2 mg/kg PO, SC,[10] repeat q14d × 3 treatments	Mites (*Chorioptes*, sarcoptic, etc; efficacy on *Demodex* is questionable); nematodes
	0.2-0.4 mg/kg PO, SC q10-14d[5,9]	Ectoparasites
Levamisole (1%)	10 mg/kg SC,[3] repeat q48h; repeat prn q14d[6]	Nematodes, including lungworms
Metronidazole	25 mg/kg PO q12h[4] × 5 days	Flagellates
Permethrin (1%)	Topical[13]	Mites; apply once via fine mist; change bedding
Praziquantel (Droncit, Mobay)	7 mg/kg PO, SC,[4] repeat q14d	Cestodes, trematodes
Sulfadimethoxine	2-20 mg/kg q24h PO,[6] SC, IM[7] × 2-5 days, off 5 days, on 2-5 days[6]	Coccidia
Sulfadimidine	100-200 mg/kg SC q24h × 3 days[3]	Coccidia

Table 41. Chemical restraint/anesthetic/analgesic agents used in hedgehogs

Agent	Dosage	Comments
Atipamezole (Antisedan, Pfizer)	0.3-0.5 mg/kg IM[14] 1.0 mg/kg IM[1]	Reversal of medetomidine
Buprenorphine (Buprenex, Reckitt & Colman)	0.01 mg/kg SC, IM q6-8h[3,12,14]	Analgesia
Butorphanol (Torbugesic, Fort Dodge)	0.05 mg/kg q8h SC prn[7] 0.2-0.4 mg/kg IM, SC q6-8h[12]	Analgesia Analgesia
Diazepam	0.5-2.0 mg/kg[10] IM	Mild sedation; may be given with ketamine for anesthesia; seizures
Fentanyl	—	See medetomidine for combination
Flunixin meglumine	No dose established - SC, IM[14]	Nonsteroidal, anti-inflammatory
Halothane	To effect	Rarely used; less preferable than isoflurane
Isoflurane	3-5%[10] induction 0.5-3.0%[12] maintenance	Anesthetic of choice; generally occurs in an induction chamber or mask Via mask or endotracheal tube
Ketamine	— 5-20 mg/kg[10] IM	See medetomidine for combinations Sedation; anesthesia; do not use in neck area where there is brown fat;[7] may use in combination with diazepam or xylazine; recovery may be prolonged and/or rough
Medetomidine (Domitor, Pfizer)	— 0.1 mg/kg IM[14]	Medetomidine combinations follow Light sedation; reverse with atipamezole
Medetomidine (M)/ ketamine (K)	(M) 0.1 mg/kg/ (K) 5 mg/kg IM[14]	Anesthesia; (M) can be reversed with atipamezole (0.3-0.5 mg/kg)
Medetomidine (M)/ ketamine (K)/ fentanyl (F)	(M) 0.2 mg/kg/ (K) 2 mg/kg/ (F) 0.1 mg/kg SC[1]	Anesthesia; good muscle relaxation; (M) can be reversed with atipamezole (1.0 mg/kg IM) and (F) can be reversed with naloxone (0.16 mg/kg IM)

Table 41. Chemical restraint/anesthetic/analgesic agents used in hedgehogs (cont.)

Agent	Dosage	Comments
Naloxone	0.16 mg/kg IM[1]	Reversal of fentanyl
Tiletamine/zolazepam (Telazol, Fort Dodge)	1-5 mg/kg[10] IM	Sedation; anesthesia; recovery may be prolonged and/or rough
Xylazine	0.5-1.0 mg/kg[10] IM	Anesthesia; may be given with ketamine

Table 42. Miscellaneous agents used in hedgehogs

Agent	Dosage	Comments
Calcium gluconate (10%)	0.5 mg/kg IM[6]	Fractures
Dexamethasone	0.1-1.5 mg/kg IM[6]	Inflammation; allergies
	5 mg/kg IM[6]	Shock
Furosemide	2.5-5.0 mg/kg q8h[14] SC, IM	Edema; diuretic
Iron dextran	25 mg/kg IM[14]	Anemia
Lactobacilli	1/2 tsp/kg q24h[6]	May aid in restoring gastrointestinal flora
Prednisolone	2.5 mg/kg SC q12h[6] prn	Allergies
	10 mg/kg SC, IM[6]	Shock
Vitamin A	400 IU/kg IM q24h × 10 days[6]	Skin disorders; excessive spine loss
Vitamin B complex	1 ml/kg IM[7]	CNS signs; paralysis of unknown origin; anorexia
Vitamin C	50-200 mg/kg PO, SC q24h[6]	Deficiency; infections; gingival disease; can use 1 g ascorbic acid/L drinking water (change daily)
Vitamins, multiple	1-2 drops/kg PO q24h[6]	Subclinical deficiency; hand-rearing orphans

267

Appendix 45. Hematologic and serum biochemical values of hedgehogs [6]

Measurement	Reference range
Hematology	
PCV (%)	36.0-38.5
RBC ($10^6/\mu l$)	7.03-7.64
Hgb (g/dl)	12.0-13.2
MCH (pg)	16.8-18.2
MCHC (g/dl)	33.3-35.2
MCV (fl)	49.1-53.2
Thrombocytes (μl)	230-430
Reticulocytes (%)	8-14
WBC ($10^3/\mu l$)	6.3-9.6
Neutrophils ($10^3/\mu l$)	1.6-2.8
Lymphocytes ($10^3/\mu l$)	3.72-6.14
Monocytes ($10^3/\mu l$)	0-0.084
Eosinophils ($10^3/\mu l$)	0.36-2.4
Basophils ($10^3/\mu l$)	0.096-0.45
Chemistries	
Calcium (mg/dl)	8.0-9.2
Phosphorus (mg/dl)	6.2-11.8
Potassium (mEq/L)	3.6-5.1
Protein, total (g/dl)	5.1-7.2
Sodium (mEq/L)	132-138
Urea (mg/dl)	37-42

Appendix 46. Biological and physiological values of hedgehogs [3,4,6,7,10,12]

Parameter	African hedgehog (*Atelerix albiventris*)	European hedgehog (*Erinaceus europaeus*)
Weight	♂ 500-600 g ♀ 250-400 g	♂ 800-1200 g ♀ 400-800 g
Temperature, rectal	36.1-37.2 °C (97-99 °F)	34-37 °C (93.2-98.6 °F)
Breeding age	♂ 6-8 mo ♀ 2-6 mo	♂ 9-10 mo ♀ 9-10 mo
Gestation	34-37 days	32 days
Litter size	1-7 (rarely to 10) (av 3)	3-5 (occasionally to 8)
Birth weight	8-13 g	8-15 g
Eyes open	13-16 days	13-16 days
Weaning age	4-5 wk	5-6 wk
Life expectancy	5-8 yr	6-10 yr
Preferred environmental temperature	25-30 °C (75-85 °F)	22-27 °C (70-80 °F)

Appendix 47. Suggested diets for hedgehogs [2,7,10]

The natural diet of hedgehogs includes insects, worms, snails, slugs, and, occasionally, small vertebrates and fruit. Because hedgehogs are insectivores and require a high-protein diet, they are commonly fed a high quality cat (or ferret) food (largely dry, but some canned or semi-moist can be provided), small amounts of diced fruits and vegetables, crickets, and mealworms. Small amounts of chicken, scrambled or hard-boiled eggs, and cottage cheese may be used. One key to balanced nutrition is to provide variety. Also, commercial hedgehog diets are available, convenient, and appropriate as the main component of the diet. Do not overfeed hedgehogs because of potential obesity; amounts can be adjusted up or down to meet special nutritional situations (ie, pregnancy, obesity). Hedgehogs are generally fed once a day in the evening. Specific diet compositions are listed below.

Diet I (for one adult hedgehog [550 g])
- 1 heaping tsp bird of prey diet or insectivore diet
- 1.5 heaping tsp high quality cat/kitten chow (ie, Hill's Science Diet, Hill's c/d cat food, Iams, Ferret Chow)
  - For younger or pregnant/lactating animals, use kitten or ferret formulations; adults may use "Lite" adult cat foods
- 1 heaping tsp fruit/vegetable mixture
  - Fruit/vegetable mix: chop together 1/2 tsp diced leafy dark greens (spinach, kale, leaf lettuce); 1/4 tsp diced carrot; 1/4 tsp diced apple; 1/4 tsp diced banana; 1/4 tsp diced grape or raisin; 1/4 tsp vitamin/mineral powder (Vionate, ARC; or crushed feline tablet)
- 6-10 small mealworms or 1-2 crickets (more if pregnant or lactating)

Diet II (for one adult hedgehog)
- 2-3 Tbs dry reduced-calorie cat food or mix of dry and canned food
- 1-2 Tbs mixed frozen vegetables
- 3-5 insects 3-4 times/wk
- Can offer limited quantities (1-2 tsp 3-4 times/wk): baby food, hard-boiled egg, wax worms, pinky mice, horsemeat

Diet III (for one adult hedgehog)
- 3 heaping tsp high quality cat/kitten chow
- 1 heaping tsp fruit/vegetable mix
- 6 small mealworms or 1-2 crickets

Diet IV (for one adult hedgehog)
- Nebraska Brand Bird of Prey Diet (Animal Spectrum) (15 g)
- Cat chow or dog kibble (10 g)
- Fruit/vegetable mixture (10 g) (diced apple [1 part]; spinach, kale, or other leafy greens [1 part]; diced bananas [1/2 part]; diced carrots [1/2 part]; sliced grapes or raisins [1/4 part]; $CaCO_3$ powder [0.03 part]; multivitamin/mineral supplement [0.015 part])
- Small amounts of items such as hard-boiled eggs, evaporated milk, cottage cheese, wax worms, small mice, and vegetable/beef baby food may occasionally be added

Appendix 48. Hand-rearing orphaned hedgehogs [11]

1. Leave neonates with mother if possible for first 24-72 hr for colostrum ingestion.

2. Feed puppy or kitten milk replacer or goat's milk (2 parts) with goat's colostrum (1 part) using a 1 cc syringe with a catheter tip or an eye dropper.

3. Neonates should be fed as much as they will eat every 2-3 hr for the first week and then the time between feedings can be gradually lengthened. The newborns should gain 1-2 g/day for the first 10 days and then 4-5 g/day for 2-3 wk and 7-9 g/day until 8-9 wk old. Solid foods should be offered after 2-3 wk and weaning should take place around 4 wk of age.

4. Manual stimulation is required for defecation and should be performed after each meal.

5. Cross-fostering to another nursing hedgehog can be performed.

Appendix 49. Literature cited - Hedgehogs

1. Arnemo JM, Soli NE. Chemical immobilization of free-ranging European hedgehogs (*Erinaceus europaeus*). *J Zoo Wildl Med* 26:246-251, 1995.

2. Crawford RL. Fact sheet: brief introduction to hedgehogs. Animal Welfare Information Center, National Agricultural Library, Beltsville, MD, 1995. 7 pp.

3. Gregory MW, Stocker L. Hedgehogs. In: Beynon PH, Cooper JE (eds). *Manual of Exotic Pets*. Brit Small Anim Vet Assoc, Gloucestershire, GB, 1991. Pp 63-68.

4. Hoefer HL. Hedgehogs. *Vet Clin N Am: Small Anim Pract* 24:113-120, 1994.

5. Hoefer HL. Clinical approach to the African hedgehog. *Proc N Am Vet Conf*: 836-838, 1999.

6. Isenbügel E, Baumgartner RA. Diseases of the hedgehog. In: Fowler ME (ed). *Zoo & Wild Animal Medicine: Current Therapy 3*. WB Saunders Co, Philadelphia, 1993. Pp 294-302.

7. Johnson-Delaney CA. Hedgehogs. In: *Exotic Companion Medicine Handbook for Veterinarians*. Wingers Publ, Lake Worth, FL, 1996.

8. Letcher JD. Amitraz as a treatment for acariasis in African hedgehogs (*Atelerix albiventris*). *J Zoo Anim Med* 19:24-29, 1988.

9. Morrisey JK. Personal communication. 1999.

10. Smith AJ. Husbandry and medicine of African hedgehogs (*Atelerix albiventris*). *J Small Exotic Anim Med* 2:21-28, 1992.

11. Smith AJ. Neonatology of the hedgehog (*Atelerix albiventris*). *J Small Exotic Anim Med* 3:15-18, 1995.

12. Smith AJ. Medical management of hedgehogs. *Proc 21st Annu Waltham/OSU Symp:* 57-61, 1997.

13. Staley EC, Staley EE. Use of permethrin as a miticide in the African hedgehog (*Atelerix albiventris*). *Vet Human Toxicol* 36:138, 1994.

14. Stocker L. Medication for use in the treatment of hedgehogs. Marshcliff, Ayelsbury, UK, 1992.

Fish

Amphibians

Reptiles

Birds

Sugar Gliders

Hedgehogs

▶ **Rodents**

Rabbits

Ferrets

Miniature Pigs

Primates

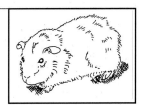

Table 43. Antimicrobial and antifungal agents used in rodents [a]

Agent	Dosage	Comments
Amikacin	2-5 mg/kg SC, IM q8-12h[18]	All/q12h in prairie dogs[44]
	15 mg/kg IM q12h[49]	High peak dosing regimen as effective as divided regimens
Ampicillin	20-100 mg/kg PO, SC, IM q12h[2]	Mice, rats
	6-30 mg/kg PO q8h[2]	Gerbils
Captan powder (Orthocide, Chevron)	1 tsp/2 cups dust[21]	Chinchillas/fungicide to prevent spread of dermatophytes between cagemates; add to dust box
Carbenicillin	100 mg/kg PO q12h[2]	Mice, rats
Ceftiofur	1 mg/kg IM q24h[17]	Guinea pigs/pneumonia
Cephalexin	50 mg/kg IM q24h[38]	Guinea pigs
Cephaloridine	10-25 mg/kg SC, IM q24h[2]	Hamsters, mice, rats
	10-25 mg/kg IM q8-24h[2]	Guinea pigs
Chloramphenicol	0.5 mg/ml drinking water[6]	Mice
	0.83 mg/ml drinking water[6]	Gerbils
	1 mg/ml drinking water[6]	Guinea pigs
	50 mg/kg PO q12h[6,11,44]	Chinchillas, guinea pigs, prairie dogs
	50-200 mg/kg PO q8h[6,11]	Gerbils, hamsters, mice, rats
	30-50 mg/kg SC, IM q12h[6,11]	All
Chloramphenicol ophthalmic ointment	Topical to eyes q6-12h[39]	All
Chlortetracycline	50 mg/kg PO q12h[1]	Chinchillas
	6-10 mg/kg SC, IM q12h[1]	Rats
	20 mg/kg SC, IM q12h[1]	Hamsters
	25 mg/kg SC, IM q12h[1]	Mice

Table 43. Antimicrobial and antifungal agents used in rodents (cont.)

Agent	Dosage	Comments
Ciprofloxacin	7-20 mg/kg PO q12h[18]	All/may cause arthropathies in young
Doxycycline	2.5 mg/kg PO q12h[1]	All
	5 mg/kg PO q12h[18]	Mice, rats/pneumonia; do not use in young and pregnant animals
Enilconazole	Dip q7d[39]	Dermatophytosis; dilute to 0.2% solution
Enrofloxacin	—	All/may cause arthropathies in young; limit SC, IM injections; SC injections can be diluted in NaCl or LRS
	2.5-5.0 mg/kg PO, SC, IM q12h[11]	
	5-10 mg/kg PO, IM q12h[18]	
	25-85 mg/kg q24h × 14 days[16]	Mice/pasteurellosis
	0.05-0.20 mg/ml drinking water × 14 days[18]	
Erythromycin	20 mg/kg PO[47]	
	0.13 mg/ml drinking water[7]	Hamsters/outbreaks of proliferative ileitis; caution: can cause enterotoxemia
Furazolidone	5.5 mg/ml drinking water[6]	Guinea pigs
	30 mg/kg PO q24h[6]	Hamsters
Gentamicin	2-4 mg/kg SC, IM q8-24h[18]	All
	5 mg/kg SC, IM q24h[2,6,11]	All
	6 mg/kg SC q24h[8]	Guinea pigs
	10 mg/kg drinking water or topical[13]	Gerbils/nasal dermatitis
Griseofulvin	—	Dermatophytosis; do not use in pregnant animals; can cause diarrhea, leukopenia, anorexia[18]

276

Table 43. Antimicrobial and antifungal agents used in rodents (cont.)

Agent	Dosage	Comments
Griseofulvin (continued)	25-50 mg/kg PO q12h × 14-60 days[18]	All
	25 mg/kg PO q24h × 30-60 days[25]	Chinchillas/use with lime sulfur dips
	15-25 mg/kg PO q24h × 14-28 days[36]	Guinea pigs/doses up to 100 mg/kg have been used
	250 mg/kg PO q10d × 4 treatments on feed[26]	Prairie dogs
	1.5% in DMSO topical × 5-7 days[18]	All
Ketoconazole	10-40 mg/kg PO q24h × 14 days[18]	Mice, rats/systemic mycoses; candidiasis
Lime sulfur dip	Dip q7d × 6 wk[2]	All/dermatophytosis; dilute 1:40 with water
Metronidazole	—	Anaerobes; add sucrose for palatability
	2.5 mg/ml drinking water × 5 days[6]	Mice
	7.5 mg/70-90 g animal PO q8h[11]	Gerbils, hamsters
	10-40 mg/animal PO q24h[6,11]	Rats
	10-40 mg/kg PO q24h[11]	Chinchillas, guinea pigs/use cautiously in chinchillas
	20-60 mg/kg PO q8-12h[18]	All
Neomycin	0.5 mg/ml drinking water[2]	Hamsters
	2.6 mg/ml drinking water[2]	Mice, rats, gerbils
	12-16 mg/kg PO q12h[2]	Guinea pigs
	15 mg/kg PO q24h[6]	Chinchillas
	100 mg/kg PO q24h[6]	Gerbils, hamsters
	50 mg/kg SC q24h[6]	Mice, rats

Table 43. Antimicrobial and antifungal agents used in rodents (cont.)

Agent	Dosage	Comments
Netilmicin	6-8 mg/kg SC, IM, IV divided q8-24h[42]	Chinchillas, guinea pigs/ *Pseudomonas*
Oxytetracycline	0.25-1.0 mg/ml drinking water[6,11]	Hamsters
	0.4 mg/ml drinking water[6,11]	Mice, rats
	0.8 mg/ml drinking water[6,11]	Gerbils
	1 mg/ml drinking water[11]	Chinchillas, guinea pigs/toxicity in guinea pigs reported[36]
	10 mg/kg PO q8h[6,11]	Gerbils
	10-20 mg/kg PO q8h[6]	Mice, rats
	50 mg/kg PO q12h[11]	Chinchillas, guinea pigs/toxicity in guinea pigs reported[36]
	5 mg/kg IM q12h[2]	Guinea pigs/toxicity in guinea pigs reported[36]
	16 mg/kg SC q24h[6,11]	Hamsters
Sulfadimethoxine	10-15 mg/kg PO q12h[18]	All
Sulfamerazine	1 mg/4 g feed[6]	Mice, rats
	0.8 mg/ml drinking water[2]	Gerbils
	1 mg/ml drinking water[2]	Chinchillas, hamsters, guinea pigs, mice, rats
Sulfamethazine	0.8 mg/ml drinking water[2]	Gerbils
	1 mg/ml drinking water[2]	Chinchillas, hamsters, guinea pigs, mice, rats
Sulfaquinoxaline	1 mg/ml drinking water[11]	Chinchillas, gerbils, guinea pigs, hamsters, mice
	0.25-1.0 mg/ml drinking water[6]	Rats
	0.05% feed[6]	Rats
Tetracycline	0.3-2.0 mg/ml drinking water[6]	Chinchillas

278

Table 43. Antimicrobial and antifungal agents used in rodents (cont.)

Agent	Dosage	Comments
Tetracycline (continued)	0.4 mg/ml drinking water[2,6,7] × 10 days	Hamsters/outbreaks of proliferative ileitis[7]
	0.7 mg/ml drinking water[6]	Guinea pigs/toxicity in guinea pigs reported[36]
	2-5 mg/ml drinking water[6]	Gerbils, mice, rats
	0.1-0.5% feed × 14 days[6]	Rats
	10-20 mg/kg PO q8-12h[6]	Gerbils, guinea pigs, hamsters, mice, rats/toxicity in guinea pigs reported[36]
	50 mg/kg PO q8-12h[6]	Chinchillas
	20 mg/kg IM q4h[2]	Gerbils
Trimethoprim/sulfa	30 mg/kg PO, SC,[11] IM[18] q12h	All/tissue necrosis may occur when given SC[18]
Tylosin (Tylan, Elanco)	0.5 mg/ml drinking water[9,11]	Gerbils, hamsters, mice, rats/PD in rats;[9] toxicity in hamsters reported[2]
	2-8 mg/kg PO, SC, IM q12h[6,11]	Hamsters
	10 mg/kg PO, SC, IM q24h[11]	Chinchillas, gerbils, guinea pigs, mice, rats/toxicity in guinea pigs reported[38]

[a] Antibiotic treatment can result in enteritis and antibiotic associated clostridial enterotoxemia, especially when antibiotics with a primary gram-positive spectrum are given. Incidence is higher when agents are given orally. Chinchillas, guinea pigs, and hamsters are most susceptible. Also, direct toxicity due to streptomycin and dihydrostreptomycin occurs in gerbils, guinea pigs, hamsters, and mice. Procaine, included in some penicillin preparations, can be toxic to mice and guinea pigs. Guinea pigs and chinchillas are highly susceptible to the ototoxic effects of chloramphenicol and aminoglycosides at dosages above those recommended clinically. Antibiotics implicated in antibiotic associated clostridial enterotoxemia include:[2,3,9,11,18,21,36,38]

- Chinchillas: penicillins (including ampicillin, amoxicillin), cephalosporins, clindamycin, erythromycin, lincomycin.
- Guinea pigs: penicillins (including ampicillin, amoxicillin), cefazolin, clindamycin, erythromycin, lincomycin, dihydrostreptomycin, streptomycin, bacitracin, chlortetracycline, oxytetracycline, tetracycline, tylosin.
- Hamsters: penicillins (including ampicillin, amoxicillin), cephalosporins, clindamycin, erythromycin, lincomycin, vancomycin, dihydrostreptomycin, streptomycin, bacitracin, oral gentamicin, tylosin.

Table 44. Antiparasitic agents used in rodents.

Agent	Dosage	Comments
Amitraz (Mitaban, Upjohn)	1.4 ml/L topical q14d × 3-6 treatments[18]	Gerbils, hamsters/demodecosis; apply with cottonball, brush; use with caution; not recommended in young
Carbaryl powder	Topical q7d x 3 wk[2] (5%)	Chinchillas, guinea pigs/ ectoparasites
Dichlorvos strip (5 cm long)	Suspend 15 cm above cage × 24 hr, then 2 ×/wk × 3 wk[2]	All/ectoparasites
Dimetridazole	1 mg/ml drinking water[2]	Mice, rats/gastrointestinal protozoa; not available in US
Fenbendazole	0.3% feed × 14 days[43]	Mice/clinical trial for cestodes, pinworms
	20 mg/kg PO q24h × 5 days[1]	All
	50 mg/kg PO × 5 days[7]	All/giardiasis
Fipronil (Frontline, Merial)	7.5 mg/kg topically q30 - 60d[39]	Hamster, mice, chipmunks/flea adulticide
Ivermectin	Spray animals or topical drops, 4-5 times/yr[5,18]	Mice/clinical trial for mite control;[5] use 1% ivermectin diluted 1:100 with 1:1 propylene glycol:water (0.1 mg/ml); topical behind ear
	0.2 mg/kg PO, SC q7d × 3 wk[2]	Chinchillas, gerbils, guinea pigs, mice, rats
	0.2-0.5 mg/kg PO, SC q14d × 3 treatments[2]	Hamsters
	0.5 mg/kg SC, repeat q14d[37]	Guinea pigs/sarcoptid mites
	8 mg/L drinking water × 4 days/wk × 5 wk[27]	Mice/pinworms
	25 mg/L drinking water 4 days/wk × 5 wk[27]	Rats/pinworms
Lime sulfur dip	Dip q7d × 6 wk[2]	All/ectoparasites; dilute 1:40 with water

Table 44. Antiparasitic agents used in rodents (cont.)

Agent	Dosage	Comments
Malathion powder (3-5%)	Topical 3 ×/wk × 3 wk[2]	Gerbils, hamsters, mice, rats/ectoparasites
Malathion spray/dip	Topical q7d × 3 wk[2]	All/ectoparasites; use 0.5% spray or 2% dip
Metronidazole	50-60 mg/kg PO q12h × 5 days[17]	Chinchillas/giardiasis; use with caution
Permethrin	0.25% dust in cage[4]	All/ectoparasites
	Cotton ball soaked in 5% solution[4]	Place in cage 4-5 wk
Piperazine adipate	0.5 mg/ml drinking water × 3 wk[2]	Rats/pinworms
	200 mg/kg PO q24h × 7 days, off 7 days, repeat[2]	Rats/pinworms
	200-600 mg/kg PO q24h × 7 days, off 7 days, repeat[2]	Gerbils
Piperazine citrate	2-5 mg/ml drinking water × 7 days, off 7 days, repeat[2]	All/pinworms
Praziquantel	6-10 mg/kg PO[18]	All/cestodes
	30 mg/kg PO q14 days × 3 treatments[7]	Gerbils, mice, rats
Pyrethrin powder	Topical 3×/wk × 3 wk[2]	Gerbils, hamsters, mice, rats/ectoparasites
	Topical q7 days × 3 wk[2]	Chinchillas, guinea pigs/ectoparasites
Pyrethrin (0.05%) shampoo	Shampoo q7 days for 4 wk[42]	Hamsters, mice, rats/flea control
Sulfadimethoxine	10-15 mg/kg PO q12h[18]	All/coccidiosis
Sulfamerazine	0.8 mg/ml drinking water[2]	Gerbils/coccidiosis
	1 mg/ml drinking water[2]	Chinchillas, hamsters, guinea pigs, mice, rats/coccidiosis
Sulfamethazine	0.8 mg/ml drinking water[2]	Gerbils/coccidiosis
	1 mg/ml drinking water[2]	Chinchillas, hamsters, guinea pigs, mice, rats/coccidiosis

Table 44. Antiparasitic agents used in rodents (cont.)

Agent	Dosage	Comments
Thiabendazole	50-100 mg/kg PO q24h × 5 days[1]	Chinchillas/ascaridiasis
	100 mg/kg PO q24h × 5 days[1]	Gerbils, guinea pigs, hamsters, mice, rats

Table 45. Chemical restraint/anesthetic/analgesic agents used in rodents

Agent	Dosage	Comments
Acepromazine	—	See ketamine combination
	0.5-1.0 mg/kg IM[18]	Chinchillas, guinea pigs, hamsters, mice, rats/preanesthetic; causes seizures in gerbils
Acetaminophen (Tylenol Syrup, McNeil)	1-2 mg/ml drinking water[24]	All/analgesia
Acetylsalicylic acid (aspirin)	50-100 mg/kg PO q4h[20]	Guinea pigs/analgesia
	100-150 mg/kg PO q4h[20]	Gerbils, hamsters, mice, rats/ analgesia
	120-300 mg/kg PO[29]	Mice
Atipamezole (Antisedan, Pfizer)	1.0-2.5 mg/kg IP[12]	Mice/medetomidine reversal
Atropine	0.05-0.10 mg/kg SC[18]	All/some rats possess serum atropinesterase
	0.4 mg/kg SC, IM[4]	Gerbils, hamsters, mice, rats
	0.1-0.2 mg/kg SC, IM[4]	Chinchillas, guinea pigs
Buprenorphine (Buprenex, Reckitt & Colman)	—	Analgesia
	0.05-2.5 mg/kg SC, IP q6-12h[18]	Mice
	0.05 mg/kg SC q8-12h[18]	Chinchillas, guinea pigs
	0.1-0.2 mg/kg SC q8h[18]	Gerbils
	0.5 mg/kg SC q8h[18]	Hamsters
	0.02-0.50 mg/kg SC, IP, IV q6-12h[18]	Rats
	0.05 mg/kg SC, IM[30]	Rats/in combination with carprofen (5-10 mg/kg)[30]
Butorphanol (Torbugesic, Fort Dodge)	—	Analgesia
	0.2 mg/kg IM[17]	Chinchillas
	2 mg/kg SC q2-4h[20]	Guinea pigs
	1-5 mg/kg SC q2-4h[20]	Gerbils, hamsters, mice, rats

283

Table 45. Chemical restraint/anesthetic/analgesic agents used in rodents (cont.)

Agent	Dosage	Comments
Carprofen (Rimadyl, Pfizer)	—	Non-steroidal, anti-inflammatory; analgesia
	4 mg/kg SC q24h[39]	Chinchillas
	5-10 mg/kg PO[30]	Rats/can give in combination with buprenorphine 0.05 mg/kg
Diazepam	—	See ketamine combination
	0.5-3.0 mg/kg IM[2]	Guinea pigs/sedation
	1-2 mg/kg IM[38]	Guinea pigs/calming effect for intense pruritus or sows apprehensive of young
	3-5 mg/kg IM[2]	Gerbils, hamsters, mice, rats/ sedation
Enflurane (Ethrane, Baxter)	To effect	Guinea pigs/chamber induction; MAC = 2.17%[41]
Fentanyl/droperidol (Innovar-Vet, Mallinckrodt)	—	Sedation; anesthesia; dilute 1:10 to reduce chance of inflammation at injection site;[2] irritation can result in self-mutilation; caution: do not use in gerbils or hamsters
	0.06-0.30 ml/kg IM[4]	Mice/sedation
	0.1-0.5 ml/kg IM[4]	Rats/sedation
	0.13-0.16 ml/kg IM[2]	Rats/sedation
	0.2-0.3 ml/kg IM[2]	Mice/sedation
	0.22-0.88 ml/kg IM[2]	Guinea pigs/sedation; inflammation at injection site at high end of dose range
	0.3-0.5 ml/kg IM[2]	Mice, rats/anesthesia
Flunixin meglumine	—	Nonsteroidal anti-inflammatory
	1-3 mg/kg SC q12h[23]	Chinchillas

Table 45. Chemical restraint/anesthetic/analgesic agents used in rodents (cont.)

Agent	Dosage	Comments
Flunixin meglumine (continued)	2.5 mg/kg SC q12-24h[20]	Gerbils, hamsters, mice, rats
	2.5-5.0 mg/kg SC q12-24h[20]	Guinea pigs
Glycopyrrolate	0.01-0.02 mg/kg SC[24]	All/excess oral or respiratory mucus
Halothane	2-5% induction; 0.25-3.0% maintenance[2,24]	All
Ibuprofen	—	Analgesia; anti-inflammatory
	7 15 mg/kg PO q4h[18]	Mice
	10 mg/kg PO q4h[18]	Guinea pigs
	10-30 mg/kg PO q4h[18]	Rats
Isoflurane	2-5% induction; 0.25-4.0% maintenance[2,24]	All/anesthetic of choice
Ketamine	—	Ketamine combinations follow
	22 mg/kg IM[2]	Mice, rats/light sedation; heavy sedation at 44 mg/kg in mice and 25-40 mg/kg in rats
	22-64 mg/kg IM[2]	Guinea pigs/light sedation; heavy sedation at 44-256 mg/kg (marked individual variation)
	40 mg/kg IM[2]	Chinchillas, hamsters/light sedation; heavy sedation at 40-150 mg/kg in hamsters (marked individual variation)
	40-60 mg/kg IM[2]	Gerbils/light sedation; heavy sedation at 70-200 mg/kg (marked individual variation)
Ketamine (K)/ acepromazine (A)	(K) 40 mg/kg/ (A) 0.5 mg/kg IM[21,25,33]	Chinchillas/anesthesia
Ketamine (K)/ diazepam (D)	(K) 20-40 mg/kg/ (D) 1-2 mg/kg IM[21]	Chinchillas/anesthesia
	(K) 20-30 mg/kg/ (D) 1-2 mg/kg IM[36]	Guinea pigs/anesthesia

Table 45. Chemical restraint/anesthetic/analgesic agents used in rodents (cont.)

Agent	Dosage	Comments
Ketamine (K)/ medetomidine (M)	(K) 50-75 mg/kg/ (M) 10 mg/kg IP[12]	Mice/anesthesia; minor procedures; use the higher dose of ketamine in females; (M) reversal of atipamezole
Ketamine (K)/ xylazine (X)	(K) 20-40 mg/kg/ (X) 2 mg/kg IM[17]	Guinea pigs/light anesthesia
	(K) 35-40 mg/kg/ (X) 4-8 mg/kg IM[2]	Chinchillas/anesthesia
	(K) 50 mg/kg/ (X) 2 mg/kg IP[2]	Gerbils/anesthesia
	(K) 50 mg/kg/ (X) 5 mg/kg IP[17]	Mice/anesthesia
	(K) 75-95 mg/kg/ (X) 5 mg/kg IM, IP[17]	Rats/anesthesia
	(K) 80 mg/kg/ (X) 5 mg/kg IM, IP[17]	Hamsters/anesthesia
Medetomidine	—	See ketamine for combination
Meperidine (Demerol, Winthrop-Breon)	20 mg/kg SC, IM q2-3h[20]	Gerbils, guinea pigs, hamsters, mice, rats/analgesia
Midazolam (Versed, Roche)	1-2 mg/kg IM[18]	All/preanesthetic
Morphine	2-5 mg/kg SC q2-4h[20]	Gerbils, hamsters, mice, rats/ analgesia
	2-5 mg/kg SC, IM q4h[20]	Guinea pigs/analgesia
Nalbuphine (Nubain, Endo Labs)	4-8 mg/kg IM q3h[20]	Gerbils, hamsters, mice, rats/ analgesia
	1-2 mg/kg IM q3h[20]	Guinea pigs/analgesia
Nalorphine	2-5 mg/kg IV[2]	All/narcotic reversal
Naloxone (Narcan, Endo Labs)	0.01-0.10 mg/kg SC, IP[24]	All/narcotic reversal
Oxymorphone	0.2-0.5 mg/kg SC, IM q6-12h[20]	Gerbils, guinea pigs, hamsters, mice, rats/analgesia
Pentazocine (Talwin, Sanofi Winthrop)	10 mg/kg SC q2-4h[20]	Gerbils, guinea pigs, hamsters, mice, rats/analgesia

Table 45. Chemical restraint/anesthetic/analgesic agents used in rodents (cont.)

Agent	Dosage	Comments
Pentobarbital	—	Anesthesia; not recommended; marginal analgesia; autonomic depression; give diluted in sterile saline (<10 mg/ml)
	30-45 mg/kg IP[18]	Guinea pigs, rats
	35-40 mg/kg IP[2]	Chinchillas
	50-90 mg/kg IP[18]	Gerbils, hamsters, mice
Pipothiazine palmitate	25 mg/kg q5wk SC[32]	Rats/long-acting neuroleptic drug; antipsychotic (experimental)
Piroxicam (Feldene, Pfizer)	3.4-20.0 mg/kg PO[46]	Mice/analgesia; non-steroidal anti-inflammatory
Propofol (Rapinovet, Mallinckrodt)	—	Anesthesia; induction
	7.5-10.0 mg/kg IV[15]	Rats
	12-26 mg/kg IV[15]	Mice
Tiletamine/zolazepam (Telazol, Fort Dodge)	—	Tiletamine/zolazepam combination follows
	20-40 mg/kg IM[14,21,25]	Chinchillas, rats/anesthesia
Tiletamine/zolazepam (T)/ xylazine (X)	(T) 30 mg/kg/ (X) 10 mg/kg IM, IP[17]	Hamsters/anesthesia
	(T) 20 mg/kg/ (X) 10 mg/kg IP[24]	Gerbils/anesthesia
Xylazine	—	See ketamine, tiletamine/zolazepam for combinations
Yohimbine (Yobine, Lloyd)	0.5-1.0 mg/kg IV[18]	All/xylazine reversal

Table 46. Emergency drugs used in rodents

Agent	Dosage	Comments
Atropine	0.05-0.10 mg/kg SC[18]	All/bradycardia; some rats possess serum atropinase
	0.4 mg/kg SC, IM[2]	Gerbils, hamsters, mice, rats
	0.1-0.2 mg/kg SC, IM[2]	Chinchillas, guinea pigs
Calcium gluconate	100 mg/kg IP[39]	Chinchillas/hypocalcemic tetany; eclampsia
	100 mg/kg IM[22]	Guinea pigs/dystocia; follow with 1 IU oxytocin (see Table 47)
Dexamethasone	4-5 mg/kg SC, IM, IP, IV[34]	Shock
Diazepam	1-2 mg/kg IM[38]	Guinea pigs/calming effect for intense pruritus
	1-5 mg/kg IM, IV, IP, IO[34]	All/treatment of seizures
Diphenylhydramine	5 mg/kg SC[28]	Guinea pigs/antihistamine; anaphylaxis
Dopamine	0.08 mg/kg IV[28]	Guinea pigs/hypotension
Doxapram	5-10 mg/kg IP, IV[17]	Chinchillas, gerbils, hamsters, mice, rats/respiratory stimulant
	2-5 mg/kg IP, IV[17]	Guinea pigs
Ephedrine (Marax, Pfizer)	1 mg/kg IV[28]	Guinea pigs/antihistamine; stimulant
Epinephrine	0.003 mg/kg IV[28]	Guinea pigs/cardiac arrest
Furosemide	1-4 mg/kg SC, IM q4-6h[19]	All/diuretic for edema, pulmonary congestion, ascites
	5-10 mg/kg SC, IM q12h[19]	All
Glycopyrrolate	0.01-0.02 mg/kg SC[24]	All/bradycardia
Lactated Ringer's solution	10-25 ml/kg IV[35]	Give slowly over 5-10 min (if unsuccessful, administer IP)
Vitamin C	50 mg/kg SC, IM[42]	Guinea pigs/ascorbic acid deficiency

Table 47. Miscellaneous agents used in rodents

Agent	Dosage	Comments
Aluminum hydroxide	20-40 mg/animal PO prn[42]	Hyperphosphatemia secondary to renal failure
Atropine	10 mg/kg SC q20min[18]	All/organophosphate toxicity; may cause cardiovascular irregularities in guinea pigs
Atropine (1%)/ phenylephrine (10%)	Topical to eyes[18]	All/mydriasis for non-albino eyes
Calcium-EDTA	30 mg/kg SC q12h[21]	Chinchillas/lead chelation
Calcium gluconate	100 mg/kg IP[39]	Chinchillas/hypocalcemic tetany; eclampsia
Cimetidine (Tagamet, SmithKline Beecham)	5-10 mg/kg q6h-q12h[1]	All/gastric, duodenal ulceration; esophagitis, gastroesophageal reflux
Cisapride (Propulsid, Janssen)	0.1-0.5 mg/kg PO q12h[34]	All/enhance gastrointestinal motility
Cyclophosphamide	300 mg/kg IP q24h[28]	Guinea pigs/anti-neoplastic
Dexamethasone	0.5-2.0 mg/kg PO, SC, then decreasing dose q12h $\times$ 3-14 days[18]	All/anti-inflammatory
	0.6 mg/kg IM[2]	All
Digoxin	0.05-0.1 mg/kg PO q12-24h[34]	Hamsters/dilated cardiomyopathy
Diphenylhydramine	5 mg/kg SC prn[28]	Guinea pigs/antihistamine; anaphylaxis
Dopamine	0.08 mg/kg IV prn[28]	Guinea pigs/hypotension, especially anesthetic related
Doxapram	—	Stimulates respiration
	5-10 mg/kg[17] IP, IV	Chinchillas, gerbils, hamsters, mice, rats
	2-5 mg/kg[17] IP, IV	Guinea pigs
Ephedrine (Marax, Pfizer)	1 mg/kg PO, IV prn[28]	Guinea pigs/antihistamine; anaphylaxis

289

Table 47. Miscellaneous agents used in rodents (cont.)

Agent	Dosage	Comments
Epinephrine	0.003 mg/kg IV prn[28]	Guinea pigs/cardiac arrest
Furosemide	—	Diuretic for edema, pulmonary congestion, ascites
	1-4 mg/kg IM q4-6h[19]	All
	5-10 mg/kg SC, IM q12h[1]	All
Heparin	5 mg/kg IV prn[28]	Guinea pigs/disseminated intravascular coagulation
Human chorionic gonadotropin (hCG)	1,000 USP units/animal IM, repeat in7 -10 days[36]	Guinea pigs/cystic ovaries
Hydralazine	1 mg/kg IV prn[28]	Guinea pigs/antihistamine
Insulin	2 U/animal SC[28]	Hamsters
Lactated Ringer's solution	50-100 ml/kg SC, IV, IO q24h[35]	All/maintenance fluid requirements
Lactobacilli	—	All/PO during antibiotic treatment period, then 5-7 days beyond cessation;[11] give 2 hr prior to or 2 hr following antibiotic treatment[11]
Loperamide (Imodium A-D, McNeil)	0.1 mg/kg PO q8h × 3 days, then q24h × 2 days[18]	All/enteropathies (diarrhea); give in 1 ml water
Metoclopromide (Reglan, Robins)	0.2-1.0 mg/kg PO, SC, IM q12h[34]	All/gastric stasis
Neomycin/ dexamethasone/ polymyxin B ophthalmic (Maxitrol, Alcon)	Topical to eyes q8-12h[34]	All/ophthalmic preparation; may cause GI stasis secondary to steroids
Oxytocin	0.2-3.0 IU/kg SC, IM, IV[2]	All/delayed parturition if unobstructed; in guinea pigs, fusion of pubic symphysis occurs if first breeding does not occur before 6-9 mo of age, resulting in dystocia—if no young produced 15 min following 1.0 IU/animal, cesarean section is indicated

Table 47. Miscellaneous agents used in rodents (cont.)

Agent	Dosage	Comments
Phenobarbital	10-20 mg/kg IP, IV[28]	Guinea pigs/seizure
Prednisone	0.5-2.2 mg/kg SC, IM[2]	All/anti-inflammatory
Pseudoephedrine (Robitussin, Robins)	1.2 mg/animal PO q12h[39]	Chinchillas/antihistamine
Sucralfate (Carafate, Hoechst Marion Roussel)	50 mg/kg PO[19]	All/oral, esophageal, gastric, and duodenal ulcers
Tropicamide (1%)	Topical to eyes[18]	All/mydriasis in albino eyes
Vitamin A	50-500 IU/100 g IM[28]	Guinea pigs, hamsters
Vitamin B complex	0.02-0.20 ml/kg SC, IM[2,40]	All/B1 (100 mg/ml), B_2 (2 mg/ml), B_{12} (0.1 mg/ml)
Vitamin C	0.2-0.4 mg/ml drinking water[36]	Guinea pigs/prevents deficiency; change daily
	20-200 mg/kg SC, IM[2]	Guinea pigs/treatment of deficiency
	50-100 mg/animal daily[36]	Guinea pigs/treatment of deficiency; start parenteral, then PO until resolution of clinical signs
Vitamin D	200-400 IU/kg SC, IM[2]	All
Vitamin E/selenium (Bo-Se, Schering)	0.1 ml/100-250 g SC[2]	All
Vitamin K_1	1-10 mg/kg IM q24h × 4-6 days[18]	All/warfarin poisoning; menadiols not used in acute cases
	2.5-5.0 mg/kg IM q24h × 3-4 wk[18]	All/brodifacom poisoning; menadiols not used in acute cases

Appendix 50. Hematologic and serum biochemical values of rodents 2,10,44

Measurement	Mouse	Rat	Gerbil	Hamster	Guinea pig	Chinchilla	Prairie dog
PCV (%)	35-40	35-45	35-45	45-50	35-45	27-54	36-54
RBC (10^6/µl)	7-11	7-10	7-8	7-8	4-7	5.6-8.4	5.9-9.4
Hgb (g%)	10-20	12-18	14-16	16.6-18.6	11-17	11.8-14.6	12.7-19.6
WBC (10^3/µl)	4-12	5-23	7.5-10.9	7-10	7-14	5.4-15.6	1.9-10.1
Neutrophils (%)	5-40	10-50	22	18-40	20-60	39-54	43-87
Lymphocytes (%)	30-90	50-70	75	56-80	30-80	45-60	8-54
Monocytes (%)	0-10	0-10	0-4	2.43	2-20	0-5	0-12
Eosinophils (%)	0-5	0-5	0-3	0-1	0-5	0-5	0-10
Basophils (%)	0-1	0-1	0-1	0-1	0-1	0-1	0-2
ALT (IU/L)	26-77	20-92	—	22-128	10-25	10-35	26-91
AP (IU/L)	45-222	16-96	—	99-186	—	6-72	25-64
AST (IU/L)	54-269	—	—	28-122	—	96	16-53
Bilirubin, total (mg/dl)	0.1-0.9	0.20-0.55	0.2-0.6	0.1-0.9	0.3-0.9	0.6-1.28	0.1-0.3
Calcium (mg/dl)	3.2-8.0	5.3-13.0	3.7-6.2	5.3-12	7.8-10.5	5.6-12.1	8.3-10.8
Chloride (mEq/L)	82-114	—	—	—	98-115	108-129	—
Cholesterol (mg/dl)	26-82	40-130	90-150	55-181	20-43	50-302	—
Creatinine (mg/dl)	0.3-1.0	0.2-0.8	0.6-1.4	0.4-1.0	0.6-2.2	0.4-1.3	0.8-2.3
Glucose (mg/dl)	62-175	50-135	50-135	37-198	60-125	109-193	120-209
Phosphorus (mg/dl)	6.0-10.4	5.8-8.2	3.7-7.0	3.0-9.9	5.3	4-8	3.6-10.0
Potassium (mEq/L)	5.1-10.4	5.9	3.3-6.3	3.9-5.5	6.8-8.9	3.3-5.7	4.0-5.7
Protein, total (g/dl)	3.5-7.2	5.6-7.6	4.3-12.5	5.2-7.0	4.6-6.2	3.8-5.6	5.8-8.1
Albumin (g/dl)	2.5-4.8	3.8-4.8	1.8-5.5	3.5-4.9	2.1-3.9	2.3-4.1	2.4-3.9
Globulin (g/dl)	0.6	1.8-3.0	1.2-6.0	2.7-4.2	1.7-2.6	0.9-2.2	3.4-4.2
Sodium (mEq/L)	112-193	135-155	141-172	128-144	146-152	142-166	144-175
Triglycerides (mg/dl)	—	26-145	—	72-227	0-145	—	—
Urea nitrogen (mg/dl)	17-28	15-21	17-27	12-26	9-32	17-45	21-44

Appendix 51. Biological and physiological data of rodents 1,2,18,44

Species	Av wt (g) ♂/♀	Age at puberty (days) ♂/♀	Life span (yr)	Temperature °C (°F)	Heart rate (BPM)	Respiratory rate/min
Mouse	20-40/25-40	50/50-60	1.5-3.0	36.5-38.0 (97.5-100.4)	325-780	60-220
Rat	450-520/250-300	65-110/65-110	2.5-3.5	35.9-37.5 (96.6-99.5)	250-450	115
Gerbil	65-100/55-85	70-85/65-85	3-4	37.0-38.5 (98.6-101.3)	360	90
Hamster	85-130/95-150	70-100/40-70	1.5-2.0	37-38 (98.6-100.4)	250-500	35-135
Guinea pig	900-1,200/700-900	90-120/60-90	4-5	37.2-39.5 (99.0-103.1)	230-380	40-100
Chinchilla	450-600/550-800	240-540/240-540[a]	8-10	36.1-37.8 (97.0-100.0)	40-100	40-80
Prairie dog	1,000-2,200/500-1,500	730-995	6-10	35.4-39.1 (95.7-102.3)	83-318	40-60

[a] Babies born in fall breed 1 yr later.

293

Appendix 51. Biological and physiological data of rodents (cont.)

Species	Estrus length (days)	Gestation (days)	Litter size	Birth weight (g)	Age eyes open (days)	Weaning age (days)	Consumption (/100 g BW/day) Food (g)	Consumption (/100 g BW/day) Water (ml)	Nutritional recommendations Min. fiber	Nutritional recommendations Carbo-hydrates (%)	Nutritional recommendations Fat (%)	Nutritional recommendations Protein (%)
Mouse	4-5	19-21	10-12	0.5-1.5	10-14	21-28	12-18	15	–	45-55	5-25	16-20
Rat	4-5	19-23	6-12	5-6	12-17	17-21	5-6	≥10-12	–	–	5-25	12-27
Gerbil	4-6	24-26	4-6	2.5-3.5	16-20	20-30	5-8	4-7	–	–	2-4	16-22
Hamster	4	15-18	4-12	2	14-16	20-28	8-12	8-10	–	8	3-5	15-25
Guinea pig	15-17	59-72	2-5	60-100	birth	14-28	6	10	16-18	16	–	18-30
Chinchilla	30-50	105-115	2-3	30-50	birth	36-48	3-6	–	–	–	–	–
Prairie dog	14-21	30	2-10	–	–	42-49	2.3-4.1	–	–	–	–	–

Appendix 52. Determining the sex of mature rodents [20]

Male	Female
• Anogenital distance is longer in the male. • Manipulate "genital papilla" (prepuce) to protrude penis. • Palpate for testicles either in a scrotal sac (if present) or subcutaneous in inguinal region. • Males have only two external openings in the inguinal area: • anus, • urethral orifice at tip of penis.	• Anogenital distance is shorter in the female. • Look for three external openings in the inguinal area: • anus (most caudal opening) • vaginal orifice (middle opening) —look carefully— and • urethral orifice at tip of urethral papilla (most anterior opening).
In very fat males, there may be a depression between the penis and anus This depression can be obliterated by manipulating the skin in that area.	The urethral papilla is located outside the vagina (unlike dogs and cats). In very fat or young females, the vaginal orifice may be either hidden by folds of skin (the former) or sealed (latter). Gentle manipulation of the skin in this area will divulge the orifice.

Appendix 53. Literature cited - Rodents

1. Allen DG, Pringle JK, Smith DA (eds). *Handbook of Veterinary Drugs*. JB Lippincott Co, Philadelphia, 1993.

2. Anderson NL. Basic husbandry and medicine of pocket pets. In: Birchard SJ, Sherding RG (eds). *Saunders Manual of Small Animal Practice*. WB Saunders Co, Philadelphia, 1994. Pp 1363-1389.

3. Battles AH. The biology, care and diseases of the Syrian hamster. *Compend Cont Educ Pract Vet* 7:815-825, 1985.

4. Bauck L, Boyer TH, Brown SA, et al. *Exotic Animal Formulary*. American Animal Hospital Assoc., Lakewood, Colorado, 1995. 46 pp.

5. Baumans V, Havenaar R, Van Herck H, et al. The effectiveness of Ivomec and Neguvon on the control of murine mites. *Lab Anim* 22:243-245, 1988.

6. Burgmann P, Percy DH. Antimicrobial drug use in rodents and rabbits. In: Prescott JF, Baggot JD (eds). *Antimicrobial Therapy in Veterinary Medicine*, 2nd ed. Iowa State University Press, Ames, 1993. Pp 524-541.

7. Burke TJ. "Wet tail" in hamsters and other diarrheas of small rodents. In: Bonagura JD (ed). *Kirk's Current Veterinary Therapy XII: Small Animal Practice*. WB Saunders Co, Philadelphia, 1995. Pp 1336-1339.

8. Campbell BG, Bartholow S, Rosin E. Bacterial killing by use of one daily gentamicin dosage in guinea pigs with *Escherichia coli* infection. *Am J Vet Res* 57:1627-1630, 1996.

9. Carter KK, Hietala S, Brooks DL, et al. Tylosin concentrations in rat serum and lung tissue after administration in drinking water. *Lab Anim Sci* 37:468-470, 1987.

10. Collins BR. Common diseases and medical management of rodents and lagomorphs. In: Jacobson ER, Kollias GV, Jr (eds). *Exotic Animals*. Churchill Livingstone, New York, 1988. Pp 261-316.

11. Collins BR. Antimicrobial drug use in rabbits, rodents, and other small mammals. In: *Antimicrobial Therapy in Caged Birds and Exotic Pets*. Veterinary Learning Systems Co, Trenton, NJ, 1995. Pp 3-10.

12. Cruz JL, Loste JM, Burzaco OH. Observations on the use of medetomidine/ketamine and its reversal with atipamezole for chemical restraint in the mouse. *Lab Anim* 32:18-22, 1998.

13. Donnelly T. Nasal lesions in gerbils. *Lab Anim* (Feb): 17-18, 1997.

14. Eisele PH. Anesthesia for small mammals. *Proc N Am Vet Conf*: 785-791, 1997.

15. Glen JB. Animal studies of the anesthetic activity of ICI 35 865. *Br J Anaesth* 56:617-627, 1980.

16. Goelz MF, Thigpen JE, Mannier J. Efficacy of various regimens in eliminating *Pasteurella pneumotropica* from the mouse. *Lab Anim Sci* 46:280-285, 1996.

17. Harkness JE. *A Practitioner's Guide to Domestic Rodents*. American Animal Hospital Association, Lakewood, CO, 1993.

18. Harkness JE, Wagner JE. *The Biology and Medicine of Rabbits and Rodents*, 4th ed. Williams & Wilkins, Philadelphia, 1995.

19. Harrenstien L. Critical care of ferrets, rabbits, and rodents. *Sem Avian Exotic Pet Med* 3:217-228, 1994.

20. Heard DJ. Principles and techniques of anesthesia and analgesia for exotic practice. *Vet Clin N Am: Small Anim Pract* 23:1301-1327, 1993.

21. Hoefer HL. Chinchillas. *Vet Clin N Am: Small Anim Pract* 24:103-111, 1994.

22. Hoefer H. Common problems in guinea pigs. *Proc N Am Vet Conf*: 831-832, 1999.

23. Hoefer H. Diagnosis and management of chinchilla diseases. *Proc N Am Vet Conf*: 833-835, 1999.

24. Huerkamp MJ. Anesthesia and postoperative management of rabbits and pocket pets. In: Bonagura JD (ed). *Kirk's Current Veterinary Therapy XII: Small Animal Practice.* WB Saunders Co, Philadelphia, 1995. Pp 1322-1327.

25. Jenkins JR. Husbandry and common diseases of the chinchilla *(Chinchilla laniger). J Small Exotic Anim Med* 2:15-17, 1992.

26. Johnson-Delaney C. Prairie dogs. *Exotic Companion Medicine Handbook for Veterinarians.* Wingers Publishing, Lake Worth, FL, 1996.

27. Klement P, Augustine JM, Delaney KM, et al. An oral ivermectin regimen that eradicates pinworms (*Syphacia* sp.) in rats and mice. *Lab Anim Sci* 46:286-290, 1996.

28. Laird KL, Swindle MM, Flecknell PA. *Handbook of Rodent and Rabbit Medicine.* Pergamon, New York, 1996.

29. Levin L. Pain control in laboratory animals. *Sci Anim Care* 5:1-4, 1994.

30. Liles JH, Flecknell PA. A comparison of the effects of buprenorphine, carprofen, and flunixin following laparotomy in rats. *J Vet Pharmacol Therap* 17:284-290, 1994.

31. McClure JT, Rosin E. Comparison of amikacin dosing regimens in neutropenic guinea pigs with *Escherichia coli* infection. *Am J Vet Res* 59:750-755, 1998.

32. McCoy J, Jori F, Stem C. Tranquillization of cane rats with a depot neuroleptic. *J Vet Pharmacol Therap* 20:233-239, 1997.

33. Morgan RJ, Eddy LB, Solie TN, et al. Ketamine-acepromazine as an anaesthetic agent for chinchillas (*Chinchilla laniger). Lab Anim* 15:282-283, 1981.

34. Morrisey JK. Personal communication. 1999.

35. Oglesbee B. Emergency medicine of pocket pets. Bonagura JD (ed). *Kirk's Current Veterinary Therapy XII: Small Animal Practice.* WB Saunders Co, Philadelphia, 1995. Pp 1328-1331.

36. Quesenberry KE. Guinea pigs. *Vet Clin N Am: Small Anim Pract* 24:67-87, 1994.

37. Quesenberry KE. Medical management of gerbils, hamsters, and guinea pigs. *Proc 21st Annu Waltham/OSU Symp*: 51-55, 1997.

38. Richardson VCG. *Diseases of Domestic Guinea Pigs.* Blackwell Scientific Publications, Oxford, 1992.

39. Richardson VCG. *Diseases of Small Domestic Rodents.* Blackwell Scientific Publications, Malden, MA, 1997.

40. Schuchman SM. Individual care and treatment of rabbits, mice, rats, guinea pigs, hamsters, and gerbils. In: Kirk RW (ed). *Current Veterinary Therapy X: Small Animal Practice.* WB Saunders Co, Philadelphia, 1989. Pp 738-765.

41. Seifen AB, Kennedy RH, Bray JP, Seifen E. Estimation of minimum alveolar concentration (MAC) for halothane, enflurane, and isoflurane in guinea pigs. *Lab Anim Sci* 39:579-581, 1989.

42. Smith DA, Burgmann PM. Formulary. In: Hillyer EV, Quesenberry KE (eds). *Ferrets, Rabbits, and Rodents: Clinical Medicine and Surgery.* WB Saunders Co, Philadelphia, 1997. Pp 392-404.

43. Taffs LF. Further studies on the efficacy of thiabendazole given in the diet of mice infected with *H nana, S obvelata*, and *A tetraptera. Vet Rec* 99:143-144, 1976.

44. Tell LA. Medical management of prairie dogs. *Proc N Am Vet Conf*: 721-724, 1995.

45. Tynes VV. Drug therapy in pet rodents. *Vet Med* (Nov): 988-991, 1998.

46. Walter T, Chan TR, Weichman BM. Effects of analgesics on bradykinin-induced writhing in mice. *Agents Actions* 27:375-377, 1989.

47. Williams BH. Diseases of rodents. *Proc N Am Vet Conf*: 690-691, 1995.

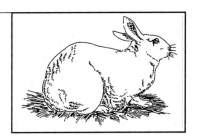

Fish

Amphibians

Reptiles

Birds

Sugar Gliders

Hedgehogs

Rodents

▶ **Rabbits**

Ferrets

Miniature Pigs

Primates

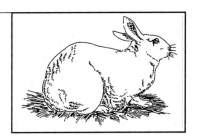

Table 48. Antimicrobial and antifungal agents used in rabbits [a]

Agent	Dosage	Comments
Alatrofloxacin (Trovan, Pfizer)	15 mg/kg IV (single dose)[68]	Bacterial meningitis
Amikacin	2 mg/kg SC, IM, IV q8h[38] 2-5 mg/kg SC, IM q8-12h[29] 10 mg/kg SC, IM q8h-q12h[1] 1.25 g/20 g methylmethacrylate[4]	Place in bone following surgical debridement of jaw abscess
Amphotericin B	1 mg/kg IV q24h[71]	Severe fungal infections; use in combination with fluconazole; potentially nephrotoxic and hepatotoxic
Cefazolin	2 g/20 g methylmethacrylate[4]	Place in bone following surgical debridement of jaw abscess
Ceftiofur (Ceftiofur, Upjohn)	2 g/20 g methylmethacrylate[4]	Place in bone following surgical debridement of jaw abscess
Ceftriaxone (Rocephin, Roche)	40 mg/kg IM q12h × 2 days[71]	
Cephalexin	11-22 mg/kg PO q8h[64]	
Cephaloridine	11-15 mg/kg IM q12h[4] 10-25 mg/kg IM, SC q24h × 5 days[32]	
Cephalothin	12.5 mg/kg q6h × 6 days[64] 2 g/20 g methylmethacrylate[4]	Place in bone following surgical debridement of jaw abscess
Chloramphenicol	25 mg/kg PO q8-12h[64] 30 mg/kg PO q12h[38] 30 mg/kg SC, IM, IV q8-12h[38,64]	

301

Table 48. Antimicrobial and antifungal agents used in rabbits (cont.)

Agent	Dosage	Comments
Chloramphenicol (continued)	50 mg/kg PO, SC, IM, IV q8h[35]	
	1.3 mg/ml drinking water[11]	Partially effective at 0.5 mg/ml in clinical trial for pasteurellosis[58]
Chlortetracycline	50 mg/kg PO q24h[11]	
Ciprofloxacin (0.3%) (Ciloxan, Alcon)	5-20 mg/kg PO q12h[64] 10-20 mg/kg PO q12h[35]	Suspension in water, stable for 14 days;[64] may cause arthropathies in young[74]
	1 drop topical OU q8-12h[27]	Nasal pasteurellosis; maintains therapeutic levels in tear film for at least 6 hr after application (tears drain into nasal sinus)
Clotrimazole (Lotrimin, Schering)	Topical[31]	Localized dermatophytosis
Doxycycline	2.5 mg/kg PO q12h[15] 4 mg/kg PO q24h[57]	
Enrofloxacin	—	May cause arthropathies in young;[74] limit SC and IM injections (may cause muscle necrosis or sterile abscesses)
	5 mg/kg PO, SC, IM, IV q12h[7,8,12]	PD;[8,12] clinical trial for pasteurellosis, × 14 days[7]
	5-10 mg/kg PO, SC, IM q12h[15]	
	5-20 mg/kg PO, IM q12h[64]	14-30 days for pasteurellosis[64]
	100 mg/L drinking water[55]	Clinical trial for pasteurellosis; successful when intake >5 mg/kg q24h[58]
	200 mg/L drinking water[7]	Clinical trial for pasteurellosis, × 14 days[7]
Fluconazole	25-43 mg/kg IV (slow) q12h[47]	Systemic fungal disease

Table 48. Antimicrobial and antifungal agents used in rabbits (cont.)

Agent	Dosage	Comments
Furazolidone	5 mg/kg PO q24h × 14 days[11] 5.5 g/L drinking water[11] 50 mg/kg feed[11]	
Gentamicin	1.5-2.5 mg/kg SC, IM, IV q8h[64] 2.5 mg/kg SC, IM, IV q8-12h[35] 4 mg/kg SC, IM q24h[11] 1 g/20 g methylmethacrylate[4]	Seldom indicated; use with caution Place in bone following surgical debridement of jaw abscess
Griseofulvin	12.5 mg/kg PO q12h × 30-45 days[39] 25 mg/kg PO q24h × 30-45 days[39] 12.5 mg/kg PO q12h × 4-6 wk[64]	Advanced cases of dermatophytosis Decrease dose by 50% with ultramicrosize form (Gris-PEG, Allergan Herbert), which has better absorption
Ketoconazole	10-40 mg/kg PO q24h × 14 days[29]	Dermatophytosis
Lime sulfur dip (2-3%)	Topical q5-7d × 4 wk[64]	Dermatophytosis; use with caution
Metronidazole	20 mg/kg PO q12h[15,35] 40 mg/kg PO q24h × 3 days[11]	
Miconazole (Conofite, Schering-Plough)	Topical q24h × 2-4 wk[29]	Localized dermatophytosis
Moxifloxacin	40 mg/kg IV q12-24h[59] (suggested frequency)	Bacterial meningitis
Neomycin	30 mg/kg PO q12h[11] 200-800 mg/L drinking water[57]	

303

Table 48. Antimicrobial and antifungal agents used in rabbits (cont.)

Agent	Dosage	Comments
Netilmicin (Netromycin, Schering)	6-8 mg/kg SC, IM, IV[76] q24h	Dilute and give over 20 min for IV use; gram negative infections
Nitrofurazone	8-11 mg/kg PO q12h[26]	
Ofloxacin (Ocuflox, Allergan)	20 mg/kg SC q8h[48]	Urogenital, skin, respiratory infections
Oxytetracycline	15 mg/kg IM q8h[50]	PD; anorexia and diarrhea at 30 mg/kg IM q8h; tissue irritation can occur
	25 mg/kg SC q24h[57]	
	50 mg/kg PO q12h[11]	
	1 mg/ml drinking water[11]	
Penicillin	40,000-60,000 IU/kg IM q12h × 5-7 days[39]	Rabbit syphilis
Penicillin G, benzathine	42,000-60,000 IU/kg IM q48h[26]	Rabbit syphilis
	42,000-84,000 IU/kg SC q7d × 3 wk[64]	
Penicillin G procaine	42,000-84,000 IU/kg SC, IM q24h[26]	
	60,000 IU/kg IM q8h[83]	PD
	40,000 IU/kg IM q24h × 5-7 days[22]	Rabbit syphilis
Rifampin (R)/ azithromycin (A)	(R) 40 mg/kg PO q12h/ (A) 50 mg/kg PO q24h[75]	*Staphylococcus* osteomyelitis
Rifampin (R)/ clarithromycin (C)	(R) 40 mg/kg/(C) 80 mg/kg PO q12h[75]	*Staphylococcus* osteomyelitis
Silver sulfadiazine cream (Silvadene cream, Marion)	Topical q24h[39]	Does not cause diarrhea if ingested
Sulfadimethoxine	10-15 mg/kg PO q12h[16]	
Sulfamethazine	1 mg/ml drinking water[11]	
	5-10 g/kg feed[11]	
Sulfamethoxine	50 mg/kg PO on day 1, then 25 mg/kg PO q24h × 10-20 days[9]	Coccidiosis

Table 48. Antimicrobial and antifungal agents used in rabbits (cont.)

Agent	Dosage	Comments
Sulfaquinoxaline	1 mg/ml drinking water[11] 0.6 g/kg feed[11]	
Tetracycline	50 mg/kg PO q8-12h[11] 50-100 mg/kg PO q8h[64] 250-1,000 mg/L drinking water[26]	Therapeutic levels not achieved even at 800-1,600 mg/L;[63] 250 mg/L not effective in clinical trial for pasteurellosis[58]
Tilmicosin (Micotil, Elanco)	25 mg/kg SC once[51]	Pasteurellosis; use cautiously: at least one death has been reported[14]
Tobramycin (Nebcin, Lilly)	1 g/20 g methylmethacrylate[4]	Place in bone following surgical debridement of jaw abscess
Trimethoprim/sulfa	15 mg/kg PO q12h[11] 30 mg/kg PO, SC, IM q12h[29,38,64] 30 mg/kg SC q24h[11]	May cause tissue necrosis SC; do not use SC[29] May cause tissue necrosis
Tylosin (Tylan, Elanco)	10 mg/kg PO, SC, IM q12h[11] 10 mg/kg PO, SC, IM q24h[17]	

[a] There is a potential for antibiotic-induced enterotoxemia following administration of some antimicrobial agents (see Appendix 32). Appetite and fecal character must be monitored closely during and following therapy.

Table 49. Antiparasitic agents used in rabbits

Agent	Dosage	Comments
Albendazole	7.5-20.0 mg/kg PO q24h[10]	Potential treatment for encephalitozoonosis
Amprolium (9.6%)	0.5 ml/pint drinking water × 10 days[29,35] 5 ml/gal drinking water × 21 days[64]	Coccidiosis
Carbaryl powder (5%)	Topical, twice weekly[29]	Ectoparasites; use sparingly
Decoquinate (Deccox, Rhone-Poulenc)	62.5 ppm in feed[29]	Coccidiosis
Diclazuril	1 ppm in feed[29]	Coccidiosis
Dimetridazole	0.2 mg/ml drinking water[11]	Protostat; not available in US
Fenbendazole	5 mg/kg PO[57] 10 mg/kg PO, repeat in 2 wk prn[35] 50 ppm in feed × 2-6 wk[57]	
Fipronil (Frontline, Merial)	Not recommended[54]	May cause neurologic disease
Imidacloprid (Advantage, Bayer)	Use cat dose; place in 2-3 areas along dorsum[54]	Flea adulticide
Ivermectin	0.1-0.2 mg/kg SC, repeat in 2 wk[6] 0.4 mg/kg PO, SC q7-14d[35] 0.4 mg/kg SC q7d × 2-3 wk[64] 0.6 mg/kg SC q14d[54]	Ear mites, clinical trial
Lasalocid	120 ppm in feed[29]	Coccidiosis
Lime sulfur (2-3%)	1-2 dips/wk × 4 wk[64] Dip q7d × 4-6 wk[64]	Ectoparasites; young animals
Lufenuron (Program, Novartis)	30 mg/kg PO monthly[54]	Flea larvicide

Table 49. Antiparasitic agents used in rabbits (cont.)

Agent	Dosage	Comments
Monensin (CoBan 60, Elanco)	0.002-0.004% in feed[29]	Coccidiosis
Piperazine	200 mg/kg PO, repeat in 2-3 wk[35,64]	
	500 mg/kg PO × 2 days[44]	Adults
	750 mg/kg PO × 2 days[44]	Young
	2-5 mg/ml drinking water × 7 days[35]	
Praziquantel	5-10 mg/kg PO, SC, IM, repeat in 10 days[1]	
Pyrantel pamoate	5-10 mg/kg PO, repeat in 2-3 wk[64]	
Pyrethrins	Use as directed for puppies/kittens[54]	Flea control
Rofenaid (Rofenaid 40, Roche)	62.5-250.0 ppm in feed[29]	Coccidiosis
Sulfadimethoxine	50 mg/kg PO once, then 25 mg/kg q24h × 10-20 days[29,35]	Coccidiosis
Sulfamerazine	100 mg/kg PO[26]	Coccidiosis
	0.05-0.15% in drinking water[26]	
Sulfamethazine	100 mg/kg PO q24h[26]	Coccidiosis
	0.5-1.0% in feed[29]	
	0.77 g/L drinking water[29]	
Sulfaquinoxaline	0.04-0.10% in drinking water[29]	Coccidiosis
	125-250 ppm in feed[29]	
	0.02-0.05% in drinking water[26]	Prevention
	0.10-0.15% in drinking water[26]	Treatment
	0.025-0.03% in feed × 4-6 wk[64]	During weaning

Table 49. Antiparasitic agents used in rabbits (cont.)

Agent	Dosage	Comments
Sulfaquinoxaline (continued)	0.025-0.10% in drinking water[64]	Alternating 2 wk periods for 4-8 wk during weaning
Thiabendazole	25-50 mg/kg PO[26] 50-100 mg/kg PO q24h × 5 days[1] 100-200 mg/kg PO[29] 0.1% in feed × 3 mo[57]	
Thiabendazole/ dexamethasone/ neomycin (Tresaderm, MSD-AgVet)	3 drops in each ear q12h[15] × 7-14 days	Ear mites; generally concurrent to ivermectin therapy

Table 50. Chemical restraint/anesthetic/analgesic agents used in rabbits

Agent	Dosage	Comments
Acepromazine	—	See ketamine, ketamine/xylazine for combinations
	0.5-1.0 mg/kg IM[29]	Preanesthetic
	0.75-1.0 mg/kg IM[39,84]	Sedative; tranquilizer
	1-5 mg/kg SC, IM[26]	Preanesthetic; lower end of dose range is generally preferred
Acetaminophen (Tylenol, McNeil)	—	Acetaminophen combination follows
	200-500 mg/kg PO[26]	Analgesia
	1-2 mg/ml drinking water[36]	
Acetaminophen/ codeine	1 ml elixir/100 ml drinking water[84]	Analgesia; non-steroidal anti-inflammatory
Acetylsalicylic acid (aspirin)	100 mg/kg PO q4h[24,38]	Non-steroidal anti-inflammatory
	100 mg/kg PO q48h[29]	
Alfentanil (Afenta, Taylor)	0.03-0.07 mg/kg IV[84]	Intraoperative analgesia for 45 min duration
Atipamezole (Antisedan, Pfizer)	0.001 mg/kg SC, IP, IV[80]	Medetomidine reversal
Atracurium	0.1 mg/kg[79] IV	Paralysis for intraophthalmic surgery; requires assisted ventilation
Atropine	0.1-3.0 mg/kg SC[29]	Many rabbits possess serum atropinase
	0.8-1.0 mg/kg IM[33]	
Buprenorphine (Buprenex, Reckitt & Colman)	0.01-0.05 mg/kg SC, IP, IV q6-12h[24,29]	Analgesia
	0.02-0.10 mg/kg SC, IV[38]	
	0.5 mg/kg per rectum q12h[36]	

309

Table 50. Chemical restraint/anesthetic/analgesic agents used in rabbits (cont.)

Agent	Dosage	Comments
Butorphanol (Torbugesic, Fort Dodge)	—	See ketamine/xylazine for combination
	0.1-0.5 mg/kg IV q4h[24,38]	Analgesia
	0.1-0.5 mg/kg SC, IM, IV q2-4h[29]	
	1-5 mg/kg SC q4-6h[3]	Lower dose preferred[14]
Carprofen (Rimadyl, Pfizer)	2.2 mg/kg PO q12h[61]	Non-steroidal anti-inflammatory; chronic joint pain
Chlorpromazine	1-10 mg/kg IM, IV[26]	Preanesthetic; lower end of dose range is generally preferred
Codeine	—	See acetaminophen combination
Diazepam	1-3 mg/kg IM[29]	Preanesthetic; tranquilizer
	1-5 mg/kg IM,[15] IV[26]	Preanesthetic; tranquilizer
	5-10 mg/kg IM[26,39]	Preanesthetic; sedative; tranquilizer; lower end of dose range is generally preferred
Enflurane	To effect	Anesthesia; MAC = 2.9%[20]
Fentanyl	0.0074 mg/kg IV[46]	Analgesia
Fentanyl patch	1/2 patch/medium-sized rabbit (3 kg) × 3 days[67]	Postoperative analgesia
Fentanyl/droperidol (Innovar-Vet, Schering-Plough)	0.15-0.44 ml/kg IM[84]	0.22 ml/kg optimal; may cause muscle necrosis at injection site
Flunixin meglumine	—	Analgesia; non-steroidal anti-inflammatory
	0.3-2.0 mg/kg PO, IM, IV q12-24h[61]	Use for no more than 3 days
	1.1 mg/kg SC, IM q12h[24,38]	
	1-2 mg/kg SC q12-24h[33]	

Table 50. Chemical restraint/anesthetic/analgesic agents used in rabbits (cont.)

Agent	Dosage	Comments
Glycopyrrolate (Robinul-V, Fort Dodge)	0.01-0.02 mg/kg SC[36]	Preanesthetic
Halothane	3-4% induction, 0.5-1.5% maintenance[26] 3-4% induction, 1-2% maintenance[29]	
Ibuprofen	— 7.5 mg/kg q6-8h PO[76] 10-20 mg/kg PO q4h[29]	Analgesia; non-steroidal anti-inflammatory; may have gastrointestinal side effects
Isoflurane	3-5% induction, 1.50-1.75% maintenance[26] 3-5% induction, 2-3% maintenance[29]	Inhalant anesthetic of choice; MAC = 2.05%
Ketamine	— 15-20 mg/kg IV[26] 20-50 mg/kg IM[26] 35-50 mg/kg IM[84]	Ketamine combinations follow; see medetomidine combination 60 min of sedation
Ketamine (K)/ acepromazine (A)	(K) 40 mg/kg/ (A) 0.5-1.0 mg/kg IM[38]	Anesthesia
Ketamine (K)/ diazepam (D)	(K) 10 mg/kg/ (D) 0.5 mg/kg IV[55] (D) 0.2-0.5 mg/kg IV, then (K) 10-15 mg/kg IV to effect[33] (K) 15 mg/kg/ (D) 0.3 mg/kg IM[52] (K) 20-30 mg/kg IM, then (D) 0.5 mg/kg IV at 5-10 min[35] (K) 20-30 mg/kg/ (D) 1-3 mg/kg IM[35]	Anesthesia; follow with isoflurane Sedation; use with isoflurane for anesthesia Anesthesia; follow with isoflurane Anesthesia; generally used with isoflurane; dentistries (with or without isoflurane) Anesthesia; use with isoflurane

311

Table 50. Chemical restraint/anesthetic/analgesic agents used in rabbits (cont.)

Agent	Dosage	Comments
Ketamine (K)/ diazepam (D) (continued)	(K) 30-40 mg/kg/ (D) 2-5 mg/kg IM[15]	Surgical anesthesia; lower end of dose range for (D) is preferred;[66] less preferable than the forementioned (K)/ (D) combinations
Ketamine (K)/ midazolam (M)	(K) 25 mg/kg/ (M) 2-5 mg/kg IM[57]	May be preferable to use (M) at <2 mg/kg[14]
Ketamine (K)/ xylazine (X)	— (K) 10 mg/kg/ (X) 3 mg/kg IV[23,38] (K) 30-40 mg/kg/ (X) 3-5 mg/kg IM[26] (K) 35 mg/kg/ (X) 5 mg/kg IM[45]	Anesthesia; may result in bradycardia; less preferable than (K)/ (D)/ isoflurane combination; seldom indicated
Ketamine (K)/ xylazine (X)/ acepromazine (A)	(K) 35 mg/kg/ (X) 5 mg/kg/ (A) 0.75 mg/kg IM[45]	Anesthesia; may result in bradycardia; less preferable than (K)/ (D)/ isoflurane combination; seldom indicated
Ketamine (K)/ xylazine (X)/ butorphanol (B)	(K) 35 mg/kg/ (X) 5 mg/kg/ (B) 0.1 mg/kg IM[49]	Anesthesia; may result in bradycardia; less preferable than (K)/ (D)/ isoflurane combination; seldom indicated
Ketoprofen (Ketofen, Fort Dodge)	1 mg/kg IM q12-24h[61]	Musculoskeletal pain; non-steroidal anti-inflammatory
Lidocaine (1.5%) (10%)	0.4 ml/kg epidural[70] Topical to glottis[36]	Epidural anesthesia Facilitates intubation
Medetomidine (Dormitor, Pfizer)	— 0.25 mg/kg IM[43] 6 mg/kg IV slowly to effect[46]	Medetomidine combinations follow Sedation Induction
Medetomidine (M)/ ketamine (K)	(M) 0.35 mg/kg IM/ (K) 5 mg/kg IV[34]	Anesthesia; surgical depth approximately 19 min

Table 50. Chemical restraint/anesthetic/analgesic agents used in rabbits (cont.)

Agent	Dosage	Comments
Medetomidine (M)/ propofol (P)	(M) 0.35 mg/kg IM/ (P) 3 mg/kg IV[34]	Anesthesia; surgical depth approximately 11 min
Meperidine (Demerol, Winthrop-Breon)	5-10 mg/kg SC, IP q2-3h[29]	Analgesia
	10 mg/kg SC, IM q2-3h[24]	Analgesia
	5-25 mg/kg SC, IM, IV[26]	
	0.2 mg/ml drinking water[36]	
Methoxyflurane	1-3% induction, 0.3-1.0% maintenance[26]	
	2-4% induction, 0.5-2.0% maintenance[29]	
Midazolam (Versed, Roche)	—	See ketamine combination; more potent, shorter action than diazepam; rapidly absorbed IM
	1-2 mg/kg IM[29]	Preanesthetic; tranquilizer
	2 mg/kg IP, IV[39]	Sedative; tranquilizer
	2-4 mg/kg IM, IP, IV[26]	Preanesthetic; seldom indicated at this dose
Morphine	1.2-5.0 mg/kg SC, IM q2-4h[84]	Analgesia
	2-5 mg/kg SC, IM q2-4h[24,38]	
	5-10 mg/kg SC, IM q4h[26]	
Nalbuphine (Nubain, Dupont)	1-2 mg/kg IM, IV q4-5h[33]	Analgesia
Nalorphine (Nalline Hydrochloride, Rhone Merieux)	1-5 mg/kg IV[26]	Narcotic reversal
Naloxone	0.01-0.10 mg/kg IM, IV[26]	Narcotic reversal

Table 50. Chemical restraint/anesthetic/analgesic agents used in rabbits (cont.)

Agent	Dosage	Comments
Oxymorphone	0.05-0.20 mg/kg SC, IM q8-12h[33] 0.2 mg/kg IM q2-4h[84]	Analgesia
Pentazocine (Talwin-V, Upjohn)	5-10 mg/kg IM, IV q2-4h[84]	Analgesia
Pentobarbital	20-45 mg/kg IP, IV[29]	Marginal analgesia; autonomic depression; not recommended
Piroxicam (Feldene, Pfizer)	0.2 mg/kg PO q8h[53]	Analgesia; non-steroidal anti-inflammatory
Promazine	1-2 mg/kg IM, IV[26]	Preanesthetic
Propofol	2-3 mg/kg IV[57] 7.5-15.0 mg/kg IV[16]	Induction after premedication; maintain with approximately 1 mg/kg IV q15min[57]
Sevoflurane	To effect	Anesthesia; MAC = 3.7%[72]
Thiamylal	15-25 mg/kg IV to effect[84]	
Thiopental	15-30 mg/kg IV to effect[84]	
Tiletamine/ zolazepam (Telazol, Fort Dodge)	3 mg/kg IM[29]	Sedation prior to gas anesthetic; caution: tiletamine causes severe renal tubular necrosis at 32 mg/kg and mild nephrosis at 7.5 mg/kg;[18] caution: not generally recommended for use in rabbits
Xylazine	— 1-3 mg/kg IM[29] 2-5 mg/kg SC, IM[21]	See ketamine for combinations Preanesthetic; tranquilizer; seldom indicated
Yohimbine (Yobine, Lloyd)	0.2-1.0 mg/kg IM, IV[26]	Xylazine reversal

Table 51. Ophthalmic drugs used in rabbits

Agent	Dosage	Comments
Atropine (1%)	Topical to eyes q12h prn[40]	Mydriasis; systemic effects are possible
Atropine (1%)/ phenylephrine (10%)	Topical to eyes[29]	Mydriasis for non-albino eyes
Betaxolol (0.5%) (Betoptic, Alcon)	Topical to eyes q12h[41]	Glaucoma; effectively decreases intraocular pressure in rabbits
Ciprofloxacin (0.3%) (Ciloxan, Alcon)	Topical to eyes q8-12h[40]	Susceptible infections
Cyclosporin A (0.2%) ointment (Optimmune, Schering-Plough)	Topical to eyes q12h[81]	Shown to increase tear production in rabbits
Dichlorophenamide (Daranide, Merck)	1-2 mg/kg PO q24h[42]	Glaucoma
Dorzolamide (Trusopt, Merck)	Topical to eyes q8-12h[40]	Glaucoma
Granulocyte macrophage colony stimulating factor (rhuGM-CSF)	Topical to eyes, 1 drop q6h[5]	Superficial corneal wounds; use 4.8% solution (16 mcg rhuGM-CSF in 33µl saline buffered to pH 7.4)
Metipranol (0.1%)/ pilocarpine (2%)	Topical to eyes q8-12h[19]	Glaucoma
Neomycin-bacitracin-polymyxin B	Topical to eyes q6h[40]	Susceptible infections; corneal ulceration
Phenylephrine (10%)	Topical to eyes	Mydriasis[37]
Prednisolone acetate (1%) ophthalmic solution	Topical to eyes q6-12h[40]	Inflammation of eye
Timolol (0.5%) (Timoptic, Merck)	Topical to eyes q12h[41]	Glaucoma
Tissue plasminogen activator	25 mcg intraocular injection[79]	Intraocular fibrin
Tropicamide (1%)	Topical to eyes[29]	Mydriasis

Table 52. Miscellaneous agents used in rabbits

Agent	Dosage	Comments
Aluminum hydroxide	30-60 mg/kg PO q8-12h[10]	Phosphorus-binder; hyperphosphatemia due to renal failure
Barium	10-14 ml/kg PO[64]	Gastrointestinal contrast studies
Bromelin enzyme	1-2 tablets/animal PO q24h × 3-5 days[64]	Trichobezoars, gastric stasis; in fresh pineapple juice
	1-2 tablets/animal PO q24h × 2-3 days[64]	Preventive for heavy hair shedders; use every few months
Ca-EDTA	27.5 mg/kg SC q6h × 20 treatments[80]	Lead toxicosis; diluted to <10 mg/ml with 0.45% NaCl/2.5% dextrose
Cellulose powder (Unifiber, Niche)	1/2-1 tsp/feeding[65]	Non-soluble fiber source for rabbits on liquid enteral diets; will pass through small diameter feeding tubes
Cholestyramine (Questran Light, Squibb)	2 g/animal PO q24h × 18-21 days[29]	Ion exchange resin for toxin absorption following inappropriate antibiotic administration; gavage with 20 ml water; may result in constipation
Chondroitin sulfate (Cosequin, Nutramax)	Used empirically at feline dose[82]	Arthritis; a neutraceutical
Cimetidine (Tagamet, SmithKline Beecham)	5-10 mg/kg q6-12h[1]	Gastric and duodenal ulcers
Cisapride (Propulsid, Janssen)	0.5 mg/kg PO q8-12h[35]	Enhances gastrointestinal motility; used for GI stasis
Dexamethasone	0.2-0.6 mg/kg SC, IM, IV[26]	Anti-inflammatory
	0.5-2.0 mg/kg PO, SC, then decreasing dose q12h × 3-14 days[29]	
	2.0 mg/kg IV, IM[15]	Shock

Table 52. Miscellaneous agents used in rabbits (cont.)

Agent	Dosage	Comments
Doxapram	2-5 mg/kg SC, IV q15min[36]	Respiratory stimulant
Epinephrine	0.2 mg/kg IV[66]	Cardiac arrest
	0.2-0.4 mg/kg IT[66]	Cardiac arrest
Epoetin alpha, recombinant (Epogen, Amgen)	50-150 IU/kg SC q2-3d[10]	Biosynthetic form of erythropoietin; treatment of anemia; use until PCV is normal, then q7d for at least 4 wk
Fecal transfaunation	Mix fresh cecotrophs with warm saline, strain through gauze, and administer via gavage[36]	Dysbiosis; placement of E-collar on donor facilitates collection of sample
Ferrous sulfate	4-6 mg/kg PO q24h[10]	Iron deficiency anemia
Furosemide	1-4 mg/kg IM q4-6h[30]	Diuretic
	5-10 mg/kg q12h[1]	
Fusafungine	Spray in nares q12h × 10 days[60]	Bacterial rhinosinusitis
Hairball laxative, feline	1-2 ml/animal PO q24h × 3-5 days[64]	Trichobezoars, gastric stasis
Hetastarch (Hespan, DuPont)	20 ml/kg IV[56]	Volume expansion in hypo-proteinemic patients; may be of benefit in endotoxemia
Human chorionic gonadotropin (hCG)	20-25 IU/animal IV[29]	Ovulation
Lactated Ringer's solution	60-90 ml/kg[2]	Treatment for shock
Lactobacilli	—	May aid in treatment of enteritis[64]
	Administer PO during antibiotic treatment period, then 5-7 days beyond cessation[17]	Give 2 hr prior to or 2 hr following antibiotic treatment

Table 52. Miscellaneous agents used in rabbits (cont.)

Agent	Dosage	Comments
Lidocaine	1-2 mg/kg IV (bolus)[67]	Cardiac arrhythmia
	2-4 mg/kg IT[67]	Cardiac arrhythmia
Loperamide (Imodium A-D, McNeil)	0.1 mg/kg PO q8h × 3 days, then q24h × 2 days[29]	Enteropathies (non-specific diarrhea); give in 1 ml water
Meclizine (Antivert, Roering)	2-12 mg/kg PO q24h[29]	Reduces disorientation and rolling with torticollis (prevents motion sickness in small animals)
	12.5-25.0 mg/kg PO q8-12h[39]	
Metoclopramide	0.5 mg/kg PO, SC q4-12h[39]	Stimulates gastrointestinal motility; gastric stasis, trichobezoars
	0.2-0.5 mg/kg PO, SC q6-8h[35]	
	0.2-1.0 mg/kg PO, SC q6-8h[29]	
Oxytocin	0.1-3.0 units/kg SC, IM[29]	Used in delayed, but unobstructed, parturition; agalactia
Papain enzyme	1-2 tablets/animal PO q24h × 3-5 days[64]	Trichobezoars, gastric stasis
	1-2 tablets/animal PO q24h × 2-3 days[64]	Preventive for heavy hair shedders; use every few months
Pineapple juice (fresh)	10 ml/medium-size animal PO q24h × 3-5 days[35,64]	Trichobezoars, gastric stasis; must use fresh juice, not canned; repeat in 3-5 days if no resolution[64]
	10 ml/medium-size animal PO q24h × 2-3 days[64]	Preventive for heavy hair shedders; use every few months
Polysulfated glycosaminoglycan (Adequan, Luitpold)	2.2 mg/kg SC, IM q3d × 21-28 days, then q14d[39]	Non-infectious, traumatic, or degenerative joint disease
Potassium citrate	33 mg/kg q8h[84]	Urinary calculi; may decrease calcium = based stone formation
Prednisolone	0.25-0.50 mg/kg PO q12h × 3 days, then q24h × 3 days, then q48h[64]	Treatment of non-responsive torticollis, when negative for pasteurellosis; give antibiotics concurrently

Table 52. Miscellaneous agents used in rabbits (cont.)

Agent	Dosage	Comments
Prednisone	0.5-2.0 mg/kg PO[1,15]	Anti-inflammatory
Sodium bicarbonate	2 mEq/kg IP, IV[30]	Ketoacidosis (pregnancy toxemia); dosage is approximate
Stanozolol (Winstrol-V, Upjohn)	1-2 mg PO once[29]	Stimulates appetite following surgery or illness
Verapamil (Isoptin, Knoll)	0.2 mg/kg SC q8h × 9 treatments[29,39] 2.5-25.0 μg/kg/hr IP[78]	Slow-channel calcium blocking agent; post-operatively to decrease adhesion formation
Viokase-V (Fort Dodge) (V)/yogurt (Y)	2-3 ml PO q12h[1]	Enzymes; trichobezoars, gastric stasis; (V) 1 tsp + (Y) 3 Tbsp, let stand 15 min; no direct effect on hair, but may be effective in digesting the matrix of the trichobezoar
Vitamin C	100 mg/kg PO q12h[9]	Nutritional supplement
Vitamin K	1-10 mg/kg IM prn[76]	Select bleeding disorders and toxicities

Appendix 54. Hematologic and serum biochemical values of rabbits [35,38]

Measurement	Normal values
Hematology	
PCV (%)	30-50
Hb (g/dl)	8.0-17.5
RBC ($10^6/\mu l$)	4-8
MCV (μm^3)	58.0-66.5
MCH (pg)	17.5-23.5
MCHC (%)	29-37
Platelets ($10^3/\mu l$)	290-650
WBC ($10^3/\mu l$)	5-12
Neutrophils (%)	35-55
Lymphocytes (%)	25-50
Monocytes (%)	2-10
Eosinophils (%)	0-5
Basophils (%)	2-7
Chemistries	
AP (IU/L)	4-16
ALT (IU/L)	14-80
AST (IU/L)	14-113
Bicarbonate (mEq/L)	16.2-31.8
Total bilirubin (mg/dl)	0-0.75
Calcium (mg/dl)	8-14
Chloride (mEq/L)	92-112
Cholesterol (mg/dl)	35-60
Creatinine (mg/dl)	0.8-2.5
Glucose (mg/dl)	75-150
LDH (IU/L)	34-129
Total lipids (mg/dl)	280-350
Phosphorus (mg/dl)	2.3-6.9
Potassium (mEq/L)	3.7-6.8
Total protein (g/dl)	5.4-7.5
Albumin (g/dl)	2.5-4.5
Globulin (g/dl)	1.9-3.5
Sodium (mEq/L)	138-155
Triglycerides (mg/dl)	124-156
Urea nitrogen (mg/dl)	15-30

Appendix 55. Biological and physiological data of rabbits [28]

Parameter	Normal values
Adult body weight of male (buck)	2-5 kg
Adult body weight of female (doe)	2-6 kg
Birth weight	30-80 g
Respiratory rate	30-60 breaths/min
Tidal volume	4-6 ml/kg
Heart rate	130-325 beats/min
Rectal temperature	38.5-40.0 °C (101.3-104.0 °F)
Life span	5-6 yr (up to 15 yr)
Food consumption	5 g/100 g/day
Water consumption	5-10 ml/100 g/day
Gastrointestinal transit time	4-5 hr
Breeding onset of male	6-10 mo
Breeding onset of female	4-9 mo
Breeding life of female	4 mo to 3 yr
Reproductive cycle	Induced ovulation
Gestation period	29-35 days
Litter size	4-10
Weaning age	4-6 wk

Appendix 56. Determining the sex of mature rabbits [73]

Male	Female
• Protrude penis by manipulating skin of prepuce. • Palpate for testicles. • Anogenital distance is longer.	• There is a common orifice for both the vagina and urethra (like dogs and cats). • No structure like a "penis" can be protruded from the urogenital orifice. • Anogenital distance is shorter.

Appendix 57. Drugs reported to be toxic in rabbits [a]

Drug	Comments
Amoxicillin[35]	Enteritis; enterotoxemia
Amoxicillin/clavulanic acid[35]	Enteritis; enterotoxemia
Ampicillin[13]	Enteritis; enterotoxemia
Cephalosporins[18]	Enteritis; enterotoxemia
Clindamycin[13]	Enteritis; enterotoxemia
Erythromycin[13]	Enteritis; enterotoxemia
Lincomycin[13]	Enteritis; enterotoxemia
Penicillin[13]	Enteritis; enterotoxemia
Procaine[28]	At doses of 0.4 mg/kg; may be fatal
Tiletamine[18]	Nephrotoxic

[a] There have also been some reports of antibiotic-related colitis in rabbits given penicillin/streptomycin, trimethoprim/sulfamethoxazole, tetracycline, and gentamicin. In general, parenteral antibiotic therapies are preferred over oral.

Appendix 58. Medical treatment for gastric stasis and trichbezoars in rabbits [a,15,29,35,55,64]

Treatment	Comments
Analgesics (see Table 50)	• Used for abdominal discomfort, thereby stimulating appetite
Antibiotics (see Table 48)	• Use when indicated; enrofloxacin or trimethoprim/sulfa are generally the drugs of choice; use parenterally until stools are passed
Exercise	• Increasing activity may aid in passage of trichobezoars
Fluid therapy	• Rehydration (via PO, SC, IV) is essential • Maintenance fluids is ≈100-120 ml/kg/day
Oral (gastric) hydration	• Important to rehydrate any material in stomach • Can use balanced electrolyte solutions, fruit juices, or water • Pineapple juice (fresh, not canned) contains the proteolytic enzyme bromelin which may be an additional benefit
Grooming	• Brushing the hair may prevent an exacerbation of the problem • Routinely brushing long-haired or heavy-shedding individuals for prevention
Nutritional support	• Important in the anorectic rabbit; helps prevent hepatic lipidosis • Force-feed ≈10-15 ml/kg q8-12h of Critical Care For Herbivores (Oxbow Pet Products) or powdered rabbit pellets in lactated Ringer's solution, and vegetable baby foods • Offer fresh greens (parsley, romaine lettuce, carrot tops, kale, etc) and timothy or grass hay ad libitum • Vitamin supplements (especially vitamin B) prn
Laxative, feline (Laxatone, Evsco)	• 1-2 ml/animal PO q24h x 3-5 days
Motility modifiers	• Promotes gastric emptying • Metoclopramide (0.2-0.5 mg/kg PO, SC q6-8h) • Cisapride (0.5 mg/kg PO q8-12h)
Enzyme supplements	• Clinical response to therapy is equivocal • Pineapple juice, fresh 　○ Aids in digestion; contains the proteolytic enzyme bromelin; enzymes have no direct effect on the hair, but presumably have a role in digesting the matrix of the trichobezoar 　○ 10 ml PO q24h x 5 days for treatment 　○ 10 ml PO q24h x 3-5 days q2-3mo may be used for the prevention of trichobezoars, but is of questionable efficacy • Papaya enzymes (papain) and Viokase-V Powder (Fort Dodge) have been used but are less efficacious than fresh pineapple juice

[a] Concurrent to treatment, it is important to correct the cause (ie, boredom, stress, excessive shedding, inadequate dietary roughage, nutritional deficiency or imbalance, obesity, etc).

Appendix 59. Literature cited - Rabbits

1. Allen DG, Pringle JK, Smith DA (eds). *Handbook of Veterinary Drugs.* JB Lippincott Co, Philadelphia, 1993.

2. Bennett RA. Rabbit and rodent orthopedics. *Proc N Am Vet Conf:* 773-774, 1998.

3. Bennett RA. Soft tissue surgery in rabbits. *Proc N Am Vet Conf:* 775-776, 1998.

4. Bennett RA. Treatment of abscesses in the head of rabbits. *Proc N Am Vet Conf:* 821-823, 1999.

5. Blair MJ, Render JA, Morreale R, et al. Granulocyte macrophage colony stimulating factor: effect on corneal wound healing. *Vet Comp Ophthalmol* 7:168-172, 1997.

6. Bowman DD, Fogelson ML, Carbone LG. Effect of ivermectin on the control of ear mites *(Psoroptes cuniculi)* in naturally infested rabbits. *Am J Vet Res* 53:105-109, 1992.

7. Broome RL, Brooks DL. Efficacy of enrofloxacin in the treatment of respiratory pasteurellosis in rabbits. *Lab Anim Sci* 41:572-576, 1991.

8. Broome RL, Brooks DL, Babish JG, et al. Pharmacokinetic properties of enrofloxacin in rabbits. *Am J Vet Res* 52:1835-1841, 1991.

9. Brown SA. Intermittent soft stools in rabbits. *Proc N Am Vet Conf:* 849-850, 1996.

10. Brown SA. Rabbit urinary tract disease. *Proc N Am Vet Conf:* 785-787, 1997.

11. Burgmann P, Percy DH. Antimicrobial drug use in rodents and rabbits. In: Prescott JF, Baggot JD (eds). *Antimicrobial Therapy in Veterinary Medicine.* Iowa State University Press, Ames, 1993. Pp 524-541.

12. Cabanes A, Arboix M, Garcia-Anton JM, et al. Pharmacokinetics of enrofloxacin after intravenous and intramuscular injection in rabbits. *Am J Vet Res* 53:2090-2093, 1992.

13. Carman RJ. Antibiotic-associated diarrhea of rabbits. *J Small Exotic Anim Med* 2:69-71, 1993.

14. Carpenter JW. Personal communication. 1999.

15. Carpenter JW, Mashima TY, Gentz EJ, et al. Caring for rabbits: An overview and formulary. *Vet Med* (April):340-364, 1995.

16. Cocksholt ID, Douglas EJ, Plummer GF, et al. The pharmacokinetics of propofol in laboratory animals. *Xenobiotica* 22:369-375, 1992.

17. Collins BR. Antimicrobial drug use in rabbits, rodents, and other small mammals. In: *Antimicrobial Therapy in Caged Birds and Exotic Pets.* Veterinary Learning Systems Co, Trenton, NJ, 1995. Pp 3-10.

18. Doerning BJ, Brammer DW, Chrisp CE, et al. Nephrotoxicity of tiletamine in New Zealand white rabbits. *Lab Anim Sci* 42:267-269, 1992.

19. Drago F, Emmi I, Marino V. Effects of beta-blockers association with pilocarpine on rabbit intraocular pressure and heart rate. *Pharmacol Res* 35:299-302, 1997.

20. Drummond JC. MAC for halothane, enflurane, and isoflurane in the New Zealand white rabbit: and a test for the validity of MAC determinations. *Anesthesiology* 62:336-338, 1985.

21. Eisele PH. Anesthesia for the rabbit. *Proc N Am Vet Conf:* 792-794, 1997.

22. Fish RE, Besch-Williford C. Reproductive disorders in the rabbit and guinea pig. In: Kirk RW, Bonagura JD (eds). *Kirk's Current Veterinary Therapy XI: Small Animal Practice.* WB Saunders Co, Philadelphia, 1992. Pp 1175-1179.

23. Flecknell PA. *Laboratory Animal Anaesthesia.* Academic Press, Inc, London, 1987.

24. Flecknell PA. Post-operative analgesia in rabbits and rodents. *Lab Anim* 20:34-37, 1991.

25. Flecknell P. Medetomidine and atipamezole: potential uses in laboratory animals. *Lab Anim:* 21-25, 1997.

26. Gillett CS. Selected drug dosages and clinical reference data. In: Manning PJ, Ringler DH, Newcomer CE (eds). *The Biology of the Laboratory Rabbit*. 2nd ed. Academic Press, San Diego, 1994. Pp 467-472.

27. Green LC, Callegan MC, Engal LS, et al. Pharmacokinetics of topically applied ciprofloxacin in rabbit tears. *Jpn J Ophthalmol* 40:123-126, 1996.

28. Harkness JE, Wagner JE. *The Biology and Medicine of Rabbits and Rodents*, 3rd ed. Lea and Febiger, Philadelphia, 1989.

29. Harkness JE, Wagner JE. *The Biology and Medicine of Rabbits and Rodents*, 4th ed. Williams & Wilkins, Philadelphia, 1995.

30. Harrenstien L. Critical care of ferrets, rabbits, and rodents. *Semin Avian Exotic Pet Med* 3:217-228, 1994.

31. Harvey C. Rabbit and rodent skin diseases. *Semin Avian Exotic Pet Med* 4:195-204, 1995.

32. Hawk CT, Leary SL. *Formulary for Laboratory Animals*. Iowa State University Press, Ames, 1995.

33. Heard DJ. Principles and techniques of anesthesia and analgesia for exotic practice. *Vet Clin N Am: Small Anim Pract* 23:1301-1327, 1993.

34. Hellebreker LJ, deBoer EJ, van Zwylen MA, et al. A comparison between medetomidine-ketamine and medetomidine-propofol anesthesia in rabbits. *Lab Anim* 31:58-69, 1997.

35. Hillyer EV. Pet rabbits. *Vet Clin N Am: Small Anim Pract* 24:25-65, 1994.

36. Huerkamp MJ. Anesthesia and postoperative management of rabbits and pocket pets. In: Bonagura JD (ed). *Kirk's Current Veterinary Therapy XII: Small Animal Practice. WB* Saunders Co, Philadelphia, 1995. Pp 1322-1327.

37. Ivey E. Personal communication. 1999.

38. Jenkins JR. Rabbits. In: Jenkins JR, Brown SA. *A Practitioner's Guide to Rabbits and Ferrets*. American Animal Hospital Association, Lakewood, CO, 1993. Pp 1-42.

39. Jenkins JR. Rabbit drug dosages. In: Bauck L, Boyer TH, Brown SA, et al. *Exotic Animal Formulary*, American Animal Hospital Association, Lakewood, CO, 1995. Pp 13-17.

40. Kern TJ. Rabbit and rodent ophthalmology. *Semin Avian Exotic Pet Med* 6:138-145, 1997.

41. Kiel JW, Patel P. Effects of timolol and betaxol on choroidal blood flow in the rabbit. *Exp Eye Res* 67:501-507, 1998.

42. Kirschner SE. Ophthalmologic diseases in small mammals. In: Hillyer EV, Quesenberry KE (eds). *Ferrets, Rabbits, and Rodents: Clinical Medicine and Surgery,* WB Saunders, Philadelphia, 1997. Pp 339-345.

43. Ko JCH, Thurman JC, Tranquilli WJ, et al. Comparison of medetomidine- propofol and medetomidine-midazolam-propofol anesthesia in rabbits. *Lab Anim Sci* 42: 503-507, 1992.

44. Kraus AL, Wesbroth SH, Flatt RE, et al. Biology and diseases of rabbits. In: Fox JG, Cohen BJ, Loew FM (eds). *Laboratory Animal Medicine*. Academic Press, Orlando, 1984. Pp 207-240.

45. Lipman NS, Marini RP, Erdman SE. A comparison of ketamine/xylazine and ketamine/xylazine/acepromazine anesthesia in the rabbit. *Lab Anim Sci* 40:395-398, 1990.

46. Lipman NS, Marini RP, Flecknell PA. Anesthesia and analgesia in rabbits. In: Kohn DF, Wixson SK, White WJ, Benson GJ (eds). *Anesthesia and Analgesia in Laboratory Animals*. Academic Press, New York, 1997. Pp 205-232.

47. Louie A, Liu QF, Drusano GL. Pharmacokinetic studies of fluconazole in rabbits characterizing doses which achieve peak levels in serum and area under the concentration-time curve values which mimic those of high-dose fluconazole in humans. *Antimicrob Agents Chemother* 42:1512-1514, 1998.

48. Marangos MN, Zhu Z, Nicolau DP, et al. Disposition of ofloxacin in female New Zealand white rabbits. *J Vet Pharmacol Therap* 20:17-20, 1997.

49. Marini RP, Avison DL, Corning BF, et al. Ketamine/xylazine/butorphanol: a new anesthetic combination for rabbits. *Lab Anim Sci* 42:57-62, 1992.

50. McElroy DE, Ravis WR, Clark CH. Pharmacokinetics of oxytetracycline hydrochloride in rabbits. *Am J Vet Res* 48:1261-1263, 1987.

51. McKay SG, Morck DW, Merrill JK, et al. Use of tilmicosin for treatment of pasteurellosis in rabbits. *Am J Vet Res* 57:1180-1184, 1996.

52. Mills DL, Walshaw R. Elective castrations and ovariohysterectomies in pet rabbits. *J Am Anim Hosp Assoc* 28: 491-498.

53. More RC, Kody MH, Kabo JM, et al. The effects of two non-steroidal anti-inflammatory drugs on limb swelling, joint stiffness, and bone torsional strength following fracture in a rabbit model. *Clin Orthoped* 247:306-312, 1989.

54. Morrisey JK. Ectoparasites of small mammals. *Proc N Am Vet Conf:* 844-845, 1998.

55. Morrisey JK. Personal communication. 1999.

56. Nielsen VG, Sidhartha T, Brix AE, et al. Hextend (hetastarch solution) decreases multiple organ injury and xanthine oxidase release after hepatoenteric ischemia-reperfusion in rabbits. *Crit Care Med* 25:1565-1574, 1997.

57. Okerman L. *Diseases of Domestic Rabbits*. 2nd ed. Blackwell Scientific Publications, Oxford, 1994.

58. Okerman L, Devriese LA, Gevaert D, et al. *In vivo* activity of orally administered antibiotics and chemotherapeutics against acute septicaemic pasteurellosis in rabbits. *Lab Anim* 24:341-344, 1990.

59. Ostergaard C, Sorensen TK, Knudsen JD, et al. Evaluation of moxifloxacin, a new 8-methoxy-quinalone, for treatment of meningitis caused by a penicillin-resistant pneumococcus in rabbits. *Antimicrob Agents Chemother* 42:1706-1712, 1998.

60. Otori N, Paydays G, Stierna P, et al. The anti-inflammatory effect of fusafungine during experimentally induced rhinosinusitis in the rabbit. *Eur Arch Otorhinolaryngol* 255:195-201, 1998.

61. Paul-Murphy J, Ramer JC. Urgent care of the pet rabbit. *Vet Clin N Am: Exotic Anim Pract* 1:127-152, 1998.

62. Paul-Murphy J. Personal communication. 1999.

63. Percy DH, Black WD. Pharmacokinetics of tetracycline in the domestic rabbit following intravenous or oral administration. *Can J Vet Res* 52:5-11.

64. Quesenberry KE. Rabbits. In: Birchard SJ, Sherding RG (eds). *Saunders Manual of Small Animal Practice*. WB Saunders Co, Philadelphia, 1994. Pp 1345-1362.

65. Quesenberry KE. Personal communication. 1999.

66. Ramer JC, Paul-Murphy J, Benson KG. Evaluating and stabilizing critically ill rabbits —Part I. *Compendium* 21:116-125, 1999.

67. Ramer JC, Paul-Murphy J, Benson KG. Evaluating and stabilizing critically ill rabbits —Part II. *Compendium* 21:30-40, 1999.

68. Rodoni D, Hanni F, Gerber CM, et al. Trovafloxacin in combination with vancomycin against penicillin-resistant pneumococci in the rabbit meningitis model. *Antimicrob Agents Chemother* 43:963-965, 1999.

69. Rosenthal K. New therapeutics in small mammals. *Proc N Am Vet Conf:* 686-687, 1995.

70. Rosenthal K. Epidural anesthesia. *Proc N Am Vet Conf:* 876, 1996.

71. Sanati H, Ramos CF, Bayer AS, et al. Combination therapy with amphotericin B and fluconazole against invasive candidiasis in neutropenic-mouse and infective-endocarditis rabbit models. *Antimicrob Agents Chemother* 41:1345-1348, 1997.

72. Scheller MS, Daidman LJ, Partridge BL. MAC of sevoflurane in humans and the New Zealand white rabbit. *Can J Anesthesiol* 35:153-156, 1988.

73. Schuchman SM. Individual care and treatment of rabbits, mice, guinea pigs, hamsters, and gerbils. In: Kirk RW (ed). *Current Veterinary Therapy X: Small Animal Practice.* WB Saunders Co, Philadelphia, 1989. Pp 738-765.

74. Sharpnack DD, Mastin JP, Childress CP, et al. Quinolone arthropathy in juvenile New Zealand white rabbits. *Lab Anim Sci* 44:436-442, 1994.

75. Shirtliff ME, Mader JT, Calhoun J. Oral rifampin plus azithromycin or clarithromycin to treat osteomyelitis in rabbits. *Clin Orthoped* 359:229-236, 1999.

76. Smith DA, Burgmann PM. Formulary. In: Hillyer EV, Quesenberry KE (eds). *Ferrets, Rabbits, and Rodents: Clinical Medicine and Surgery.* WB Saunders Co, Philadelphia, 1997. Pp 392-403.

77. Smith RL, Kajiyama G, Schurman DJ. Staphylococcal septic arthritis: antibiotic and nonsteroidal anti-inflammatory drug treatment in a rabbit model. *J Orthoped Res* 15:919-926, 1997.

78. Steinleitner A, Lambert H, Kazensky C, et al. Reduction of primary post-operative adhesion formation under calcium channel blockade in the rabbit. *J Surg Res* 48:42-45, 1990.

79. Stiles J, Didier E, Ritchie B, et al. *Encephalitozoon cuniculi* in the lens of a rabbit with phacoclastic uveitis: confirmation and treatment. *Vet Comp Ophthalmol* 7:233-238, 1997.

80. Swartout MS, Gerken DF. Lead-induced toxicosis in two domestic rabbits. *J Am Vet Med Assoc* 191:717-719, 1987.

81. Toshida H, Nakaysu K, Kanai A. Effect of cyclosporin A eyedrops on tear secretion in the rabbit. *Jpn J Ophthalmol* 42:168-173, 1998.

82. Uebelhart D, Thonar EJ, Zhang J, et al. Protective effect of exogenous chondroitin 4,6-sulfate in the acute degradation of articular cartilage in the rabbit. *Osteoarth Cartil* 6 Suppl A:6-13, 1998.

83. Welch WD, Lu Y-S, Bawdon RE. Pharmacokinetics of penicillin-G in serum and nasal washings of *Pasteurella multocida* free and infected rabbits. *Lab Anim Sci* 37:65-68, 1987.

84. Wixson SK. Anesthesia and analgesia. In: Manning PJ, Ringler DH, Newcomer CE (eds). *The Biology of the Laboratory Rabbit.* 2nd ed. Academic Press, San Diego, 1994. Pp 87-109.

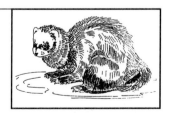

Table 53. Antimicrobial and antifungal agents used in ferrets

Agent	Dosage	Comments
Amikacin	10-15 mg/kg SC, IM q12h[3]	
Amoxicillin	—	Can use with metronidazole and bismuth subsalicylate for *Helicobacter*
	10-20 mg/kg PO q12h[3]	
	20 mg/kg PO, SC q12h[24]	
	30 mg/kg PO q8h[19] × 21 days	*Helicobacter*
Amoxicillin/ clavulanate (Clavamox, Pfizer)	12.5 mg/kg q12h PO[4] 13-25 mg/kg PO q8-12h[24]	
Amphotericin B	0.4-0.8 mg/kg IV q7d[2]	Blastomycosis; monitor for azotemia; total dose 7-25 mg
Ampicillin	5 mg/kg PO q6h[2] 5-30 mg/kg SC, IM, IV q12h[4]	
Cefadroxil (Cefa-drops, Fort Dodge)	15-20 mg/kg PO q12h[4]	
Cephalexin (Keflex, Dista)	15-25 mg/kg PO q12h[4] 15-30 mg/kg PO q8h[24]	
Cephaloridine	10-15 mg/kg SC, IM q24h × 5-7 days[3] 10-25 mg/kg SC, IM q24h × 5-7 days[46]	Dermatitis
Chloramphenicol	25-50 mg/kg PO q12h[3] 30-50 mg/kg SC, IM, IV q12h[3,9] 50 mg/kg PO, SC, IM, IV q12h[23,24]	2 wk minimum for proliferative bowel disease[23,24]
Ciprofloxacin	— 5-15 mg/kg PO q12h[4] 10-30 mg/kg PO q24h[4]	Mix 500 mg tablet in 10 ml water (50 mg/ml)

Table 53. Antimicrobial and antifungal agents used in ferrets (cont.)

Agent	Dosage	Comments
Clarithromycin (Biaxin, Abbott)	50 mg/kg PO q24h or divided q12h × 14d[34]	*Helicobacter*; use with omeprazole (or ranitidine) and metronidazole
Clindamycin	5.5-10.0 mg/kg PO q12h[4]	Anaerobic infections; bone and dental disease
Cloxacillin	10 mg/kg PO, IM, IV q6h[2]	
Enrofloxacin	5-10 mg/kg PO, SC, IM q12h[4] 10-20 mg/kg PO, SC, IM q24h[4]	IM for short term; injectable form can be given PO in palatable liquid;[4] liquid for PO can also be compounded commercially
Erythromycin	10 mg/kg PO q6h[2] 220 g/ton feed[17]	Controlling *Campylobacter* diarrhea in large groups
Gentamicin	5 mg/kg SC, IM q24h[9] 2 mg/kg PO q12h × 10-14 days[11] 2-4 mg/kg SC, IM, IV q12h[4]	Parenteral form can be given PO; proliferative colitis that is non-responsive to chloramphenicol[3,11] If given IV, dilute with saline and administer over 20 min
Griseofulvin	25 mg/kg PO q24h[24]	Refractory dermatomycosis; with lime-sulfur dips q7d[24]
Ketoconazole	10-30 mg/kg PO q8h[2]	
Lime sulfur	Dip q7d[24]	Dermatomycosis; see griseofulvin
Lincomycin	11 mg/kg PO q8h[2]	
Metronidazole	— 15-20 mg/kg PO q12h[3] 20 mg/kg PO q12h[23,24] 50 mg/kg PO q24h[9] 75 mg/kg PO q24h[34] × 14 days	Anaerobic infections; can use with amoxicillin and bismuth subsalicylate for *Helicobacter* *Helicobacter;* use with clari-thromycin and omeprazole

Table 53. Antimicrobial and antifungal agents used in ferrets (cont.)

Agent	Dosage	Comments
Neomycin	10-20 mg/kg PO q6h[2,9]	
Netilmicin (Netromycin, Schering)	6-8 mg/kg SC, IM, IV q24h[47]	Severe staphylococcal infections
Oxytetracycline	20 mg/kg PO q8h[2,3,9]	
Penicillin G (sodium or potassium)	40,000-44,000 IU/kg IM q24h[2-4]	
Sulfadimethoxine	25 mg/kg PO, SC, IM q24h[4] 30-50 mg/kg PO q12-24h[9]	
Sulfamethazine	1 mg/ml drinking water[9]	
Sulfasoxazole	50 mg/kg PO q8h[4]	
Tetracycline	20 mg/kg PO q8h[9] 25 mg/kg PO q12h[3]	
Trimethoprim/sulfa	5 mg/kg PO q24h[20] 15-30 mg/kg PO, SC q12h[24]	Pyelonephritis
Tylosin (Tylan, Elanco)	10 mg/kg PO q8-12h[4,9] 5-10 mg/kg IM, IV q12h[9]	

Table 54. Antiparasitic agents used in ferrets

Agent	Dosage	Comments
Amitraz (Mitaban, Upjohn)	Topical to affected area 3-6 times q14d[47]	Demodecosis; use full concentration
Amprolium	19 mg/kg PO q24h[4]	Coccidiosis
Carbaryl (5%)	Topical q7 days × 3-6 treatments[4]	Ectoparasites
Diethylcarbamazine	5-11 mg/kg PO q24h[2,24]	Heartworm preventative; rarely used; ivermectin preferred
Fipronil (Frontline, Rhone Merieux)	1 pump of spray or 1/5-1/2 of cat pipette topical q60d[33]	Flea adulticide
Imidacloprid (Advantage, Bayer)	1 cat dose divided onto 2-3 spots along dorsum q30d[33]	Flea adulticide
Ivermectin	0.4 mg/kg PO, SC, repeat in 2-4 wk[24,41]	
	0.2-0.5 mg/kg SC, repeat q2wk × 3 treatments[24]	Sarcoptic mange
	0.5-1.0 mg/kg in ears, repeat in 2 wk[4,24]	Ear mites; half dose in each ear; treat cats and dogs in house
	0.05 mg/kg PO monthly[24]	Heartworm preventative
	0.05 mg/kg PO, SC[24]	Heartworm microfilaricide; 3-4 wk post-adulticide treatment
	0.055 mg/ferret PO monthly[34]	Heartworm preventative; Heartgard, MSD-Ag Vet;[1] use small cat dose
Lufenuron (Program, Novartis)	30-45 mg/kg PO monthly[33]	Flea larvicide
Melarsomine dihydrochloride (Immiticide, Rhone Merieux)	2.5 mg/kg IM once, repeat in 1 mon with 2 treatments 24 hr apart[4]	Heartworm adulticide; possible therapeutic option in place of thiacetarsemide
Metronidazole	15-20 mg/kg PO q12h × 2 wk[3]	Gastrointestinal protozoa
Milbemycin oxime (Interceptor, Novartis)	1.15-2.33 mg/kg PO monthly[47]	Heartworm preventative
Piperazine	50-100 mg/kg PO q14d[4]	Intestinal nematodes
Praziquantel	5-10 mg/kg PO, SC, repeat in 2 wk[3]	Cestodes

Table 54. Antiparasitic agents used in ferrets (cont.)

Agent	Dosage	Comments
Pyrantel pamoate	4.4 mg/kg PO, repeat in 2 wk[4]	
Pyrethrins	Topical q7d prn[33]	Fleas; use products safe for puppies and kittens
Sulfadimethoxine	20-50 mg/kg PO q24h[3] 50 mg/kg PO, then 25 mg/kg q24h × 9 days[3]	Coccidia
Thiacetarsemide (Caparsolate, Rhone Merieux)	2.2 mg/kg IV q12h × 2 days[16,24,49]	Heartworm adulticide; follow 3-4 wk later with ivermectin;[24] use heparin (100 U/animal [0.45-1.35 kg] SC q24h × 21 days) concurrently to reduce risk of thromboemboli formation; after 3 wk, change heparin to aspirin (22 mg/kg PO q24h × 3 mo[49]); not commonly used

Table 55. Chemical restraint/anesthetic/analgesic agents used in ferrets

Agent	Dosage	Comments
Acepromazine	—	See ketamine for combination
	0.10-0.25 mg/kg SC, IM[3,14,45]	Preanesthetic; light sedation
	0.2-0.5 mg/kg SC, IM[14,45]	Tranquilization
Acetylsalicylic acid (aspirin)	0.5-22.0 mg/kg PO q8-24h[24]	Analgesia; anti-inflammatory; antipyretic
Alphaxalone/ alphadalone (Saffan, Glaxovet)	6-8 mg/kg IM[29]	Anesthesia; used mostly in laboratory situations; not available in US
Atipamezole (Antisedan, Pfizer)	1 mg/kg SC, IP, IV[13]	Medetomidine reversal
Atropine	0.04-0.05 mg/kg SC, IM, IV[14,21,24,45]	Preanesthetic; bradycardia; hypersalivation
Buprenorphine (Buprenex, Reckitt & Colman)	0.01-0.03 mg/kg SC, IM, IV q8-12h[21]	Analgesia
Butorphanol (Torbugesic, Fort Dodge)	—	See ketamine, medetomidine for combinations
	0.05-0.5 mg/kg SC, IM q8-12h[4]	Analgesia
Carprofen (Rimadyl, Pfizer)	1 mg/kg PO q12-24h[4]	Nonsteroidal, anti-inflammatory; use with caution in animals with enteritis or gastritis
Diazepam	—	See ketamine for combination
	1-2 mg/kg IM[3,14]	Tranquilization; seizure control[3]
	1 mg/animal IV[24]	Seizure control; 1-2 boluses
	1.0-1.5 mg/hr continuous IV[24]	Status epilepticus control
	≤ 1 mg/kg IM[3]	Stimulates appetite
Enflurane	2% maintenance[10]	Anesthesia

Table 55. Chemical restraint/anesthetic/analgesic agents used in ferrets (cont.)

Agent	Dosage	Comments
Fentanyl/droperidol (Innovar-Vet, Schering Plough)	0.15 ml/kg IM[12]	Minor surgical procedures; deep sedation
Flunixin meglumine	0.3 mg/kg PO, SC q24h[4] 0.5-2.0 mg/kg SC, IV q12-24h[21]	Nonsteroidal anti-inflammatory; use with caution in animals with enteritis or gastritis; use caution in using drug more than 5 days continuously; injectable form in palatable syrup for PO
Glycopyrrolate	0.01 mg/kg IM[21]	Preanesthetic; bradycardia; hypersalivation
Halothane	3.0-3.5% induction; 0.5-2.5% maintenance[14]	Anesthesia
Isoflurane	5% induction; 2-3% maintenance[3]	Anesthetic agent of choice
Ketamine	— 10-20 mg/kg IM[14] ≤20 mg/kg IM[21] 30-60 mg/kg IM[14]	Ketamine combinations follow Tranquilization Induction; higher doses may cause apnea Anesthesia
Ketamine (K)/ acepromazine (A)	(K) 20-35 mg/kg/ (A) 0.20-0.35 mg/kg SC, IM[24,45]	Anesthesia
Ketamine (K)/ diazepam (D)	(K) 10-20 mg/kg/ (D) 1-2 mg/kg IM[24] (K) 25-35 mg/kg/ (D) 2-3 mg/kg IM[3,32] 0.1 ml/kg IV[10]	Anesthesia; poor analgesia[32] Induction; will allow intubation with premedication; use equal volumes of (K) at 100 mg/ml and (D) at 5 mg/ml
Ketamine (K)/ medetomidine (M)	(K) 5 mg/kg/ (M) 0.08 mg/kg IM[10] (K) 8 mg/kg/ (M) 0.1 mg/kg[13] IM	Induction Anesthesia; analgesia; may result in hypotension and respiratory depression

Table 55. Chemical restraint/anesthetic/analgesic agents used in ferrets (cont.)

Agent	Dosage	Comments
Ketamine (K)/ medetomidine (M)/ butorphanol (B)	(K) 5 mg/kg/ (M) 0.08 mg/kg/ (B) 0.1 mg/kg IM[10]	Induction
Ketamine (K)/ midazolam (M)	0.1 ml/kg IV[10]	Induction; use equal volumes of (K) at 100 mg/ml and (M) at 5 mg/ml
Ketamine (K)/ xylazine (X)	(K) 10-25 mg/kg/ (X) 1-2 mg/kg IM[24,32]	Anesthesia; avoid in sick animals;[24] may result in cardiac arrhythmias[32]
Ketoprofen	1 mg/kg PO, IM q24h[4]	Nonsteroidal anti-inflammatory; use with caution in animals with enteritis or gastritis; use caution in using drug more than 5 days continuously
Medetomidine (Dormitor, Pfizer)	—	Medetomidine combination follows; see ketamine for combinations
	0.1 mg/kg SC, IM[13]	Light sedation
Medetomidine (M)/ butorphanol (B)	(M) 0.08 mg/kg/ (B) 0.1 mg/kg IM[29]	Anesthesia; monitor blood pressure and ventilation
Meperidine (Demerol, Winthrop-Breon)	5-10 mg/kg SC, IM, IV q2-4h[21]	Analgesia
Methoxyflurane	1-3% induction[14]	Anesthesia
Midazolam (Versed, Roche)	—	See ketamine for combination
	0.3-1.0 mg/kg SC, IM[6]	Mild sedation; premedication
Morphine	0.5-5.0 mg/kg SC, IM q2-6h[21]	Analgesia
Nalbuphine (Nubain, Endo Labs)	0.5-1.5 mg/kg IM, IV q2-3h[21]	Analgesia
Naloxone (Narcan, Dupont)	0.04 mg/kg SC, IM, IV[5]	Reversal of opioids
Oxymorphone	0.05-0.20 mg/kg SC, IM, IV q8-12h[21]	Analgesia

336

Table 55. Chemical restraint/anesthetic/analgesic agents used in ferrets (cont.)

Agent	Dosage	Comments
Pentazocine (Talwin, Sanofi Winthrop)	5-10 mg/kg IM q4h[21]	Analgesia
Pentobarbital	30-50 mg/kg IP[53]	Anesthesia; minimal analgesia; respiratory depression; prolonged recovery; other agents preferred
	1-2 mg/kg PO q12h[4]	Seizure control; use oral elixir
Tiletamine/ zolazepam (Telazol, Fort Dodge)	12-22 mg/kg IM[37]	Minor surgical procedures at 22 mg/kg
Xylazine	—	See ketamine for combination
	1 mg/kg SC, IM[14]	Tranquilization
Yohimbine (Yobine, Lloyd)	0.5 mg/kg IM[51]	Xylazine reversal

Table 56. Cardiopulmonary agents used in ferrets

Agent	Dosage	Comments
Aminophylline	4 mg/kg PO, IM, IV q12h[4] 4.4-6.6 mg/kg PO, IM q12h[24]	Bronchodilation
Atenolol (Tenormin, ICI)	6.25 mg/animal PO q24h[4,48]	Beta adrenergic blocker for hypertrophic cardiomyopathy
Atropine	0.02-0.04 mg/kg SC, IM[4]	Bradycardia
Captopril (Capoten, Squibb)	1/8 of 12.5 mg tablet/animal PO q48h[24]	Vasodilator; starting dose, gradually increase to q12-24h; can cause lethargy
Digoxin (Cardoxin, Evsco)	0.005-0.01 mg/kg PO q12-24h[4,41] 0.01 mg/kg PO q12h, start at 75% lean BW[24]	Positive inotrope for dilated cardiomyopathy; monitor serum levels
Diltiazem (Cardizem, Marion Merrill Dow)	1.5-7.5 mg/kg PO q12h[4,48]	Calcium channel blocker for hypertrophic cardiomyopathy
Doxapram	1-2 mg/kg IV[12] 5-11 mg/kg IV[2]	Respiratory stimulant
Enalapril (Enacard, Merck)	0.25-0.5 mg/kg PO q24-48h[4,41,48] 1/8 of 2.5 mg tablet/animal PO q24h[24]	Vasodilator for dilated cardiomyopathy; do not use with concurrent renal disease[4]
Epinephrine	0.02 mg/kg SC, IM, IV,[39] IT	Cardiac arrest; anaphylactic reactions
Furosemide	2 mg/kg PO, SC, IM, IV q8-12h[24,48] 1-4 mg/kg PO, SC, IM, IV q8-12h[4]	Diuretic
Nitroglycerin 2% ointment (Nitrol, Savage)	1/16-1/8 inch/animal q12-24h[3]	Vasodilator for cardiomyopathy; apply to shaved inner thigh or pinna
Propranolol (Inderal, Wyeth-Ayerst)	0.2-1.0 mg/kg PO q8-12h[24] 2 mg/kg PO, SC q12h[2,3]	Beta blocker for hypertrophic cardiomyopathy; may cause lethargy, loss of appetite[3]
Theophylline	4.25 mg/kg PO q8-12h[47]	Bronchodilator; use elixir

Table 57. Miscellaneous agents used in ferrets [a]

Agent	Dosage	Comments
Acetylsalicylic acid (aspirin)	22 mg/kg PO q24h × 3 mo[49]	Heartworm treatment; see thiacetarsemide (Table 54)
Amantadine (Symmetrel, Endo Labs)	6 mg/kg as aerosol q12h[44]	Influenza; experimental antiviral
Aminophylline	4 mg/kg PO, IM, IV q12h[4]	Bronchodilation
	4.4-6.6 mg/kg PO, IM q12h[24]	
Apomorphine	0.7 mg/kg SC[18]	Emetic
	5 mg/kg SC[2]	Emetic; may cause excitation
Atropine	5-10 mg/kg[4] SC, IM	Organophosphate toxicity
Barium (20%)	15 ml/kg PO[23,24]	Gastrointestinal contrast study
Bismuth subsalicylate (Pepto-Bismol, Procter & Gamble)	0.25 ml/kg PO q4-6h[23,24]	Gastrointestinal ulcers; may help prevent *Helicobacter* colonization[23,24]
	17.5 mg/kg PO q8h[19]	
Chlorpheniramine (Chlor-Trimeton, Squibb)	1-2 mg/kg PO q8-12h[4,24]	Antihistamine; control sneezing and coughing when interferes with eating or sleeping[24]
Cimetidine (Tagamet, SmithKline Beecham)	5-10 mg/kg PO, SC, IM q8h[4,28]	H_2 blocker; inhibits acid secretion; gastrointestinal ulcers; unpalatable; give IV slowly
	10 mg/kg PO, IV q8h[23,24]	
Cisapride (Propulsid, Janssen)	0.5 mg/kg PO q8-12h[38]	Antiemetic; motility enhancer
Dexamethasone	0.5-2.0 mg/kg SC, IM, IV[4]	
	1 mg/kg IM[24]	Post-adrenalectomy; follow with prednisone
Dexamethasone NaPO4	4-8 mg/kg IM, IV[4]	Shock therapy
	6-8 mg/kg IV[24]	Prior to blood transfusion

Table 57. Miscellaneous agents used in ferrets (cont.)

Agent	Dosage	Comments
Diazoxide (Proglycem, Medical Market Specialties)	10 mg/kg/day PO divided q8-12h[22,24] 10-20 mg/kg PO q12h[3]	Insulinoma; insulin-blocker; gradually increase to 30[43]-60[22,24] mg/kg q24h prn; can cause hypertension, lethargy, depression, nausea;[24] some consider it minimally effective
Diphenhydramine (Benadryl; Parke-Davis)	0.5-2.0 mg/kg PO, IM, IV q8-12h[4,24]	Antihistamine; control sneezing and coughing when interferes with eating or sleeping;[24] give at high dose IM prevaccination where previous reaction encountered[4]
Doxapram	1-2 mg/kg IV[12] 5-11 mg/kg IV[2]	Respiratory stimulant
Epinephrine	0.02 mg/kg SC, IM, IV,[39] IT	Severe vaccine reaction; cardiac arrest
Epoetin alfa (Epogen, Amgen)	50-150 IU/kg PO, IM q48h[4]	Stimulates erythropoiesis; after desired PCV is reached, administer q7d for maintenance
Famotidine (Pepcid, Merck)	0.25-0.50 mg/kg PO, IV q24h[4]	Inhibits acid secretion; gastrointestinal ulcers
Flunixin meglumine (Banamine, Schering)	— 1 mg/kg SC, IM[18] 2.5 mg/animal SC, IM q12h prn[20]	Nonsteroidal, anti-inflammatory; see also Table 55 Prevention of prostaglandin-mediated hypotension of endotoxemia Reduce inflammation in mastitis
Flutamide	10 mg/kg PO q12h[4]	Antiandrogenic drug used to alleviate signs of adrenal disease; reduces enlarged periurethral prostate tissue; lifetime treatment
Furosemide	2 mg/kg PO, SC, IM, IV q8-12h[24,48] 1-4 mg/kg PO, SC, IM, IV q8-12h[4]	Diuretic

340

Table 57. Miscellaneous agents used in ferrets (cont.)

Agent	Dosage	Comments
Gonadotropin-releasing hormone (GnRH; Cystorelin, Sanofi)	20 µg/animal SC, IM[22,24]	Termination of estrus after 10th day of estrus; repeat in 2 wk prn[24]
Hairball laxative, feline	1-2 ml/animal PO q48h[3]	Trichobezoar prophylaxis
Heparin	100 µ/animal (0.45-1.35 kg) SC q24h × 21 days[49]	Heartworm treatment; see thiacetarsemide (Table 54)
	200 U/kg SC, IM q12h × 5 days[24]	Decreases thromboembolism; start day prior to heartworm adulticide treatment
Human chorionic gonadotropin (hCG; Pregnyl, Organon)	—	Use 10 or more days after onset of estrus to induce ovulation; repeat in 1-2 wk prn[22,24]
	50-100 IU/animal IM[20]	
	100 IU/animal IM[22,24,31]	
	100-200 IU/animal IM[3]	
Hydrocortisone Na succinate	25-40 mg/kg IV[2]	Shock
Hydroxyzine (Atarax, Roerig)	2 mg/kg q8h PO[47]	Antihistamine; pruritus; may cause drowsiness
Insulin, NPH	0.5-6.0 IU/kg, or to effect SC[2]	Diabetes mellitus; diabetic ketoacidosis; monitor blood glucose
	0.1 IU/animal SC q12h[42]	
Insulin, Ultralente	0.1 IU/animal SC q24h[47]	Diabetes mellitus; monitor blood glucose
Ipecac (7%)	2.2-6.6 ml/animal PO[18]	Emetic
Iron dextran	10 mg/animal IM[4]	Iron deficiency anemia; hemorrhage
Kaolin/pectin	1-2 ml/kg PO q2-6h prn[4]	Gastrointestinal protectant
Lactulose syrup (Cephulac, Merrill Dow)	0.15-0.75 ml/kg PO q12h[4]	Absorption of blood ammonia in hepatic disease; may cause soft stools at higher dose

Table 57. Miscellaneous agents used in ferrets (cont.)

Agent	Dosage	Comments
Leuprolide (Lupron Depot 30 day, TAP)	100 µg/kg IM q4-8wk[1] 100-200 µg/kg IM q4wk[34] or prn	Long-acting GnRH analog which may cause an initial stimulation then suppression of LH and FSH; palliative treatment of adrenal disease (will not resolve tumor); administer q4wk until clinical signs regress, then treatment interval can be up to q8wk; need to give for life of ferret; may lose efficacy over time; must be prepared in aliquots and frozen until used; very expensive
Loperamide	0.2 mg/kg PO q12h[4]	Antidiarrheal; useful in treatment of epizootic catarrhal gastro-enteritis
Melatonin	0.5-1.0 mg/animal q24h[40] prn	Symptomatic treatment for hairloss associated with hyperadrenocorticism; may not affect tumor growth
Metoclopramide (Reglan, Robins)	0.2-1.0 mg/kg q6-8h[44] PO, SC, IM	Antiemetic; motility enhancer
Misoprostol (Cytotech, Searle)	1-5 µg/kg PO q8h[34]	Gastric ulcers
Mitotane (o,p'-DDD; Lysodren, Bristol-Myers)	50 mg/animal PO q24h × 7 days, then q72h[22,24]	Hyperadrenocorticism; variable results and not a reliable alternative to adrenalectomy; treat until resolution of signs; may be toxic; pharmacist can prepare aliquots with cornstarch in #1 capsules[22,24]
Nutri-Cal (Evsco)	1-3 ml/animal PO q6-8h[24]	Nutritional supplement
Omeprazole (Prilosec, Astra Merck)	0.7 mg/kg PO q24h[19] 1/2 capsule/animal PO q24h × 28 days[34]	Proton-pump inhibitor; decreases gastric secretion of HCl *Helicobacter;* use with clarithromycin and metronidazole
Oxytocin	0.2-3.0 IU/kg SC, IM[3] 5-10 IU/animal IM[2]	Expels retained fetuses; stimulates lactation[3]
Pet-Tinic (SmithKline Beecham)	0.2 ml/kg PO q24h[24]	Nutritional/iron supplement for anemia
Prednisone	0.6 mg/kg PO q24h[2]	Gradually taper dose

Table 57. Miscellaneous agents used in ferrets (cont.)

Agent	Dosage	Comments
Prednisone (continued)	1.25-2.50 mg/kg PO q24h[36]	Eosinophilic gastroenteritis; treat until clinical signs abate; gradually decrease to q48h[36]
	1 mg/kg PO q24h × 7-14 days[24]	Use following heartworm adulticide treatment; thrombo-embolism
	0.25-1.0 mg/kg/day PO divided q12h[22,24]	Insulinoma; gradually increase to 4 mg/kg/day prn; up to 2 mg/kg/day when given with diazoxide[22,24]
	0.25 mg/kg PO q12h × 5 days, then 0.1 mg/kg q12h × 10 days[24]	Post-operative adrenalectomy; after initial dose of dexamethasone
	0.5 mg/kg PO q12h × 7-10 days, then q24h × 7-10 days, then q48h × 7-10 days[35]	Post-operative adrenalectomy
Prednisolone Na succinate	22 mg/kg IV[24]	Prior to blood transfusion; give slowly
Prostaglandin F$_2$-α (Lutalyse, Upjohn)	0.1-0.5 mg/animal IM prn[3,4]	Metritis; expels necrotic debris
Ranitidine (Zantac, Glaxo Wellcome)	24 mg/kg PO q8h × 2 wk[17]	Inhibits acid secretion; gastro-intestinal ulcers; *Helicobacter* treatment (with clarithromycin)
Stanozolol (Winstrol, Upjohn)	0.5 mg/kg PO, SC q12h[3]	Anemia; anabolic steroid; use with caution in hepatic disease
Sucralfate (Carafate, Hoechst Marion Roussel)	25 mg/kg PO q8h[28]	Gastrointestinal ulcers
	1/8 of 1 g tablet/animal PO q6h[23,24]	Gastrointestinal ulcers
Theophylline elixir	4.25 mg/kg PO q8-12h[4]	Bronchodilator
Vitamin B complex	1-2 mg/kg IM prn[4]	Dose based on thiamine content
Vitamin K	—	Use feline dosage[34]
Yeast, brewer's	1/8-1/4 tsp PO q12h[24]	Source of chromium to stabilize glucose and insulin for animals with insulinomas

[a] See Appendix 65 for chemotherapy protocols for lymphoma.

Appendix 60. Hematologic values of ferrets 15,52

Measurements	Albino ferrets		Fitch ferrets	
	Male	Female	Male	Female
PCV (%)	55 (44-61)	49 (42-55)	43 (36-50)	48 (47-51)
RBC (10⁶/μl)	10.2 (7.3-12.2)	8.1 (6.8-9.8)	—	—
Hgb (g/dl)	17.8 (16.3-18.2)	16.2 (14.8-17.4)	14.3 (12.0-16.3)	15.9 (15.2-17.4)
WBC (10³/μl)	9.7 (4.4-19.1)	10.5 (4.0-18.2)	11.3 (7.7-15.4)	5.9 (2.5-8.6)
Neutrophils (%)	57.0 (11-82)	59.5 (43-84)	40.1 (24-78)	31.1 (12-41)
Bands (%)	—	—	0.9 (0-2.2)	1.7 (0-4.2)
Lymphocytes (%)	35.6 (12-54)[a]	33.4 (12-50)	49.7 (28-69)	58.0 (25-95)
Monocytes (%)	4.4 (0-9)	4.4 (2-8)	6.6 (3.4-8.2)	4.5 (1.7-6.3)
Eosinophils (%)	2.4 (0-7)	2.6 (0-5)	2.3 (0-7)	3.6 (1-9)
Basophils (%)	0.1 (0-2)	0.2 (0-1)	0.7 (0-2.7)	0.8 (0-2.9)
Platelets (10³/μl)	453 (297-730)	545 (310-910)	—	—
Reticulocytes (%)	4.0 (1-12)	5.3 (2-14)	—	—

[a] May be as high as 75% in young ferrets.[25]

344

Appendix 61. Serum biochemical values of ferrets [15,26,52]

Measurements	Albino ferrets	Fitch ferrets
ALT (IU/L)	—	170 (82-289)
AP (IU/L)	23 (9-84)	53 (30-120)
AST (IU/L)	65 (28-120)	—
Bilirubin, total (mg/dl)	<1.0	—
BUN (mg/dl)	22 (10-45)	28 (12-43)
Calcium (mg/dl)	9.2 (8.0-11.8)	9.3 (8.6-10.5)
Carbon dioxide	—	24.9 (20-28)[a]
Chloride (mmol/L)	116 (106-125)	115 (102-121)
Cholesterol (mg/dl)	165 (64-296)	—
Creatinine (mg/dl)	0.6 (0.4-0.9)	0.4 (0.2-0.6)
GGT (IU/L)	—	5
Glucose (mg/dl)	136 (94-207)	101 (63-134)
LDH (IU/L)	—	460 (241-752)[a]
Lipase (U/L)	—	0-200
Phosphorus (mg/dl)	5.9 (4.0-9.1)	6.5 (5.6-8.7)
Potassium (mmol/L)	5.9 (4.5-7.7)	4.9 (4.3-5.3)
Protein, total (g/dl)	6.0 (5.1-7.4)	5.9 (5.3-7.2)
Albumin (g/dl)	3.2 (2.6-3.8)	3.7 (3.3-4.1)
Globulin (g/dl)	—	2.2 (2.0-2.9)[a]
Albumin:globulin	—	1.8 (1.3-2.1)[a]
Sodium (mmol/L)	148 (137-162)	152 (146-160)
Triglycerides (mg/dl)	—	18 (10-32)[a]

[a] From males only; cardiac sample.

Appendix 62. Urinalysis values of ferrets [b,39,52]

Parameter	Male	Female
Volume (ml/24 hr)	26 (8-48)	28 (8-140)
Sodium (mmol/24 hr)	1.9 (0.4-6.7)	1.5 (0.2-5.6)
Potassium (mmol/24 hr)	2.9 (1.0-9.6)	2.1 (0.9-5.4)
Chloride (mmol/24 hr)	2.4 (0.7-8.5)	1.9 (0.3-7.8)
pH	6.5-7.5[a]	6.5-7.5[a]
Protein (mg/dl)	7-33	0-32
Exogenous creatinine clearance (ml/min/kg)	—	3.32 ± 2.16
Insulin clearance (ml/min/kg)	—	3.02 ± 1.78

[a] Urine pH can vary according to diet; normal urine pH in ferrets on a high-quality, meat-based diet is approximately 6.0.
[b] Endogenous creatinine clearance (ml/min/kg) = 2.50 ± 0.93.

Appendix 63. Proposed schedule of vaccinations and routine prophylactic care for ferrets [3,7,8,45]

Age	Recommendation
4-6 wk	CDV[a] vaccination if dam is unvaccinated
6-8 wk	CDV[a] vaccination; physical examination; fecal examination
≈ 10 wk	CDV[a,b] vaccination; physical examination; fecal examination
12-14 wk	CDV[a,b] vaccination; rabies vaccination;[c] physical examination; fecal examination (optional); see [d]
4-6 mo	Spay/castrate (some recommend these surgeries between 6-8 mo of age); fecal examination; remove musk glands (optional); see [d]
1 yr	CDV[a,e] booster; rabies booster;[c] physical examination including dental prophylaxis; fecal examination if indicated; CBC; see [d]
2 yr	CDV[a,e] booster; rabies booster;[c] physical examination including dental prophylaxis; fecal examination if indicated; CBC; see [d]
3 yr and older (every 6 mo)	CDV[a,e] booster (annual); rabies booster[c] (annual); physical examination including dental prophylaxis; fecal examination if indicated; CBC; serum chemistries, including fasting blood glucose; see [d]

[a] CDV = canine distemper vaccine (nonferret origin; MLV of chick-embryo origin is recommended); Fervac-D (United Vaccine) is the only CDV vaccine approved for use in ferrets; although not approved for use in ferrets, Galaxy-D (Solvay) has also been used.

[b] Vaccinations are generally administered at 2-3 wk intervals until the ferret is 12-14 wk of age.

[c] Only a killed virus vaccine (Imrab 3, Rhone Merieux, Inc) should be used.

[d] Heartworm prevention may be indicated in ferrets in endemic areas.

[e] In previously unvaccinated adults, an initial series of two vaccinations given 2-4 wk apart should be given.

Appendix 64. Clinical signs and treatment of ferret endocrine diseases [27,34]

Disease	Clinical signs	Sex/age predilection
Hyperestrogenism (generally related to protracted estrus/ovarian remnant; also see hyperadrenocorticism)	• Severity varies: pale mucous membranes, vulvar enlargement, weakness, anorexia, weight loss, alopecia of tail and abdomen, melena, petechiae • Systolic murmur, weak pulses, posterior paresis, and systemic infections as disease progresses • Progression of disease slower in adrenocortical vs protracted estrus/ovarian remnant related disease	• Can occur following protracted estrus (ie, >3 wk) • Can occur in spayed ferrets if remnant ovarian tissue present
Adrenocortical disease (hyperadrenocorticism)	• See hyperestrogenism • Bilaterally symmetric alopecia starting on tail and progressing cranially • Vulvar enlargement in >90% of spayed females with this disease • Occasional pruritus • Prostatomegaly (resulting in dysuria, anuria) • Adrenal gland(s) may be palpably enlarged (left gland more commonly affected)	• Adult spayed females and neutered males; one report in intact ferret • Average onset 2-4 yr of age
Pancreatic endocrine neoplasia (insulinoma)	• Episodic weakness, lethargy, hypersalivation, ataxia, posterior paresis, seizures • Episodes frequently follow periods of exercise or fasting	• No reported sex predilection • Usually >3 yr of age
Diabetes mellitus	• Some unpublished reports in domestic ferrets • Polyuria, polydipsia, polyphagia, dehydration, weight loss	• Unknown

Disease	Diagnostic indicators	Treatment	Prognosis
Hyper-estrogenism	• Nonregenerative anemia • Thrombocytopenia • Leukopenia	• Supportive care and ovariohyster-ectomy, or surgical excision of remnant ovarian tissue • Some recommend initial conservative medical treatment (ie, hCG, GnRH, supportive care) prior to surgery	• Fair to good if PCV >20% • Guarded if PCV 14-19% • Grave if PCV <14%
Adreno-cortical disease	• CBC, biochemistry para-meters usually WNL • Enlarged adrenal glands are rarely seen radio-graphically • Ultrasonography can be diagnostic in most cases • Elevated serum estradiol, androstenedione, and 17-OH progesterone are diagnostic • Although seldom needed, skin biopsy may show signs consistent with endocrine disease (hyperkeratosis, epidermal thinning) • ACTH stimulation and dexamethasone suppression tests not diagnostic	• Adrenalectomy of affected gland if unilateral; complete removal of larger gland and debulk-ing of smaller gland if bilateral disease; right adrenal gland difficult to remove; bilateral adrenal-ectomies have been performed with encouraging results • Leuprolide may decrease clinical signs, but will not alter tumor growth; mitotane is not a reliable treatment	• Histologic diagnoses are generally adre-nocortical ade-noma or hyper-plasia; rarely, adeno-carcinoma • Prognosis good with adrenalectomy • Metastasis is rare
Insulinoma	• Blood glucose ≤60-70 mg/dl (and frequently much lower) on multiple samples • CBC, biochemistry values (except glucose), radiographs, and ultrasound usually within normal limits • Blood insulin concentrations are not reliable, but values above 250-300 pmol/L are probably abnormal	• Objective is to achieve euglycemia • Combination of surgical excision of pancreatic nodules and medical thera-py (prednisone, diazoxide) usually required for optimal stabilization • Client compliance critical for effective home management	• Stabilization possible with treatment, but disease is usually chronic and eventually fatal • Tendency is to slowly metastasize (primarily within pancreas)
Diabetes mellitus	• Hyperglycemia, glycos-uria, ketonuria	• Insulin (follow feline protocols)	• Fair with treatment

Appendix 65. Chemotherapy protocols for lymphoma in ferrets [a]

Protocol I[a,3]			
Week	Day	Agent	Dosage
1	1	Prednisone	1 mg/kg PO q12h and continued throughout therapy
	1	Vincristine	0.12 mg/kg IV
	3	Cyclophosphamide	10 mg/kg PO, SC
2	8	Vincristine	0.12 mg/kg IV
3	15	Vincristine	0.12 mg/kg IV
4	22	Vincristine	0.12 mg/kg IV
	24	Cyclophosphamide	10 mg/kg PO, SC
7	46	Cyclophosphamide	10 mg/kg PO, SC
9	—	Prednisone	Gradually decrease dose to 0 over the next 4 wk

Protocol II[b,41]		
Week	Agent	Dosage
1	Vincristine	0.07 mg/kg IV
	Asparaginase	400 IU/kg IP
	Prednisone	1 mg/kg PO q24h and continued throughout therapy
2	Cyclophosphamide	10 mg/kg SC
3	Doxorubicin	1 mg/kg IV
4-6	As weeks 1-3 above, but discontinue asparaginase	—
8	Vincristine	0.07 mg/kg IV
10	Cyclophosphamide	10 mg/kg SC
12	Vincristine	0.07 mg/kg IV
14	Methotrexate	0.5 mg/kg IV

[a] CBCs should be checked weekly during therapy. After therapy is discontinued, continue to monitor CBCs and do physical examination at 3-mo intervals.

[b] Protocol is continued in sequence biweekly after week 14, making the therapy protocol less intensive.

Appendix 66. Literature cited - Ferrets

1. Antinoff N. Neoplasia in ferrets. In: Bonagura JD (ed). *Kirk's Current Veterinary Therapy XIII: Small Animal Practice.* WB Saunders Co, Philadelphia, 2000. Pp 1149-1152.

2. Besch-Williford CL. Biology and medicine of the ferret. *Vet Clin North Am: Small Anim Pract* 17:1155-1183, 1987.

3. Brown SA. Ferrets. In: Jenkins JR, Brown SA. *A Practitioner's Guide to Rabbits and Ferrets.* American Animal Hospital Association, Lakewood, CO, 1993. Pp 43-111.

4. Brown SA. Ferret drug dosages. In: Antinoff N, Bauck L, Boyer TH, et al. *Exotic Formulary.* 2nd ed. AAHA Press, Lakewood, CO, 1999. Pp 43-61.

5. Brown SA. Clinical techniques in the ferret. *Semin Avian Exotic Pet Med* 6:75-85, 1997.

6. Brunson D. Personal communication. 1999.

7. Burke TJ. Common diseases and medical management of ferrets. In: Jacobson ER, Kollias GV, Jr (eds). *Exotic Animals.* Churchill Livingstone, New York, 1988. Pp 247-260.

8. Carpenter JW, Harms CA, Harrenstien L. Biology and medicine of the domestic ferret: an overview. *J Small Exotic Anim Med* 2:151-162, 1994.

9. Collins BR. Antimicrobial drug use in rabbits, rodents, and other small mammals. In: *Antimicrobial Therapy in Caged Birds and Exotic Pets.* Veterinary Learning Systems Co, Trenton, NJ, 1995. Pp 3-10.

10. Evans AT, Springsteen KK. Anesthesia of ferrets. *Semin Avian Exotic Pet Med* 7:48-52, 1998.

11. Finkler MR. Ferret colitis. In: Kirk RW, Bonagura JD (eds). *Kirk's Current Veterinary Therapy XI: Small Animal Practice.* WB Saunders Co, Philadelphia, 1992. Pp 1180-1181.

12. Flecknell PA. *Laboratory Animal Anesthesia.* Academic Press, San Diego, 1987.

13. Flecknell P. Medetomidine and atipamezole: potential uses in laboratory animals. *Lab Anim*: 21-25, 1997.

14. Fox JG. Anesthesia and surgery. In: Fox JG (ed). *Biology and Diseases of the Ferret.* Lea and Febiger, Philadelphia, 1988. Pp 289-302.

15. Fox JG. Normal clinical and biological parameters. In: Fox JG (ed). *Biology and Diseases of the Ferret.* Lea and Febiger, Philadelphia, 1988. Pp 159-173.

16. Fox JG. Parasitic diseases. In: Fox JG (ed). *Biology and Diseases of the Ferret.* Lea and Febiger, Philadelphia, 1988. Pp 235-247.

17. Fox JG. Bacterial and mycoplasmal diseases. In: Fox JG (ed). *Biology and Diseases of the Ferret.* Williams & Wilkins, Philadelphia, 1998. Pp 321-354.

18. Fox JG. Diseases of the gastrointestinal system. In: Fox JG (ed). *Biology and Diseases of the Ferret.* Williams & Wilkins, Philadelphia, 1998. Pp 273-290.

19. Fox JG, Lee A. The role of *Helicobacter* species in newly recognized gastrointestinal diseases of animals. *Lab Anim Sci* 47:222-227, 1997.

20. Fox JG, Pearson RC, Bell JA. Disease of the genitourinary system. In: Fox JG (ed). *Biology and Diseases of the Ferret.* Williams & Wilkins, Philadelphia, 1998. Pp 247-272.

21. Heard DJ. Principles and techniques of anesthesia and analgesia for exotic practice. *Vet Clin North Am: Small Anim Pract* 23:1301-1327, 1993.

22. Hillyer EV. Ferret endocrinology. In: Kirk RW, Bonagura JD (eds). *Kirk's Current Veterinary Therapy XI: Small Animal Practice.* WB Saunders Co, Philadelphia, 1992. Pp 1185-1188.

23. Hillyer EV. Gastrointestinal diseases of ferrets (*Mustela putorius furo*). *J Small Exotic Anim Med* 2:44-45, 1992.

24. Hillyer EV, Brown SA. Ferrets. In: Birchard SJ, Sherding RG (eds). *Saunders Manual of Small Animal Practice.* WB Saunders Co, Philadelphia, 1994. Pp 1317-1344.

25. Hoover JP, Baldwin CA. Changes in physiologic and clinicopathologic values in ferrets from 12 to 47 weeks of age. *Comp Anim Pract* 2:40-44, 1998.

26. Kawasaki TA. Laboratory parameters in disease states in ferrets. *Proc N Am Vet Conf*: 663-667; 1992.

27. Kolmstetter CM, Carpenter JW, Morrisey JK. Diagnosis and treatment of ferret endocrine diseases. *Vet Med* (Dec.): 1104-1110.

28. Lightfoot TL. Common ferret syndromes. *Proc N Am Vet Conf*: 839-842, 1999.

29. Marini RP, Fox JG. Anesthesia, surgery, and biomethodology. In: Fox JG (ed). *Biology and Diseases of the Ferret*. Williams & Wilkins, Philadelphia, 1998. Pp 449-484.

30. Marini RP, Ryden EB, Rosenblad WD, et al. Functional islet cell tumor in six ferrets. *J Am Vet Med Assoc* 202:430-433, 1993.

31. Mead RA, Joseph MM, Neirinckx S. Optimal dose of human chorionic gonadotropin for inducing ovulation in the ferret. *J Zoo Biol* 7:263-267, 1988.

32. Moreland AF, Glaser C. Evaluation of ketamine, ketamine-xylazine and ketamine-diazepam anesthesia in the ferret. *Lab Anim Sci* 35:287-290, 1985.

33. Morrisey JK. Ectoparasites of ferrets and rabbits. *Proc N Am Vet Conf*: 844-845, 1998.

34. Morrisey JK. Personal communication. 1999.

35. Neuwirth L, Isaza R, Bellah J, et al. Adrenal neoplasia in seven ferrets. *Vet Radiol Ultrasound* 34:340-346, 1993.

36. Palley LS, Fox JG. Eosinophilic gastroenteritis in the ferret. In: Kirk RW, Bonagura JD (eds). *Kirk's Current Veterinary Therapy XI: Small Animal Practice*. WB Saunders Co, Philadelphia, 1992. Pp 1182-1184.

37. Payton AJ, Pick JR. Evaluation of a combination of tiletamine and zolazepam as an anesthetic for ferrets. *Lab Anim Sci* 39:243-246, 1989.

38. Quesenberry KE. Gastrointestinal disorders of ferrets. *Proc N Am Vet Conf*: 870-871, 1996.

39. Quesenberry KE. Basic approach to veterinary care. In: Hillyer EV, Quesenberry KE (eds). *Ferrets, Rabbits, and Rodents: Clinical Medicine and Surgery*. WB Saunders Co, Philadelphia, 1997. Pp 14-25.

40. Ramer J. Personal communication. 1998.

41. Rosenthal K. Ferrets. *Vet Clin North Am: Small Anim Pract* 24:1-23, 1994.

42. Rosenthal KL. Endocrine diseases. In: Hillyer EV, Quesenberry KE (eds). *Ferrets, Rabbits, and Rodents: Clinical Medicine and Surgery*. WB Saunders Co, Philadelphia, 1997. Pp 91-98.

43. Rosenthal K. Endocrine disorders of ferrets: insulinoma and adrenal gland disease. *21st Annu Waltham/OSU Symp Treat Small Anim Dis: Exotics*: 35-38, 1997.

44. Rosenthal KL. Respiratory diseases. In: Hillyer EV, Quesenberry KE (eds). *Ferrets, Rabbits, and Rodents: Clinical Medicine and Surgery*. WB Saunders Co, Philadelphia, 1997. Pp 77-84.

45. Ryland LM, Bernard SL, Gorham JR. A clinical guide to the pet ferret. *Compend Cont Educ Pract Vet* 5:25-31, 1983.

46. Scott D. Dermatoses of pet rodents, rabbits, and ferrets. In: Scott D, Miller W, Ariffen C (eds). *Small Animal Dermatology*. 5th ed. Philadelphia, WB Saunders Co, 1995. Pp 1127-1137.

47. Smith DA, Burgmann PM. Formulary. In: Hillyer EV, Quesenberry KE (eds). *Ferrets, Rabbits, and Rodents: Clinical Medicine and Surgery*. WB Saunders Co, Philadelphia, 1997. Pp 394-395.

48. Stamoulis ME. Cardiac disease in ferrets. *Semin Avian Exotic Pet Med* 4:43-48, 1995.

49. Stamoulis ME, Miller MS, Hillyer EV. Cardiovascular diseases. In: Hillyer EV, Quesenberry KE (eds). *Ferrets, Rabbits, and Rodents: Clinical Medicine and Surgery*. WB Saunders Co, Philadelphia, 1997. Pp 63-76.

50. Supakorndej P, McCall JW, Lewis RE, et al. Biology, diagnosis, and prevention of heartworm infection in ferrets. *Proc Heartworm Symp*: 59-69, 1992.

51. Sylvina TJ, Berman NG, Fox JG. Effects of yohimbine on bradycardia and duration of recumbency in ketamine/xylazine anesthetized ferrets. *Lab Anim Sci* 40:178-182, 1990.

52.Thornton PC, Wright PA, Sacra PJ, et al. The ferret, *Mustela putorius furo,* as a new species in toxicology. *Lab Anim* 13:119-124, 1979.

53. Wixson SK. Anesthesia and analgesia in ferrets. In: Kohn DF, Wixson SK, White WJ, Benson GJ (eds). *Anesthesia and Analgesics in Laboratory Animals*. Academic Press, New York, 1997. Pp 274-279.

Fish

Amphibians

Reptiles

Birds

Sugar Gliders

Hedgehogs

Rodents

Rabbits

Ferrets

▶ **Miniature Pigs**

Primates

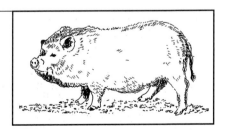

Table 58. Antimicrobial agents used in miniature pigs [a]

Agent	Dosage	Comments
Amoxicillin	10 mg/kg PO q12h[17]	
Amoxicillin/ clavulanate (Clavamox, Pfizer)	11-13 mg/kg PO q24h[8]	
Ampicillin	4-10 mg/kg IM, IV[10] 10-20 mg/kg IM q6-8h[8]	
Apramycin (Apralan, Elanco)	10-20 mg/kg PO q12-24h[8] 100 mg/L drinking water[8]	
Ceftiofur (Naxcel, Pharmacia & Upjohn)	3-10 mg/kg IM q24h[8] 1.1-2.2 mg/kg q24h × 7 days[5]	Rhinitis
Ceftriaxone (Rochephin, Roche)	50-75 mg/kg IM q24h[17]	
Cephalexin	20 mg/kg PO q12h[18]	
Cephradine	25-50 mg/kg PO q12h[17]	
Chloramphenicol[a]	10-25 mg/kg IM q12h[8]	
Enrofloxacin	2.5-5.0 mg/kg IM q24h[8]	
Gentamicin	2-4 mg/kg IM q8-12h[8]	
Lincomycin	11 mg/kg IM q24h[8]	
Metronidazole	66 mg/kg PO q24h[17]	
Neomycin	7-12 mg/kg PO q12h[10] 10 mg/kg PO q6h[8]	
Oxytetracycline	6-11 mg/kg IM, IV[10] 10-20 mg/kg PO q6h[10] 100 mg/animal on day 1, then 200 mg q7d × 3 treatments[5]	Rhinitis
Penicillin G, procaine	22,000- 45,000 IU/kg IM q24h[8]	

Table 58. Antimicrobial agents used in miniature pigs [a] (cont.)

Agent	Dosage	Comments
Penicillin G (procaine/benzathine combination)	40,000 IU/kg[10] IM	
Spectinomycin (Spectam, Merial)	10 mg/kg PO q12h[10]	
Trimethoprim/sulfa	5 mg/kg IM q24h[17] 25-50 mg PO q24h[17]	
Tylosin (Tylan, Elanco)	5.0-8.8 mg/kg[5] IM 2-4 mg/kg IM[10]	

[a] Not to be used in animals for human consumption.

Table 58. Antiparasitic agents used in miniature pigs [a]

Agent	Dosage	Comments
Amprolium	100 mg/kg in food or water q24h[10]	
Dichlorvos	20 mg/kg PO[1]	
Fenbendazole	10 mg/kg PO q24h × 3 days[5]	Whipworms
Ivermectin	0.3 mg/kg PO, SC, IM[5] 0.2 mg/kg IM[17]	Repeat in 10-14 days for sarcoptic mange
Levamisole	10 mg/kg PO[1]	
Metronidazole	66 mg/kg PO q24h[17]	
Piperazine	200 mg/kg PO[1]	
Pyrantel	6.6 mg/kg PO, repeat prn[5]	
Sulfadimethoxine	25 mg/kg PO[1]	

[a] Not to be used in animals for human consumption.

Table 60. Chemical restraint/anesthetic/analgesic agents used in miniature pigs [a]

Agent	Dosage	Comments
Acepromazine	—	See ketamine combination
	0.03-0.10 mg/kg IM[5]	Facilitates catheter placement
	0.2-1.1 mg/kg IM[5]	Tranquilization
	0.1-0.2 mg/kg IM[5]	Calm sow to allow nursing
Aspirin	10-20 mg/kg PO q6h[17]	Analgesia; anti-inflammatory; antipyretic; enteric coated
	10 mg/kg PO q12h[9]	
Atropine	—	See detomidine combination
	0.04 mg/kg SC, IM, IV[6]	Preanesthetic; bradycardia; hypersalivation
Azaperone (Stresnil, Schering-Plough)	0.25-0.50 mg/kg IM[5]	Relaxation, sedation, without ataxia
	2 mg/kg IM[5]	Sedation, with ataxia
	2-8 mg/kg IM[6,9]	Sedation; immobilization
	2.2 mg/kg IM[5]	Calm sow to allow nursing
Buprenorphine (Buprenex, Reckitt & Colman)	0.05-0.10 mg/kg IM, IV q8-12h[17]	Analgesia
	0.005-0.010 mg/kg IM q12h[9]	
Butorphanol (Torbutrol, Torbugesic, Fort Dodge)	—	See detomidine, ketamine for combinations
	0.1-0.3 mg/kg IM, IV q8-12h[17]	Analgesia
	0.05-0.20 mg/kg SC, IV q3-4h[9]	
Detomidine (Dormosedan, Pfizer)(D)/ butorphanol (B)/ midazolam (M)/ atropine (A)	(D) 0.125 mg/kg/ (B) 0.3 mg/kg/ (M) 0.3 mg/kg/ (A) 0.06 mg/kg IM[6]	Anesthesia; reverse with naloxone and yohimbine; also reverse with flumazenil, if needed
Diazepam	—	See ketamine combination
	0.5-3.0 mg/kg IM[4]	Tranquilization, minor procedures

Table 60. Chemical restraint/anesthetic/analgesic agents used in miniature pigs [a] (cont.)

Agent	Dosage	Comments
Diazepam (continued)	0.5-8.5 mg/kg IM[6] 0.5-10.0 mg/kg IM[18] 0.5-1.5 mg/kg IV[18]	Sedation
Droperidol	— 0.1-0.4 mg/kg IM[5,6]	See fentanyl/droperidol Tranquilization, minor procedures
Fentanyl/droperidol (Innovar-Vet, Schering-Plough)	1 ml/12-25 kg IM[5] 1 ml/9-14 kg[11] IM	Tranquilization, minor procedures Sedation
Flumazenil (Romazicon, Hoffman-LaRoche)	1 mg/10-15 mg midazolam IV[6]	Midazolam reversal
Flunixin meglumine (Banamine, Schering-Plough)	0.5-1.0 mg/kg SC, IV q12-24h[9]	Analgesia
Glycopyrrolate (Robinul-V, Fort Dodge)	0.005-0.010 mg/kg SC, IM, IV[6]	Preanesthetic; bradycardia; hypersalivation
Guaifenesin (G)/ ketamine (K)/ xylazine (X)	0.5-1.0 ml/kg IV to effect[11]	(G) (5%) with (K) (1-2 mg/ml) and (X) (1 mg/ml); induction; maintain at 2.2 ml/kg/hr
Halothane	4-5% induction[5]	
Isoflurane	4-5% induction[5]	
Ketamine	— — 5-20 mg/kg IM[9]	Ketamine combinations follow; see guaifenesin, tiletamine/ zolazepam for combinations Poor muscle relaxation; poor visceral analgesia; rough recoveries, especially IM; use with other agents[5] Sedation; immobilization
Ketamine (K)/ acepromazine (A)	(K) 10-20 mg/kg/ (A) 0.05-0.50 mg/kg IM[6]	Anesthesia

Table 60. Chemical restraint/anesthetic/analgesic agents used in miniature pigs [a] (cont.)

Agent	Dosage	Comments
Ketamine (K)/ diazepam (D)	(D) 1-2 mg/kg IM, then (K) 12-20 mg/kg IM[5]	Short-term anesthesia; prolong with (K) 2-4 mg/kg IV prn
	(K) 7 mg/kg/ (D) 0.5 mg/kg IV[11]	Sedation
Ketamine (K)/ xylazine (X)	(K) 5-20 mg/kg/ (X) 1-2 mg/kg IM[6]	Anesthesia
	(X) 2.2 mg/kg IM, followed by (K) 12-20 mg/kg IM[5]	Short-term anesthesia; prolong with (K) 2-4 mg/kg IV prn
	(K) 1-2 mg/kg/ (X) 0.5 mg/kg IV[11]	Tranquilization
	(K) 2 mg/kg/ (X) 2 mg/kg IV[11]	Sedation
	(K) 1.5 mg/kg/ (X) 0.75 mg/kg IV[11]	Sedation for cesarian section, with local anesthetic at incision
Ketamine (K)/ xylazine (X) butorphanol (B)	(K) 11 mg/kg/ (X) 2 mg/kg/ (B) 0.22 mg/kg IM[6]	Anesthesia
Meperidine (Demerol, Winthrop-Breon)	2-10 mg/kg IM q4h[9]	Analgesia
Midazolam (Versed, Roche)	—	See detomidine combination
	0.1-0.5 mg/kg[17] IM	Sedation
Morphine	0.2 mg/kg IM q4h[9]	Analgesia; ≤ 20 mg total
Naloxone (P/M Naloxone, Schering-Plough)	4 mg total dose IV[6]	Narcotic reversal
Nitrous oxide	—	Nitrous oxide and oxygen at equal levels (1-2 L/min), prior to isoflurane induction; may help calm animal during mask induction[18]
Pentazocine (Talwin-V, Pharmacia & Upjohn)	2 mg/kg IM q4h[9]	Analgesia

Table 60. Chemical restraint/anesthetic/analgesic agents used in miniature pigs [a] (cont.)

Agent	Dosage	Comments
Phenylbutazone	4-8 mg/kg PO q12h[17]	Anti-inflammatory; analgesia; antipyretic
Promazine hydrochloride	0.5-2.0 mg/kg IM[11]	Tranquilization
	0.4-1.0 mg/kg IV[11]	Tranquilization
Thiamylal	1.5-2.5 mg/kg IV[11]	Induction
Tiletamine/ zolazepam (Telazol, Ft. Dodge)	—	Tiletamine/zolazepam combinations follow
	—	Poor muscle relaxation; may cause rough recoveries[5]
	4-6 mg/kg IM[6,9]	Sedation; immobilization
Tiletamine/ zolazepam/ ketamine (K)/ xylazine (X)	—	Reconstitute Telazol (500 mg) with 2.5 ml xylazine (100 mg/ml) and 2.5 ml ketamine (100 mg/ml), instead of water; mix has 50 mg/ml each of tiletamine, zolazepam, ketamine, xylazine
	0.006-0.013 ml/kg IM[12]	Tranquilization; sedation
	0.020-0.026 ml/kg IM[12]	Prior to intubation; surgical anesthesia
	0.022-0.044 ml/kg IM[5]	Induction; maintain with 0.022 ml/kg IV prn
Tiletamine/ zolazepam (T)/ xylazine (X)	(T) 6 mg/kg/ (X) 2.2 mg/kg IM[5,6]	Anesthesia
	(T) 2 mg/kg/ (X) 2 mg/kg IV[5]	Rapid induction
	(X) 2.2 mg/kg, then (T) 2-4 mg/kg IM[11]	Anesthesia
Xylazine	—	See guaifenesin, ketamine, tiletamine/zolazepam for combinations
	0.5-3.0 mg/kg IM[4]	Sedation; tranquilization; deep sedation seldom encountered
	1-2 mg/kg IM[9]	Sedation; immobilization

**Table 60. Chemical restraint/anesthetic/analgesic agents used in
miniature pigs [a] (cont.)**

Agent	Dosage	Comments
Yohimbine (Antagonil, Wildlife Laboratories)	0.125 mg/kg IV[5] 0.3 mg/kg IV[6]	Xylazine reversal

[a] Not to be used in animals for human consumption.

361

Table 61. Miscellaneous agents used in miniature pigs [a]

Agent	Dosage	Comments
Attapulgite (Kaopectate, Upjohn)	2.2 ml/kg PO[1]	Gastrointestinal protectant; diarrhea
Dantrolene sodium (Dantrium, Procter & Gamble)	2-5 mg/kg PO, IV q8h[7]	Malignant hyperthermia
Gleptoferrin	50 mg/animal IM in first few days of life, repeat in 2-3 wk[5]	Iron deficiency in baby pigs
Glucose	20-40 ml/kg of 5% solution IP[5] 10-20 ml/kg of 10% solution IP[5]	Hypoglycemic neonate
Hydrogen peroxide	1 ml/ 5 kg PO[18]	Induce vomiting; some animals may require larger dose
Ipecac	7-15 ml/animal PO[18]	Induce vomiting
Iron dextran	50 mg/animal IM in first few days of life, repeat in 2-3 wk[5]	Iron deficiency in baby pigs
Oxytocin	10-20 IU/animal[3] IM	Dystocia, if not obstructed
Prostaglandin F$_{2\alpha}$ (Lutalyse, Upjohn)	5 mg/animal[3] IM	Induces parturition in 24-30 hr when given within 3 days of expected parturition; abortion after 12 days of gestation
Ranitidine (Zantac, Glaxo Wellcome)	150 mg/animal PO q12h[1]	Antisecretory for gastric acid

[a] Not to be used in animals for human consumption.

Appendix 67. Hematologic and serum biochemical values of miniature pigs [a,13]

Measurement	Mean (reference range)
Hematology	
PCV (%)	45 (36-53)
RBC ($10^6/\mu l$)	7.0 (5.4-8.6)
Hgb (g/dl)	14.9 (12.5-17.3)
MCH (pg)	21.4 (18.8-24.0)
MCHC (g/dl)	33.2 (31.6-34.8)
MCV (fl)	64 (57-72)
Platelets (μl)	441 (201-680)
WBC ($10^3/\mu l$)	12.6 (6.6-18.6)
Neutrophils (%)	42 (18-66)
Bands (%)	0.2 (0.0-1.2)
Lymphocytes (%)	46 (19-72)
Monocytes (%)	8 (1-13)
Eosinophils (%)	4 (0-10)
Basophils (%)	0.5 (0.0-2.5)
Chemistries	
ALT (IU/L)	34 (20-47)
AST (IU/L)	28 (10-56)
Bilirubin, total (mg/dl)	0.1 (0.0-0.3)
Calcium (mg/dl)	10.6 (9.6-11.6)
Chloride (mEq/L)	104 (94-114)
Cholesterol (mg/dl)	102 (38-165)
CPK (IU/L)	168 (48-288)
Creatinine (mg/dl)	1.6 (1.2-2.0)
Glucose (mg/dl)	80 (36-123)
Phosphorus (mg/dl)	6.9 (5.1-8.1)
Potassium (mEq/L)	4.6 (4.0-5.2)
Protein, total (g/dl)	7.5 (6.1-8.9)
Albumin (g/dl)	4.7 (3.9-5.5)
Globulin (g/dl)	2.8 (1.6-4.0)
A:G ratio	1.8 (0.8-2.8)
Sodium (mEq/L)	147 (144-153)
BUN (mg/dl)	19 (9-29)

[a] n = 30 healthy, mature Yucatan miniature pigs.

Appendix 68. Biological and physiological data of miniature pigs [2-5]

Parameter	Values
Life expectancy	20-25 years
Respiratory rate (bpm)	
• Newborn	50-60
• Weaned pigs	25-40
• 10-15 wk	30-40
• 15-26 wk	25-35
• Sows, boars	13-18
Heart rate (bpm)	
• Newborn	200-250
• Weaned pigs	90-100
• 10-15 wk	80-90
• 15-26 wk	75-85
• Sows, boars	70-80
Temperature	
• Newborn	39.0 °C (102.2 °F)
• Weaned pigs	39.3 °C (102.7 °F)
• 10-15 wk	39.1 °C (102.3 °F)
• 15-26 wk	38.8 °C (101.8 °F)
• Sows, boars	38.6 °C (101.4 °F)
Weight	
• Birth	250-450 g
• Adult male	9-39 kg (20-85 lb)
• Adult female	11-55 kg (25-120 lb)
Reproduction	
• Puberty	
○ Boars	3 mo of age
○ Gilts	3.5-4.0 mo of age
• Estrous cycle	18-24 (av 21) days
• Standing heat duration	1-3 days
• Ovulation	
○ Gilts	24-36 hr after onset of estrus
○ Sows	30-44 hr after onset of estrus
• Gestation length	112-116 (av 114) days
• Litter size	4-15 (av 6-8) piglets

Appendix 69. Preventive medicine recommendations for miniature pigs [14-16]

Minimum recommended vaccinations	
• Pet pigs	
◦ Erysipelas	8-12 wk of age; repeat in 3 wk; revaccinate semiannually or annually
◦ Leptospirosis	8-12 wk of age; repeat in 3 wk; revaccinate semiannually or annually
• Breeder pigs	
◦ Erysipelas	8-12 wk of age; repeat in 3 wk; revaccinate 3 wk before breeding
◦ Leptospirosis	8-12 wk of age; repeat in 3 wk; revaccinate 3 wk before breeding
◦ Parvovirus	5-6 mo of age; repeat in 3 wk; revaccinate 3-8 wk before breeding; boars should be revaccinated semiannually
Selected disease vaccinations	
• Colibacillosis (baby pig scours) *(E. coli)*	Sows: 5 and 2 wk before first farrowing, and 2 wk before each subsequent farrowing
• Other enteritides (rotavirus, TGE virus, *Clostridium, Salmonella*)	Sows: 5 and 2 wk before farrowing
• Atrophic rhinitis *(Bordetella bronchiseptica, Pasteurella multocida* [types A and D])	Sows: 7 and 3 wk before first farrowing, and 3 wk before each subsequent farrowing Piglets: 1 wk of age; repeat in 3 wk Boars: semiannually or annually
• Pneumonia *(Mycoplasma hyopneumoniae)*	Sows: 5 and 2 wk before first farrowing, and 2 wk before each subsequent farrowing Piglets: 1 wk of age; repeat in 2-3 wk Boars: semiannually or annually
• Pneumonia *(Actinobacillus pleuropneumoniae)*	Sows: 5 and 2 wk before farrowing Piglets: 3-8 wk of age; repeat in 3 wk

Appendix 69. Preventive medicine recommendations for miniature pigs [14-16] (cont.)

Neonatal care	
• Preferred environmental temperature at 1-7 days of age	33-35 °C (92-95 °F); may be lowered 1.7-2.8 °C (3-5 °F) each wk for 4-6 wk until weaned
• Colostrum	15-20 ml in 2-3 feedings within 1st 12 hr of life
• Iron dextran or gleptoferron supplementations	50 mg IM at 1 day of age; repeat at 3 wk of age
• Other care	Cut umbilical cord and dip in tincture of iodine; trim needle teeth (canines) at 1 day of age
Castration	<3 mo of age
Ovariohysterectomy/Ovariectomy	>3.5-4.0 mo of age, but may be performed as early as 6 wk of age
Tusk (canine) removal	Breeding boars (only if necessary)
Fecal examination	
• Young (6 wk to 6 mo of age)	Bimonthly
• Adults	Biannually (minimum)

Appendix 70. Literature cited - Miniature pigs

1. Boldrick L. *Veterinary Care of Pot-bellied Pet Pigs.* All Publishing Co, Orange, CA, 1993.

2. Braun W, Jr. Helping your clients raise healthy potbellied pigs. *Vet Med* 88(5):414-428, 1993.

3. Braun W, Jr. Reproduction in the potbellied pigs. *Vet Med* 88(5):429-434, 1993.

4. Braun WF, Jr. Potbellied pigs: general medical care. In: Bonagura JD (ed). *Kirk's Current Veterinary Therapy XII—Small Animal Practice.* WB Saunders Co, Philadelphia, 1995. Pp 1388-1392.

5. Braun WF, Jr, Casteel SW. Potbellied pigs—miniature porcine pets. *Vet Clin N Am: Small Anim Pract* 23:1149-1177, 1993.

6. Calle PP, Morris PJ. Anesthesia for nondomestic suids. In: Fowler ME, Miller RE (eds). *Zoo & Wild Animal Medicine: Current Therapy 4.* WB Saunders Co, Philadelphia, 1999. Pp 639-646.

7. Claxton-Gill MS, Cornick-Seahorn JL, Gamboa JC, et al. Suspected malignant hyperthermia syndrome in a miniature pot-bellied pig anesthetized with isoflurane. *J Am Vet Med Assoc* 203:1434-1436, 1993.

8. Friendship RM. Antimicrobial drug use in swine. In: Prescott JF, Baggot JD (eds). *Antimicrobial Therapy in Veterinary Medicine*, 2nd ed. Iowa State University Press, Ames, 1993. Pp 477-489.

9. Heard DJ. Principles and techniques of anesthesia and analgesia for exotic practice. *Vet Clin N Am: Small Anim Pract* 23:1301-1327, 1993.

10. Howard JL. Table of common drugs: approximate doses. In: Howard JL. *Current Veterinary Therapy 3—Food Animal Practice.* WB Saunders Co, Philadelphia, 1993. Pp 930-933.

11. Johnson L. Physical and chemical restraint of miniature pet pigs. In: Reeves DE (ed). *Care and Management of Miniature Pet Pigs.* Veterinary Practice Publishing Co, Santa Barbara, CA, 1993. Pp 59-66.

12. Ko JCH, Thurman JC, Tranquilli GJ, et al. Problems encountered when anesthetizing potbellied pigs. *Vet Med* 88(5):435-440, 1993.

13. Radin MJ, Weiser MG, Fettman MJ. Hematologic and serum biochemical values for Yucatan miniature swine. *Lab Anim Sci* 36:425-427, 1986.

14. Reeves DE. Neonatal care of miniature pigs. In: Reeves DE (ed). *Care and Management of Miniature Pet Pigs.* Veterinary Practice Publishing Co, Santa Barbara, CA, 1993. Pp 41-45.

15. Reeves DE. Parasite control in miniature pet pigs. In: Reeves DE (ed). *Care and Management of Miniature Pet Pigs.* Veterinary Practice Publishing Co, Santa Barbara, CA, 1993. Pp 101-107.

16. Reeves DE. Vaccination schedule for miniature pigs. In: Reeves DE (ed). *Care and Management of Miniature Pet Pigs.* Veterinary Practice Publishing Co, Santa Barbara, CA, 1993. Pp 109-111.

17. Swindle MM. Minipigs as pets. *Proc North Am Vet Conf:* 648-649, 1993.

18. Tynes VV. Emergency care for potbellied pigs. Vet *Clin N Am: Exotic Anim Pract* 1:177-189, 1998.

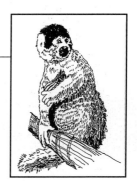

Table 62. Antimicrobial and antifungal agents used in primates

Agent	Dosage	Comments
Amikacin	2.3 mg/kg IM q24h[21,49]	Lemurs[49]
Amoxicillin	11 mg/kg PO q12h[9]	
	11 mg/kg SC, IM q24h[9]	
Amphotericin B	0.25-1.0 mg/kg IV q24h[20]	
Ampicillin	20 mg/kg PO, IM, IV q8h[20]	
	50-100 mg/kg IM q12h × 7-10 days[21]	
Cefazolin sodium	25 mg/kg IM, IV q12h × 7-10 days[21]	
Cefotaxime (Claforan, Hoechst Marion Roussel)	100-200 mg/kg IV q6-8h[36]	Great apes/bacterial meningitis; excellent penetration into CSF
Ceftazidime	50 mg/kg IM, IV q8h[5]	Lemurs
Ceftizoxime (Cefizox, Fujisawa)	75-100 mg/kg IM q12h × 7 days[21]	
Ceftriaxone (Rocephin, Roche)	50-100 mg/kg IM q12-24h[36]	Great apes/bacterial meningitis; excellent penetration into CSF; transient, self-limiting diarrhea is a side effect
Cephalexin	20 mg/kg PO q12h[6]	
Cephaloridine	20 mg/kg IM q12h[6]	
Chloramphenicol	50 mg/kg PO q12h[6]	
	50-100 mg/kg PO, SC, IV q8h[20]	
	20 mg/kg IM q12h[6]	
Ciprofloxacin	250 mg/animal PO once, then 125 mg q12h[25]	Rhesus macaques/PD (5.1-13.0 kg animals)
	16-20 mg/kg PO q12h[21]	Based on PD dosage above;[25] suspension of crushed tablets in water

Table 62. Antimicrobial and antifungal agents used in primates (cont.)

Agent	Dosage	Comments
Doxycycline	60 mg/animal PO once, then 30 mg q12h[25]	Rhesus macaques/PD (5.1-13.0 kg animals)
	3-4 mg/kg PO q12h[21]	Based on PD dosage above[25]
Enrofloxacin	5 mg/kg PO, IM q24h × 10 days[1]	Shigella flexneri; injectable form given PO
Erythromycin	75 mg/kg PO q12h × 10 days[21]	
	5 mg/kg IM q12h × 7-14 days[9]	*Campylobacter*-associated diarrhea
Erythromycin ethyl-succinate (EryPed Drops, Abbott)	20 mg/kg PO q12h[39]	Tamarins/clostridial enteritis
Ethambutol	22.5 mg/kg PO q24h[50]	Rhesus macaques/myco-bacteriosis; treat concurrently with isoniazid and rifampin; reduce to 15 mg/kg after 6 wk; continue treatment for 1 yr
Fluconazole (Diflucan, Roerig)	18 mg/kg PO q24h[2]	Swamp monkeys/systemic mycoses; treat concurrently with flucytosine; may be effective as sole agent
Flucytosine (Ancobon, Roche)	143 mg/kg PO q24h[2]	Swamp monkeys/systemic mycoses; treat concurrently with fluconazole
Furazolidone	5 mg/kg PO q6h × 7 days[21]	
	20-40 mg/kg PO q6h[20]	
Gentamicin	1-2 mg/kg IM, IV q8h × 5-7 days[21]	
	2-3 mg/kg IM, IV q12h × 5-7 days[21]	
	3 mg/kg IM q6-8h[48]	Baboons/PD
Griseofulvin	20 mg/kg PO q24h[20]	
	200 mg/kg PO q10d[20]	

Table 62. Antimicrobial and antifungal agents used in primates (cont.)

Agent	Dosage	Comments
Isoniazid	15 mg/kg PO q24h[50]	Rhesus macaques/mycobacteriosis; treat concurrently with ethambutol and rifampin; reduce to 10 mg/kg after 6 wk; continue treatment for 1 yr; supplement with pyridoxine
Itraconazole	10 mg/kg PO q24h[19]	Fungal (yeast) gastroenteritis
Kanamycin	7.5 mg/kg IM q12h[20]	
Lincomycin	5-10 mg/kg IM q12h[21]	
Metronidazole	25 mg/kg PO q12h[31]	Gastroenteritis
	12.5-15.0 mg/kg PO q12h[19]	Clostridial infections
Minocycline (Minocin, Lederle)	15 mg/kg PO q12h × 7 days[21,23]	Lemurs[23]
Neomycin	10 mg/kg PO q12h[6]	
Nitrofurantoin	2-4 mg/kg IM, IV q8h[20]	
Norfloxacin (Noroxin, Roberts)	25-30 mg/kg PO q12h[39]	Tamarins
Nystatin	200,000 units/animal PO q6h[9]	Gastrointestinal candidiasis; continue 48 hr after clinical recovery
Oxytetracycline	10 mg/kg SC, IM[6]	
Penicillin G, benzathine	40,000 IU/kg IM q72h[20]	
Penicillin G, procaine	20,000 IU/kg IM q12h[20]	
Piperacillin (Pipracil, Lederle)	80-100 mg/kg IM, IV q8h × 7-10 days[21]	
	100-150 mg/kg IM, IV q12h[21]	
Rifampin (Rifadin, Hoechst Marion Roussel)	22.5 mg/kg PO q24h[50]	Rhesus macaques/mycobacteriosis; treat concurrently with ethambutol and isoniazid; reduce to 15 mg/kg after 6 wk; continue treatment for 1 yr
Sulfamethazine	66 mg/kg PO q12h[4]	
Sulfasalazine (Azulfidine, Pharmacia)	30 mg/kg PO q12h[18]	

Table 62. Antimicrobial and antifungal agents used in primates (cont.)

Agent	Dosage	Comments
Tetracycline	20-25 mg/kg PO q8-12h × 7-10 days[21] 25 mg/kg IM, IV q12h[21]	
Trimethoprim/sulfa	24 mg/kg PO q12h[9] 27 mg/kg SC q24h[9] 50 mg/kg PO q12h[5] 25 mg/kg SC, IM q24h[5]	 Lemurs Lemurs
Tylosin (Tylan, Elanco)	5 mg/kg PO q12h[19]	Clostridial infections

Table 63. Antiparasitic agents used in primates

Agent	Dosage	Comments
Albendazole	25 mg/kg PO q12h × 5 days[51]	*Filaroides*
Chloroquine (Aralen, Sanofi)	10 mg/kg PO, IM once, then 5 mg/kg 6 hr later, then 5 mg/kg q24h × 2 days[51]	*Plasmodium;* treat concurrently with primaquine
Clindamycin (Antirobe, Upjohn)	12.5-25.0 mg/kg q12h[51]	*Toxoplasma*
Dichlorvos	10-15 mg/kg PO q24h × 2-3 days[14]	Gastrointestinal nematodes
Diethylcarbamazine	6-20 mg/kg PO q24h × 6-15 days[51] 20-40 mg/kg PO q24h × 7-21 days[21]	*Dipetalonema*
Doxycycline	5 mg/kg PO q12h × 1 day, then 2.5 mg/kg q24h[51]	*Balantidium*
Fenbendazole	50 mg/kg PO q24h × 3 days[5] 50 mg/kg PO q24h × 14 days[51]	Lemurs *Filaroides*
Furazolidone	— 5 mg/kg PO q6h × 7 days[46] 100 mg/animal PO q6h × 7 days[46]	Great apes/*Giardia;* more palatable, but less effective than other agents Juveniles Adults
Iodoquinol (diiodohydroxyquin; Yodoxin, Glenwood)	— 12-16 mg/kg PO q8h[46] 650 mg/animal PO q8h[46] 20 mg/kg PO q12h × 3 wk[20]	Great apes/minimal absorption, use with other agents for invasive disease; 14-21 days for *Balantidium coli;* 21 days for *Entamoeba* Infants, juveniles Adults Intestinal amebiasis; *Balantidium*

Table 63. Antiparasitic agents used in primates (cont.)

Agent	Dosage	Comments
Ivermectin	0.2 mg/kg PO, SC, IM[5,21,51]	
Levamisole	5mg/kg PO, repeat in 3 wk[14] 10 mg/kg[51] PO	*Strongyloides, Filaroides, Trichuris*
Mebendazole	15 mg/kg PO q24h × 3 days[51] 22 mg/kg PO q24h × 3 days, repeat in 2 wk[9]	*Strongyloides, Necator, Pterygodermatitis, Trichuris*
Metronidazole	17.5-25.0 mg/kg PO q12h × 10 days[51] 30-50 mg/kg PO q12h × 5-10 days[29,51]	Enteric flagellates and amoebas *Balantidium coli*
Oxytetracycline	1,500 mg/kg/day IV, continuous infusion[46]	Gorillas/*Balantidium coli*; non-ambulatory animals
Paromomycin (Humatin, Park Davis)	12.5-15.0 mg/kg PO q12h × 5-10 days[51] 10 mg/kg PO q8h × 5-10 days[46] 10-20 mg/kg PO q12h × 5-10 days[29]	Amoeba; minimal absorption; use with other agents for invasive disease Great apes/*Entamoeba* *Balantidium coli*
Pentamidine isethionate (NebuPent, Fujisawa)	4 mg/kg IM, IV q24h × 14 days[46]	Great apes/*Pneumocystis*; IV by slow infusion; may cause hypotension, cardiac arrhythmias
Piperazine	65 mg/kg PO q24h × 10 days[14]	
Praziquantel	40 mg/kg PO, IM[51] 15-20 mg/kg PO, IM[51]	Trematodes Some cestodes
Primaquine (Primaquine phosphate, Sanofi)	0.3 mg/kg PO q24h × 14 days[51]	*Plasmodium;* treat concurrently with chloroquine
Pyrantel pamoate	6 mg/kg PO[5] 11 mg/kg PO, once[51]	Lemurs *Necator;* pinworms

376

Table 63. Antiparasitic agents used in primates (cont.)

Agent	Dosage	Comments
Pyrimethamine (Daraprim, Glaxo Wellcome)	2 mg/kg q24h × 3 days, then 1 mg/kg q24h × 4 wk[46,51]	*Toxoplasma;* in great apes, maximum dosages of 100 mg/animal q24h for days 1-3 and 25 mg/animal q24h for 4 wk; treat concurrently with sulfadiazine; supplement with folinic acid
Quinacrine (Atabrine, Winthrop)	2 mg/kg PO q8h × 7 days[46]	Great apes/*Giardia*; maximum dose of 300 mg/day
Sulfadiazine	—	*Toxoplasma;* treat concurrently with pyrimethamine
	25-50 mg/kg PO q6h[46]	Great apes/maximum dose of 6 g/animal/treatment
	100 mg/kg/day[51] PO	
Sulfadimethoxine	50 mg/kg/day PO × 1 day, then 25 mg/kg/day[51]	Coccidiosis
Tetracycline	15 mg/kg PO q8h × 10-14 days[46]	Great apes/*Balantidium coli*; infants, juveniles
	500-1,000 mg/animal PO q8h × 10-14 days[46]	Great apes/*Balantidium coli;* adults
Thiabendazole	50 mg/kg PO q24h × 2 days[51]	*Strongyloides, Necator*
	75-100 mg/kg PO, repeat in 3 wk[14]	
Trimethoprim/sulfa	30 mg/kg PO q6h × 14 days[46]	Great apes/*Pneumocystis carinii*

Table 64. Chemical restraint/anesthetic/analgesic agents used in primates

Agent	Dosage	Comments
Acepromazine	—	See acepromazine for combination
	0.5-1.0 mg/kg PO, SC, IM[20]	Preanesthetic; tranquilizer
Acetaminophen	5-10 mg/kg PO q6h[20]	Analgesic; anti-inflammatory; anti-pyretic
Acetylsalicylic acid (aspirin)	5-10 mg/kg PO q4-6h[13]	Analgesic; anti-inflammatory; anti-pyretic
	100 mg/kg PO q24h[4] 25 mg/kg rectal suppository[35]	Anti-inflammatory; analgesic
Alphaxalone/ alphadolone (Saffan, Glaxo)	—	Injectable anesthetic; available in Europe
	5 mg/kg IV bolus[8]	
	10 mg/kg/hr IVinfusion[8]	
Atipamezole (Antisedan, Pfizer)	—	Medetomidine reversal
	0.2 mg/kg IV[35]	Squirrel monkeys
	0.15-0.30 mg/kg IV[27]	Chimpanzees
Atropine	0.02-0.05 mg/kg IM[35]	Macaques, baboons/preanesthetic; bradycardia; hypersalivation
	0.04 mg/kg SC, IM, IV[14]	
Buprenorphine (Buprenex, Reckitt & Colman)	0.01 mg/kg IM, IV q12h[13]	Analgesia
	0.01-0.03 mg/kg IM q6-12h[40]	Most useful of opioid agonist-antagonists[40]
Butorphanol (Torbugesic, Fort Dodge)	0.1-0.2 mg/kg IM q12-48h[13]	Analgesia
Carprofen (Rimadyl, Pfizer)	2-4 mg/kg PO, SC q12-24h[37]	Analgesia; anti-inflammatory
Chlorpromazine	1-6 mg/kg PO, IM[20]	Preanesthetic

Table 64. Chemical restraint/anesthetic/analgesic agents used in primates (cont.)

Agent	Dosage	Comments
Diazepam	—	See ketamine for combination
	0.5-1.0 mg/kg PO[13]	Sedation; give in small amount of food or drink 30-60 min prior to anesthesia; degree of sedation variable; recovery prolonged
	0.25-0.50 mg/kg IM, IV[17]	Seizures; muscle relaxation during anesthesia
	0.1-0.5 mg/kg IM[13]	Lemurs/prevents ketamine-induced seizures
Fentanyl	5-10 µg/kg IV bolus[35]	Use with isoflurane anesthesia
	10-25 µg/kg/hr continuous infusion[35]	Use with isoflurane anesthesia
Fentanyl/droperidol (Innovar-Vet, Janssen)	0.05-0.10 ml/kg IM, IV[20]	Preanesthetic
	0.3 ml/kg IM[6]	Heavy sedation
Fentanyl patch (Duragesic, Janssen)	4-8 µg/kg/hr, change patch q72h[38]	Analgesia; do not cut patch; cover portion not in use
Flumazenil (Romazicon, Hoffman-LaRoche)	0.025 mg/kg IV[15]	Benzodiazepine reversal
Flunixin meglumine	0.3-1.0 mg/kg SC, IV q12-24h[13]	Analgesia
Glycopyrrolate	0.005-0.010 mg/kg IM[35]	Macaques, baboons/preanesthetic; bradycardia; hypersalivation
	0.013-0.017 mg/kg IM[21]	
Ibuprofen	20 mg/kg/day PO[33]	Analgesia; anti-inflammatory
	1% solution, sub-gingival irrigation[10]	Periodontitis
Ketamine	—	Ketamine combinations follow; tranquilization; anesthesia; mg/kg dose increases as size of animal decreases; caution: causes seizures in lemurs when used as sole agent (see diazepam, midazolam, ketamine/acepromazine)

379

Table 64. Chemical restraint/anesthetic/analgesic agents used in primates (cont.)

Agent	Dosage	Comments
Ketamine (continued)	5 mg/kg IM[13]	Great apes/immobilization; follow with inhalant anesthetic
	10-15 mg/kg IM[13]	Medium-size primates (10-30 kg)/ immobilization; follow with inhalant anesthetic
	20 mg/kg IM[13]	Marmosets, tamarins/ immobilization; follow with inhalant anesthetic
	5-40 mg/kg IM[21]	All
Ketamine (K)/ acepromazine (A)	(K) 4 mg/kg/ (A) 0.04 mg/kg IM[5]	Lemurs
Ketamine (K)/ diazepam (D)	(K) 15 mg/kg/ (D) 1 mg/kg IM[6]	Anesthesia
Ketamine (K)/ medetomidine (M)	(K) 2-6 mg/kg/ (M) 0.03-0.06 mg/kg IM[27]	Chimpanzees
	(K) 5.0-7.5 mg/kg/ (M) 0.033-0.075 mg/kg IM[44]	Use higher dosages for smaller primates
Ketamine (K)/ xylazine (X)	(K) 10 mg/kg/ (X) 0.5 mg/kg IM[6]	Anesthesia
Ketoprofen (Ketofen, Fort Dodge)	5 mg/kg IM q6-8h[37]	Analgesia; anti-inflammatory
Ketorolac (Torador, Syntex)	15-30 mg/animal[37]	Macaques, baboons/nonsteroidal, anti-inflammatory
Medetomidine (Domitor, Pfizer)	—	See ketamine for combination
	0.05-0.10 mg/kg PO[24]	Induction; followed by ketamine
	0.1 mg/kg SC, IM[35]	Squirrel monkeys
Meperidine (Demerol, Winthrop-Breon)	2-4 mg/kg IM q3-4h[13]	Analgesia; caution: sudden death reported in healthy animals[40]
Midazolam (Versed, Roche)	0.1-0.5 mg/kg IM[13]	Lemurs/prevents ketamine-induced seizures
Morphine	1-2 mg/kg PO, SC, IM, IV q4h[40]	Analgesia

Table 64. Chemical restraint/anesthetic/analgesic agents used in primates (cont.)

Agent	Dosage	Comments
Nalbuphine	0.5 mg/kg IM, IV q3-6h[13]	Analgesia
Naloxone	0.01-0.05 mg/kg IM, IV[6]	Narcotic reversal
Naproxen (Naprosyn, Syntex)	10 mg/kg PO q12h[21,23]	Lemurs[23]/analgesic; anti-inflammatory; antipyretic
Oxymorphone	0.03-0.20 mg/kg SC, IM, IV q6-12h[13]	Analgesia
	0.075 mg/kg SC, IM, IV q4-6h[40]	New world primates
	0.15 mg/kg SC, IM, IV q4-6h[40]	Old world primates
Pancuronium (Pavulon, Organon)	0.08-0.1 mg/kg IV[35]	Paralytic agent; requires assisted ventilation
Pentazocine (Talwin-V, Upjohn)	2-5 mg/kg IM q4h[13]	Analgesia
Propofol	1-2 mg/kg IV as initial bolus, followed by infusion to effect[35]	Chimpanzees
	2.0-4.0 mg/kg IV for induction prn[35]	Baboons
	2.5-5.0 mg/kg IV bolus, followed by infusion 0.3-0.4 mg/kg/min[42]	Macaques/intubation and ventilatory support suggested
	5 mg/kg IV bolus, followed by 25 mg/kg/h infusion for maintenance[8]	Rhesus macaques
Succinylcholine	2 mg/kg IV[12]	Paralytic agent; requires ventilatory support; use with caution
Thiamylal	25 mg/kg IV to effect[20]	Anesthesia
Thiopental	25 mg/kg IV to effect[20]	Anesthesia
Tiletamine/ zolazepam (Telazol, Fort Dodge)	1-20 mg/kg IM[45]	Anesthesia; wide range of dosages for different species
	1.5-3.0 mg/kg IM[3]	Macaques
	2-6 mg/kg IM[17]	
	4-10 mg/kg IM[13]	

Table 64. Chemical restraint/anesthetic/analgesic agents used in primates (cont.)

Agent	Dosage	Comments
Tubocurarine	0.09 mg/kg IV[12]	Paralytic agent; requires ventilatory support; use with caution
Vecuronium (Norcuron, Organon)	0.04-0.06 mg/kg IV[35]	Paralytic agent; requires assisted ventilation
Xylazine	—	See ketamine for combination

Table 65. Miscellaneous agents used in primates

Agent	Dosage	Comments
Acetylcysteine (Mucomyst, Apothecon)	50-60 ml/hr via inhalation × 30-60 min q12h[20]	Mucolytic
Aminophylline	25-100 mg/animal PO q12h[20]	Bronchodilation
	10 mg/kg IV[5]	Lemurs/bronchodilation
Bismuth subsalicylate (Pepto-Bismol, Procter & Gamble)	1 ml/kg PO q6-8h[21]	Intestinal protectant; gastrointestinal ulcers
Calcium chloride	10-20 mg/kg IV slowly[41]	Severe hypocalcemia (monitor heart rate closely); to reverse aminoglycoside induced shock
Calcium gluconate	200 mg/kg SC, IM, IV[41]	Prophylaxis and therapy of nutritional secondary hyper-parathyroidism
Captopril (Capoten, Squibb)	1 mg/kg PO[41]	Angiotensin converting enzyme (ACE) inhibitor; vasodilator
Cherry flavored drink (Koolaid)	PO prn[7]	Mix with medication to enhance flavor; mix at 4 × normal concentration
Chlorpheniramine (Chlor-Trimeton, Squibb)	0.5 mg/kg/day PO, in divided doses[20]	Antihistamine
Cisapride (Propulsid, Janssen)	0.2 mg/kg PO q12h[16]	Macaques/promotes gastrointestinal motility
Dexamethasone	≤ 2 mg/kg PO, IM, IV[20]	
Dimercaptosuccinic acid (DMSA; Chemet, McNeil)	10 mg/kg PO q8h × 5 days, then q12h × 2 wk[52]	Chimpanzees/lead chelation
Diphenhydramine (Benadryl, Parke-Davis)	5 mg/kg IM[5]	Lemurs/antihistamine
Diphenoxylate/ atropine (Lomotil, Searle)	1 ml/animal PO q8h[14]	Opiate antidiarrheal
Doxapram	2 mg/kg IV[6]	Respiratory stimulant
Enalapril (Enacard, Merck)	0.3 mg/kg PO, IV[41]	Angiotensin converting enzyme (ACE) inhibitor; balanced vasodilator

Table 65. Miscellaneous agents used in primates (cont.)

Agent	Dosage	Comments
Ephedrine	12 mg/kg PO q4h[20]	Nasal congestion; bronchoconstriction
Famotidine (Pepcid, Merck)	0.5-0.8 mg/kg PO q24h[31]	Mild gastroenteritis; gastrointestinal ulcers
Fluoxetine (Prozac, Eli Lilly)	0.45 mg/kg PO q24h[47]	Anti-anxiety
Folic acid	0.04-0.20 mg/kg PO q24h[21]	Supplement during pyrimethamine therapy
Furosemide	2 mg/kg PO[20]	Diuretic
Glipizide (Glucotrol, Pfizer)	1.1 mg/kg PO q24h[11]	Titi monkeys/diabetes mellitus (non-insulin-dependent)
Grape flavored syrup (Syrpalta, Emerson)	PO prn[32]	Mix as needed to flavor liquid medications and crushed tablets
Haloperidol (Haldol, McNeil)	0.5-2.0 mg/kg IM[41]	Vervet, green monkeys/anti-anxiety
Human chorionic gonadotropin (hCG)	250 units IM[41]	Squirrel monkeys/induces ovulation in 40% of animals
Insulin, NPH	0.25-0.50 units/kg/day SC starting dose[21]	Diabetes mellitus; diabetic ketoacidosis
Kaolin/pectin	0.5-1.0 ml/kg PO q2-6h[20]	Intestinal protectant
Levothyroxine	0.01 mg/kg PO q12h[26]	Hypothyroidism
Oxytocin	5-20 units (total dose) IM, IV[30]	Uterine inertia
Paroxetine (Paxil, SmithKline Beecham)	0.3 mg/kg PO q12h[47]	Anti-anxiety
Phenylephrine (Neo-Synephrine, Winthrop)	Intranasal q6h[20]	Nasal congestion; follow directions on label
Prednisolone sodium succinate (Solu-Delta Cortef, Upjohn	10 mg/kg IV[5] 1-15 mg/kg IV[30]	Lemurs/shock All/shock
Prednisone	0.5-1.0 mg/kg PO q12h × 3-5 days, then q24h × 3-5 days, then q48h × 10 days, then 1/2 dose q48h[18,21]	Lower doses for pain, inflammation; higher for autoimmune, inflammatory bowel disease, etc

Table 65. Miscellaneous agents used in primates (cont.)

Agent	Dosage	Comments
Pyridoxine	3.5 mg/kg in feed[14]	Supplement during isoniazid therapy
Trimeprazine	1-2 mg/kg PO q6h[20]	Antihistamine
Vitamin C (ascorbic acid)	4-10 mg/kg PO q24h[21]	
Vitamin D[3]	2,000 IU/kg in feed q24h[21]	
Vitamin E (E)/ selenium (S)	(E) 3.75 IU/kg/ (S) 1.15 mg/kg IM q3d × 1 mo[43]	(E)/(S) responsive myopathy, neuropathy

385

Appendix 71. Hematologic and serum biochemical values of primates 21

Measurement	Baboon (*Papio* sp.)	Capuchin monkey (*Cebus* sp.)	Chimpanzee (*Pan troglodytes*)	Common marmoset (*Callithrix* sp.)	Lemur (*Lemur* sp.)
Hematology					
PCV (%)	44.7	45-53	39.7-44.1	45-48	48-53
RBC ($10^6/\mu$l)	4.5-4.8	6	5.03-6.05	6.9	6.2-9.8
Hgb (g/dl)	13	14-17	12.5-14.5	15.1-15.5	15.6-20.2
WBC ($10^3/\mu$l)	14.1	5-24	7.4-17.6	7-12	6.2-16.9
Neutrophils (%)	60.5	55	37.4-66.6	28-55	14-40
Lymphocytes (%)	36	41	29-57	43-67	49-81
Monocytes (%)	1.5	1.8	0-2.3	0.4-2.1	4
Eosinophils (%)	1.5	1.6	0-5.8	0.5-0.6	0-4
Basophils (%)	0.4	<1	0-0.7	0.3-1.3	<1
Platelets ($10^3/\mu$l)	406	108-187	216-482	390-490	—
Chemistries					
ALT (IU/L)	12-20	—	1.4-10.0	9.5-10.2	54.6
AST (IU/L)	22-28	—	4-13.4	160-182	20.3
Bilirubin (mg/dl)	0.3-0.4	—	0.06-0.28	0.5-0.6	—
BUN (mg/dl)	8-14	24-44	9.0-19.0	27	18.1
Calcium (mg/dl)	8-10	10	8.0-10.0	9.5-10.2	10.0-12.3
Cholesterol (mg/dl)	60-134	170-254	161-257	53-248	—
Glucose (mg/dl)	80-95	44-94	62-94	126-150	—
LDH (IU/L)	244-1100	—	—	799	180-210
Phosphorus (mg/dl)	5.5-8.5	7	3.6-6.0	1.6-10.4	4.3-7.6
Protein, total (g/dl)	6-7	7.5-8.7	6.7-8.1	7	7.8

Appendix 71. Hematologic and serum biochemical values of primates (cont.)

Measurement	Rhesus macaque (*Macaca mulatta*)	Spider monkey (*Ateles* sp.)	Squirrel Monkey (*Saimiri sciureus*)	Tamarin (*Saguinus* sp.)
Hematology				
PCV (%)	39-43	35-40	43-56	45
RBC ($10^6/\mu l$)	4.5-6.0	5.5	7.1-10.9	6.6
Hgb (g/dl)	12.7	16	12.9-17.0	15.5
WBC ($10^3/\mu l$)	11.5-12.4	10-12	5.1-10.9	12.6-14.4
Neutrophils (%)	20-56	52	36-66	43-64
Lymphocytes (%)	40-76	40	27-55	34-49
Monocytes (%)	0-2	3	0-6	2-5
Eosinophils (%)	1-3	5	0-11	1.0-1.2
Basophils (%)	0-1	0-1	<1	0.1
Platelets ($10^3/\mu l$)	130-144	239-343	112	331-650
Chemistries				
ALT (IU/L)	145-171	—	59-99	7-14
AST (IU/L)	20-34	—	56-118	49-59
Bilirubin (mg/dl)	0.10-0.66	—	0.10-0.53	0.14-0.26
BUN (mg/dl)	14.2-19.6	25.9	23-39	6-12
Calcium (mg/dl)	8.1-11.3	12.8	8.3-9.7	10
Cholesterol (mg/dl)	94-162	—	127-207	69
Glucose (mg/dl)	53-87	82.3	52-108	125-189
LDH (IU/L)	201-665	—	271-490	—
Phosphorus (mg/dl)	4-6	—	3.3-7.7	3-6
Protein, total (g/dl)	6.1-7.1	10.2	6.9-8.1	6.2-8.6

Appendix 72. Biological and physiological data of primates 21

Species	Temperature °C (°F)	Respiratory (rate/min)	Heart rate (BPM)	Av wt (kg) ♂/♀	Estrus length (days)	Gestation (days)	Weaning age (days)	Life span (max yr)
Baboon (*Papio* sp.)	36.0-39.0 (96.8-102.2)	29	80-200	21/12-15	31	175-180	180-456	40-45
Capuchin monkey (*Cebus* sp.)	37.0-38.5 (98.6-101.3)	30-50	165-225	3.8/2.7	16-20	160	270	46
Chimpanzee (*Pan troglodytes*)	35.5-37.8 (95.9-100.0)	35-60	80-150	42/31	36	228	547-1460	53
Common marmoset (*Callithrix* sp.)	35.4-39.7 (95.7-103.5)	20-50	240-350	0.31/0.29	16	148	60-180	12
Lemur (*Lemur* sp.)	37.9-38.1 (100.2-100.6)	—	168-210	2.9/2.5	39	135	105	27
Rhesus macaque (*Macaca mulatta*)	36.0-40.0 (96.8-104.0)	10-25	150-333	6.2/3.0	28	167	210-425	30
Spider monkey (*Ateles* sp.)	36.0-39.4 (96.8-102.9)	18-30	160-210	6.2/5.8	26	229	365	20
Squirrel monkey (*Saimiri sciureus*)	33.5-38.8 (92.3-101.8)	20-50	225-350	0.75/0.58	18	170	182	20
Tamarin (*Saguinus* sp.)	39.3-40.1 (102.7-104.2)	—	—	0.45/0.51	16	145	60-90	13

Appendix 73. Preventive medicine recommendations for primates [21,22,28,34]

Procedure	Schedule	Comments
Physical examination	Annually, or prn	Include CBC, serum biochemistry, dentistry, etc
Tuberculin testing (Tuberculin, mammalian, human isolates, intradermic; Cooper's Animal Health)	0.1 ml ID via 25-27 ga needle; examine at 24, 48, 72 hr; test annually	Positive reaction is erythema and/or edema persisting for >48 hr; tuberculin products with at least 1,500 units per test dose are recommended; intrapalpebral test site can be examined without restraint; alternate sites include the abdomen, thorax, forearm; Old World primates ideally should be tested q3mo if they are in contact with humans whose tuberculosis status is not known; false positives (especially orangutans) and false negatives (anergic animals) can occur; refer to detailed recommendations in references if a positive reaction is obtained
Fecal parasite examination	q3-12mo	Direct wet mount of fresh feces for protozoa; flotation and/or sedimentation procedures for parasite ova; trichrome stains can be used to identify protozoal cysts
Fecal culture	Initial screen, then prn	Culture for *Salmonella, Shigella, Campylobacter, Yersinia;* may take ≥ 3 samples to identify carriers of *Salmonella* or *Shigella;* can be asymptomatic carriers; stain direct fecal smears to identify WBCs and RBCs if infectious enteritis suspected
Serology	Initial screen and serum banking, then prn	Herpes B: all macaques; virus is shed intermittently and sero-negative animals may still be latent carriers; all macaques should be handled as carriers irrespective of serologic status because of fatal potential in humans Others (eg, retroviruses, para-influenza, measles, cytomegalo-virus, hepatitis B); based on species and history (especially origin)

Procedure	Schedule	Comments
Tetanus vaccination	—	All species/human tetanus toxoid can be used; although combination vaccinations containing diphtheria and pertussis are frequently used, vaccination for these diseases is not necessary; give IM because SC deposition of aluminum adjuvants may cause sterile abscesses
	0.5 ml IM at 5-7 and 13-15 mo of age, then booster q5yr[34]	
	3, 6, 9 mo of age, then booster q3-5yr, or in case of injury[22]	
	2, 4, 6, 18 mo of age, then 4-6 yr and 14-16 yr of age, then booster q10yr[21,28]	Based on human schedule
Measles vaccination	—	Modified-live vaccine; do not vaccinate pregnant animals
	6 mo of age, then booster in 5-7 mo[22]	Monkeys
	15 mo of age, booster at 10-12 yr of age[21,22,28]	Great apes,[22] all species[21,28]/based on human schedule[21,28]
	0.5 ml SC at >6 mo of age, ± booster at 13-15 mo of age[34]	
Poliovirus vaccination	—	Great apes only/modified-live oral vaccine; shedding of the vaccine virus may occur
	2, 4, 18 mo of age, then 4-6 yr and 14 16 yr of age[21,28]	Based on human schedule; follow current human pediatric recommendations for route and frequency
	3, 6, 9, 24 mo of age[22]	Juveniles
	q2mo × 3 vaccinations[22]	Adults

Procedure	Schedule	Comments
Poliovirus vaccination (continued)	2, 4, 15 mo of age, then 4-6 yr of age[34]	
Rabies vaccination	—	Not sanctioned by the American Veterinary Medical Association; used by some institutions in rabies-endemic areas; use only killed virus preparations

Appendix 74. Literature cited - Primates

1. Banish LD, Sims R, Bush M, et al. Clearance of *Shigella flexneri* carriers in a zoologic collection of primates. *J Am Vet Med Assoc* 203:133-136, 1993.

2. Barrie MT, Stadler CK. Successful treatment of Cryptococcus neoformans infection in an Allen's swamp monkey (*Allenopithecus nigroviridus*) using fluconazole and flucytosine. *J Zoo Wildl Med* 26:109-114, 1995.

3. Booker JL, Erickson HH, Fitzpatrick EL. Cardiodynamics in the rhesus macaque during dissociative anesthesia. *Am J Vet Res* 43:671-676, 1982.

4. Canadian Council on Animal Care. *Guide to the Use of Experimental Animals.* Vols. I and II. Canadian Council on Animal Care, Ontario, Canada, 1984.

5. Feeser P, White F. Medical management of *Lemur catta, Varecia variegata,* and *Propithecus verreauxi* in natural habitat enclosures. *Proc Am Assoc Zoo Vet/ Am Assoc Wildl Vet:* 320-323, 1992.

6. Flecknell PA. *Laboratory Animal Anaesthesia.* Academic Press, London, 1987.

7. Foltin RW. Getting cynomolgus to take their medicine. *Lab Primate Newsl* 36:4-5, 1997.

8. Foster A, Zeller W, Pfannkuch H. Effect of thiopental, saffan, and propofol anesthesia on cardiovascular parameters and bronchial smooth muscle in the Rhesus monkey. *Lab Anim Sci* 46:327-334, 1996.

9. Fraser CM, Bergeron JA, Mays A, et al. (eds). Diseases of nonhuman primates. In: *The Merck Veterinary Manual,* 7th ed. Merck & Co, Rathway, NJ, 1991. Pp 1032-1036.

10. Gaffar A, Afflitto J, Coleman EJ, et al. Efficacy of ibuprofen rinse in a subgingival irrigator on periodontitis in primates. *J Dental Res* 68:970, 1989.

11. Gilardi KVK, Valverde CR. Glucose control with glipizide therapy in a diabetic dusky titi monkey (Callicebus moloch). *J Zoo Wildl Med* 26:82-86, 1995.

12. Hawk CT, Leary SL (eds). *Formulary for Laboratory Animals.* Iowa State University Press, Ames, 1995.

13. Heard DJ. Principles and techniques of anesthesia and analgesia for exotic practice. *Vet Clin N Am: Small Anim Pract* 23:1301-1327, 1993.

14. Holmes DD. *Clinical Laboratory Animal Medicine.* Iowa State University Press, Ames, 1984.

15. Horne WA, Wolfe BA, Norton TM, Loomis MR. Comparison of the cardio-pulmonary effects of medetomidine-ketamine and medetomidine-Telazol induction on maintenance isoflurane anesthesia in the chimpanzee. *Proc Am Assoc Zoo Vet:* 22-25, 1998.

16. Hotchkiss CE. Use of cisapride for the treatment of intestinal pseudo-obstruction in a stumptail macaque (*Macaca arctoides*). *J Zoo Wildl Med* 26:98-101, 1995.

17. Ialeggio DM. Practical medicine of primate pets. *Compend Cont Educ Pract Vet* 11:1252-1258, 1989.

18. Isaza R, Baker B, Dunker F. Medical management of inflammatory bowel disease in a spider monkey. *J Am Vet Med Assoc* 200:1543, 1992.

19. James SB, Calle PP, Raphael BL, et al. A survey for fecal *Clostridium* toxins in primate feces at the Wildlife Conservation Park/Bronx Zoo. *Proc Am Assoc Zoo Vet:* 119-121, 1998.

20. Johnson DK, Russell RJ, Stunkard JA. *A Guide to Diagnosis, Treatment and Husbandry of Nonhuman Primates.* Veterinary Medicine Publishing Co, Edwardsville, KS, 1981.

21. Johnson-Delaney CA. Primates. *Vet Clin N Am: Small Anim Pract* 24:121-156, 1994.

22. Junge RE. Preventative medicine recommendations. A report of the American Association of Zoo Veterinarians Infectious Disease Committee, Philadelphia, 1991.

23. Junge RE, Mehren KG, Meehan TP, et al. Periarticular hyperostosis and renal disease in six black lemurs of two family groups. *J Am Vet Med Assoc* 205:1024-1029, 1994.

24. Kearns KS, Afema J, Duncan A. Dosage trials using medetomidine as an oral preanesthetic agent in chimpanzees. *Proc Am Assoc Zoo Vet:* 511, 1998.

25. Kelly DJ, Chulay JD, Mikesell P, et al. Serum concentrations of penicillin, doxycycline, and ciprofloxacin during prolonged therapy in rhesus monkeys. *J Infect Dis* 166:1184-1187, 1992.

26. Lamberski N. Hypothyroidism in white-faced saki monkeys (*Pithecia pithecia*). *Proc N Am Vet Conf:* 876, 1998.

27. Lewis JCM. Medetomidine-ketamine anaesthesia in the chimpanzee (*Pan troglodytes*). *J Vet Anaesthesiol* 20:18-20, 1993.

28. Loomis MR. Update of vaccination recommendations for nonhuman primates. *Proc Am Assoc Zoo Vet:* 257-260, 1990.

29. Marks SK. Disease review: balantidiasis. A report of the American Association of Zoo Veterinarians Infectious Disease Committee, Philadelphia, 1994.

30. Melby EC, Altman NH (eds). *CRC Handbook of Laboratory Animal Science.* Vol 3. CRC Press, Cleveland, OH, 1976.

31. Morris PJ. Clinical update: gastrointestinal disease syndromes in colobinae. *Proc N Am Vet Conf:* 903-904, 1996.

32. Orkin JL. Getting cynomolgus to take their medicine. *Lab Primate Newsl* 36:4-5, 1997.

33. Patton DL, Sweney YC, Bohannon NJ, et al. Effects of doxycycline and anti-inflammatory agents on experimentally induced chlamydial upper genital tract infection in female macaques. *J Infect Dis* 175:648-654, 1997.

34. Paul-Murphy J. Preventative medicine program for non-human primates. *Proc N Am Vet Conf:* 736-738, 1992.

35. Popilskis SJ, Kohn DF. Anesthesia and analgesia in nonhuman primates. In: Kohn DF, Wixson SK, White WJ, Benson GJ (eds). *Anesthesia and Analgesia in Laboratory Animals.* Academic Press, New York, 1997. Pp 233-255.

36. Pernikoff DS, Orkin J. Bacterial meningitis syndrome: an overall review of the disease complex and considerations of cross infectivity between great apes and man. *Proc Am Assoc Zoo Vet:* 235-241, 1991.

37. Ramer JC, Emerson C, Paul-Murphy J. Analgesia in nonhuman primates. *Proc Am Assoc Zoo Vet:* 480-483, 1998.

38. Raphael B. Personal communication. 1999.

39. Rolland RM, Chalifoux LV, Snook SS, et al. Five spontaneous deaths associated with *Clostridium difficile* in a colony of cotton-top tamarins. *Lab Anim Sci* 47:472-476, 1997.

40. Rosenberg DP. Nonhuman primate analgesia. *Lab Anim* (Oct):22-32, 1991.

41. Rossoff IS (ed). *Handbook of Veterinary Drugs and Chemicals.* Pharatox Publishing Co, Taylorville, IL. 1994.

42. Sainsbury AW, Eaton BD, and Cooper JE. An investigation into the use of propofol in long-tailed macaques (*Macaca fasicularis*). *J Vet Anaesthesiol* 18:223-228, 1991.

43. Salles CJ, Valls X, Marco A, et al. Anemia, myopathy, and/or steatitis in new world monkeys. *Proc Am Assoc Zoo Vet:* 74-78, 1998.

44. Schaftenaar W. Evaluation of four years experience with medetomidine-ketamine anaesthesia in zoo animals. *Eur Assoc Zoo Wildl Vet:* 32-38, 1996.

45. Schobert E. Telazol use in wild and exotic animals. *Vet Med* (Oct): 1080-1088, 1987.

46. Swenson RB. Protozoal parasites of great apes. In: Fowler ME (ed). *Zoo & Wild Animal Medicine: Current Therapy 3.* WB Saunders Co, Philadelphia, 1993. Pp 352-355.

47. Wallace RS, Bell B, Prosen H, Clyde V. Behavioral and medical therapy for self-mutilation and generalized anxiety in a bonobo. *Proc Am Assoc Zoo Med:* 393-395, 1998.

48. Watson JR, Stoskopf MK, Rozmiarek H, et al. Kinetic study of serum gentamicin concentrations in baboons after single-dose administration. *Am J Vet Res* 52:1285-1287, 1991.

49. Wissman M, Parsons B. Surgical removal of a lipoma-like mass in a lemur (Lemur fulvus fulvus). *J Small Exotic Anim Med* 2:8-12, 1992.

50. Wolf RH, Gibson SV, Watson EA, et al. Multidrug chemotherapy of tuberculosis in rhesus monkeys. *Lab Anim Sci* 38:25-33, 1988.

51. Wolff PL. Parasites of the new world primates. In: Fowler ME (ed). *Zoo & Wild Animal Medicine: Current Therapy 3.* WB Saunders Co, Philadelphia, 1993. Pp 378-389.

52. Young LA, Lung NP, Isaza R, et al. Anemia in a chimpanzee (*Pan troglodytes*) associated with lead toxicity and uterine leiomyoma. *Proc Am Assoc Zoo Vet:* 287, 1994.

Selected
Appendices

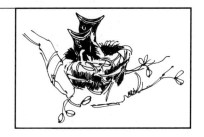

Appendix 75. Checklist for the care of sick, injured, or orphaned wildlife [a]

- Veterinarian's main responsibility is to provide the primary medical care, and qualified personnel (rehabilitators) provide the aftercare and training for release.

- Medical problems are frequently similar to those found in domestic animals; the wild animal's behavior and the restraint procedures required are different.

- Rehabilitators can provide initial supportive care recommendations. Contact the International Wildlife Rehabilitation Council (707-864-1761) or the National Wildlife Rehabilitators Association (320-259-4086) for rehabilitators near you.

- Check with state and federal officials on permit requirements if you hospitalize wildlife.

- Impact at the population level of releasing rehabilitated animals to the wild is minimal; may be important education opportunity for public; on rare occasions, a non-releasable animal can be placed in a conservation education or captive breeding program. Most importantly, perhaps, is that wildlife presented for rehabilitation are "windows" into potentially greater environmental problems.

- When a patient is submitted, ask yourself the following questions:
  1. What is medically wrong with the animal and can it be treated?
  2. If treated, is the animal releasable or can it be placed in an education program? Unfortunately, euthanasia is often required.
  3. If treatment is possible, can the animal survive the rehabilitation period (which may be months)?

- Obtaining a history:
  1. Is the "orphan" truly an orphan? If not, return to nest or site found (natural parents provide the best care). Rabbits and deer, in particular, leave their young unattended for much of the day. It's also important to know that the "scent of man" will not cause rejection of the young by the mother. Although such events are not common, some birds and mammals have been known to reclaim young even after several days. The public, therefore, should be encouraged to call you or a rehabilitator before they move the animal.
  2. When was animal found? Where?
  3. Get name, address, and phone number of the rescuer.
  4. Has any medical or supportive care been provided?

- Initial patient evaluation:
  1. Determine species and age. What is its natural history (herbivore/carnivore/frugivore/insectivore? migratory? etc)?
  2. Zoonotic (rabies, etc) potential?
  3. Generally only a cursory examination (to minimize stress) should be performed until an animal (especially orphan) is hydrated and warm. Assume a minimum 5% dehydration for all sick or injured wildlife.
  4. Administer hydrating solutions for the first 24 hours (parenteral: $1/_2$ strength LRS and $2^1/_2$% dextrose, LRS, or Normosol [Abbott]; PO: Pedialyte [Ross], Gatorade [Gatorade], or Biolyte [Upjohn].

Appendix 75. Checklist for the care of sick, injured, or orphaned wildlife (cont.)

- Initial patient evaluation (cont.):
  5. Treat hypothermia (provide an initial temperature range of ≈ 80-90 °F [27-32 °C]). If a heating pad is used, it should be placed only on the low setting.
  6. Following the rewarming phase, meet energy requirements (dextrose, Emeraid I [Lafeber], etc).
  7. Other medications and therapy as indicated.
  8. Place in appropriate-size incubator, cage, etc; provide proper substrate.

- Problems of hand-rearing:
  1. Runting, aspiration pneumonia, stress, malnutrition, enteropathies, and secondary diseases.
  2. Behavioral problems (avoid taming or imprinting). In general, minimize exposure to humans and domestic animals.

- General feeding guidelines for orphans:
  1. Recommended diets are presented in the following appendixes.
  2. Neonatal animals may refuse to eat (management problems? inappropriate environmental temperature? inappropriate size, consistency, taste, or amount of diet?).
  3. Determine appropriate method of feeding (eg, baby opossums must be fed via a stomach tube; not all baby birds gape; etc).
  4. Attempt to determine the amount of calories required for each day's feeding.
  5. Neonatal mammals must be stimulated to urinate and defecate by gently brushing anal and urogenital areas with moist cotton or clean tissue after each feeding.

[a] See references in following appendices.

Species	Diet	Frequency	Weaning
Armadillo	Esbilac (Pet-Ag) or Zoologic 33/40 (Pet-Ag) and water 2:3	2-4 × daily	Wean at 6-8 wk onto cat/dog or kitten/puppy chow or canned food and native foods. Adding grubs, insects, and insect eggs to their diet will gradually adapt them to natural foods. Supplemental vitamin K_1 is required. They enjoy swimming in dishpans. To reintroduce into the wild, take them outside to forage for insects.
Badger	Esbilac or Zoologic 33/40 and water 4:7	2-3 × daily	Wean at 8-10 wk onto canned or dry dog or cat food and native foods. Release at 5 mo.
Bat	Bat milk: • Zoologic 33/40 and water 1:2:3 • 1 drop Avitron (Lamber K) and 2 drops Avimin (Lamber K) to every 35 ml of formula	Feed via 1-3 ml syringe 3-4 × daily	Insectivorous bats: add mealworms and crickets until ready to be housed with adults and/or trained for release. Feed in a head-down and sternal position. Frugivorous bats: add pureed bananas, grapes, melon, papaya, and apples. Wean at 3-4 wk.
Beaver	Esbilac and Multi-Milk (Pet-Ag) 2:1 or Esbilac and Zoologic 30/55 (Pet-Ag) and water 2:2:3	3-4 × daily	Wean at 8 wk onto rodent pellets and native foods (shrubs, twigs, branches, etc.).
Bobcat	KMR (Pet-Ag) or Zoologic 42/25 (Pet-Ag) and water 2:3	3-4 × daily	Wean at 8-9 wk onto canned or dry kitten food and rodents. May begin nibbling on pureed rodents (or cat food) at 10 days of age. Gradually add live rodents for them to kill. Release at 4-5 mo in a similar manner to that for the fox and coyote.

Appendix 76. Recommended diets and weaning considerations for orphaned wild mammals (cont.)

Species	Diet	Frequency	Weaning
Coyote	Esbilac or Zoologic 33/40 and water 4:5	2-4 × daily	Wean at 5-7 wk onto puppy or ferret diet and rodents (ie, pureed mice). May begin nibbling on pureed rodents (or dog or ferret food) at 10 days of age. Gradually introduce live rodents for them to kill. A litter can be released at 5-6 mo. Very difficult to rear and release single animals.
Deer (white-tailed)	Lamb, kid (goat), or doe (deer) milk replacer	2-4 × daily (generally 1 oz/lb 2 × daily) with a lamb's nipple. Can use goat or cow colostrum if the neonate hasn't nursed.	Gradually decrease the number of feedings by 1/day over a period of ≈ 1 wk as the fawn starts nibbling grass. Wean at 8-12 wk on a wild ruminant diet (16-25% protein), hay, and browse. Be careful handling fawns; they panic easily and may injure themselves in escape attempts. Best to raise with conspecifics (do not raise alone).
Fox (red or gray)	Esbila or Zoologic 33/40 and water 4:7	2-3 × daily	Wean at 7-8 wk onto puppy canned or dry food, rodents (ie, pureed mice) and 5% fruit. May begin nibbling on pureed rodents (or dog food) at 10 days of age. Gradually introduce live rodents for them to kill. A litter can be released at 5-6 mo. Very difficult to rear and release single animals.
Opossum	Esbilac and Multi-Milk 4:1 or Esbilac and Zoologic 30/55 and water 2:1:4	3-6 × daily (must tube feed max 1.5 ml/28 g BW)	Wean at 13-15 wk onto canned or dry dog food and native foods. Supplemental calcium is required. House carefully (because they may get out, crawl behind things, and not come out even to eat). Feed in a sitting position with forefeet elevated.

Species	Diet	Frequency	Weaning [a]
Rabbit	Esbilac and Multi-Milk 3:2 or Zoologic 30/55 and Zoologic 42/25 and water 3:2:5	2-4 × daily	Begin weaning at 2-3 wk by gradually adding native forage, hay grass clippings, rabbit pellets, apples, carrots, and grain. Avoid over-handling (shock). Acidophilus (ie, yogurt) may be a useful supplement; small amount of honey may promote eating if they initially reject the milk. Place them in wire mesh bottom cages outside; release at 3-5 wk (when eating anatural diet).
Raccoon	KMR or Zoologic 42/25 and water 1:2	3-5 × daily (needs to be burped)	Wean at 8-10 wk onto dry dog food and native foods. They become aggressive with age. Feed in sitting position with forefeet elevated.
Skunk	Esbilac or Zoologic 33/40 and water 4:5	2-4 × daily depending on the age	Wean at 6-8 wk onto dry dog food, rodent pellets, and native foods.
Squirrel	• 3 oz Esbilac or Unilac (Foremost McKesson) • 1 tsp baby cereal	At least q2h (feed with animal on belly)	Wean by 6 wk onto rodent pellets, vegetables, crackers, apples, and a variety of nuts and grain. Adapt easily to the wild once weaned. Release at 12-14 (occasionally 10) wk.
Woodchuck (groundhog) and marmot	Esbilac or Zoologic 33/40 and water 4:5	2-4 × daily	Wean at 6-8 wk onto rodent pellets and native forage (vegetables, grains, fruit, seeds, and nuts). They enjoy playing in sand.

[a] Although this outline is intended to provide general guidelines for the care of orphaned wildlife, the veterinarian is strongly encouraged to transfer these animals to experienced rehabilitators as soon as possible and/or to contact rehabilitators if questions arise. In addition, any individual working with wildlife should check with state and federal officials on permit requirements.

[b] Avoid overfeeding of orphaned wild mammals.

Appendix 76. Recommended diets and weaning considerations for orphaned wild mammals (cont.)

1 _____. Zoologic milk matrix formulation and mixing guide. Pet-Ag, Hampshire, IL.
2 Evans RH. Care and feeding of orphan mammals and birds. In: Kirk RB (ed). *Current Veterinary Therapy IX: Small Animal Practice*. WB Saunders Co, Philadelphia, 1986. Pp 775-787.
3 Johnson V, Adams P, Goodrich P, et al. *Wild Animal Care and Rehabilitation Manual*. Beech Leaf Press, Kalamazoo, MI, 1991.
4 Lollar A, Schmidt-French B. *Captive Care and Medical Reference for the Rehabilitation of Insectivorous Bats*. Bat World, Mineral Wells, TX, 1998.
5 Marcum D. *Rehabilitation of North American Wild Mammals: Feeding and Nutrition*. International Wildlife Rehabilitation Council, Suisun, CA, 1997.
6 Moore AT, Joosten S. *Principles of Wildlife Rehabilitation*. National Wildlife Rehabilitation Association, St Cloud, MN, 1997.

Appendix 77. Feeding frequency and temperature recommendations for hand-rearing orphaned, altricial birds [a,1,2]

Age class	Characteristics	Feeding frequency	Temperature[b]
Hatchling (days 0 to 4)	• No feathers or small amount of down • Bulbous body • Frail appendages • Unable to sit up • Eyes closed	q15min (7 am - 9 pm)	80-90 °F (26-32 °C)
Nestling (days 4 to 10)	• Quills show • Feathers sprout • Downy feathers on head • Cannot perch • Eyes open	q20-30min (7 am - 9 pm)	80-85 °F (26-29 °C)
Fledgling (days 10 to 14)	• Feathered • Short tail feathers • First attempts to fly • Can perch • Will preen	q40-60min (7 am - 9 pm)	70-80 °F (21-26 °C)
Juveniles/immatures (>15 days to adult)	• Feathered • Normally imprinted • Defensive • Able to fly • Still being fed by parents	q2-4h Provide items for self-feeding (7 am - 9 pm until self-feeding)	70-80 °F (21-26 °C)
Adults	• Adult plumage • Aggressive • Normally arrive injured	Self-feeding or force-feeding	70-80 °F (21-26 °C)

a Although this outline is intended to provide general guidelines for the care of orphaned wildlife, the veterinarian is strongly encouraged to transfer these animals to experienced rehabilitators as soon as possible and/or to contact rehabilitators if questions arise. In addition, any individual working with wildlife should check with state and federal officials on permit requirements.

b After the bird is healthy and normothermic.

1 Evans RH. Care and feeding of orphan mammals and birds. In: Kirk RB (ed). *Current Veterinary Therapy IX: Small Animal Practice*. WB Saunders Co, Philadelphia, 1986. Pp 775-787.

2 Moore AT, Joosten S. *Principles of Wildlife Rehabilitation*. National Wildlife Rehabilitation Association, St Cloud, MN, 1997.

Appendix 78. Suggested diets used in hand-rearing orphaned, altricial wild birds a,1-5

Species	Diet[1]	Diet[b,2]	Diet[3]
Ground insectivores (eg, robins, thrushes, towhees, wrens)	1 cup Hill's Science Diet p/d dog food (or Purina Hi-Pro dog food) softened in water 1/2 cup mynah bird food/turkey pellets 2 soft-boiled eggs; berries 1/3 cup cooked Roman Meal cereal 1 tsp dark loam, 1 tsp dolomite vit/min mix Mix above diet 1:1 with earthworms	1 part Hill's Science Diet Feline Growth 1 part Gerber's High Protein Cereal 1 tsp bone meal water for proper consistency add: crickets, mealworms, earthworms, grubs, grasshoppers, and some berries	See below[c]
Aerial insectivores (eg, swallows, kingbirds, phoebes, swifts, nighthawks)[d]	1 cup high-protein pablum; 1 soft-boiled egg 1/4 cup cooked Roman Meal cereal 1 cup dried insect mix (fish food) Mix above diet 1:1 with live insects; feed in small bites	1 part Hill's Science Diet Feline Growth 2 parts Gerber's High Protein Cereal Ca supplement; water for proper consistency supplement with crickets, mealworms, grubs, waxworms, grasshoppers	—
Insectivorous omnivores (eg, blackbirds, mockingbirds, orioles, thrashers, warblers, tanagers)	Same as for ground insectivores, except cooked Roman Meal cereal is increased to cup and insects or worms can be used	1 cup ZuPreem Dry Omnivore Chow 1/3 cup Gerber's High Protein Cereal 3 Tbs brewer's yeast *Lactobacillus* spp, *Streptococcus faecium*[f] vitamin/bone meal; water for consistency supplement with fresh, thawed crickets	See below[c]
Insectivorous frugivores (eg, waxwings, flickers, wood-peckers)	Same as for insectivorous omnivores, but 20% of diet is berries	—	—

Species	Diet[1]	Diet[b,2]	Diet[3]
Omnivores (eg, jays, shrikes, crows, grackles)	Same as for insectivorous omnivores, but chopped, skinned mice and insects can be added (not more than 10% of diet)	1 part Hill's Science Diet Feline Growth 1 part Gerber's High Protein Cereal (or ZuPreem) Dry Omnivore Chow, soaked) *Lactobacillus* spp, *Streptococcus faecium*[f] vitamin/bone meal; water for consistency add: crickets, grubs, flies, small pieces of fruit or Gerber's strained fruit	See below[c]
Granivores (eg, finches, chickadees, juncos)	Same as for insectivorous omnivores; at day 10, 20% of diet is seeds	1/4 cup Hill's Science Diet Feline Growth 1/2 cup Gerber's High Protein Cereal 2 Tbs Gerber's strained peas (or Heinz dehydrated peas/carrots) *Lactobacillus* spp, *Streptococcus faecium*[f] vitamin/bone meal; water for consistency	See below[e]
Columbiformes (eg, pigeons, doves)	Exact (Kaytee), Nutristart (Lafeber), or other commercial psittacine hand-rearing diet; must tube feed 2-4 × daily until crop is full	—	—

a Although this outline is intended to provide general guidelines for the care of orphaned wildlife, the veterinarian is strongly encouraged to transfer these animals to experienced rehabilitators as soon as possible and/or to contact rehabilitators if questions arise. In addition, any individual working with wildlife should check with state and federal officials on permit requirements.

b Hatchlings of all species can be fed diet consisting of 1 part hard-boiled egg yolk, 1 part Gerber's High Protein Cereal, 1 part soaked Feline Growth, mixed with warm water.

c Use a combination of a commercially prepared psittacine hand-rearing formula and Science Diet p/d (Hill's).

d These birds are very difficult to raise and generally require the skills of experienced rehabilitators.

e Use a commercially prepared psittacine hand-rearing formula (eg, Exact [Kaytee], Nutristart [Lafeber]).

f Bird Bene-Bac Gel, Pet-Ag.

Appendix 78. Suggested diets used in hand-rearing orphaned, altricial wild birds (cont.)

1 Evans RH. Care and feeding of orphan mammals and birds. In: Kirk RB (ed). *Current Veterinary Therapy IX: Small Animal Practice*. WB Saunders Co, Philadelphia, 1986. Pp 775–787.
2 Project Wildlife, San Diego, California.
3 Carpenter JW, Rupiper DJ. Personal communication. 1999.
4 Baicich PJ, Harrison C. *A Guide to the Nests, Eggs, and Nestlings of North American Birds*. 2nd ed. Academic Press Natural World, San Diego, 1997.
5 Ehrlich PR, Dobkin DS, Wheye D. *The Birder's Handbook*. Simon and Schuster/Fireside, New York, 1988.

Appendix 79. Suggested diets used in hand-rearing precocial, semi-precocial, and semi-altricial orphaned wild birds [a,1,2]

Species	Diet
Galliformes (eg, pheasants, quail, grouse, turkeys)	Commercial gamebird, turkey, or chicken starter and growing ration (use small size ration for quail); supplement with insects; small amount of grit
Anseriformes (eg, ducks, geese)	Duck starter pellets (wk 1-4) and duck grower/finisher pellets (until mature); alternatively can use commercial "all purpose pellets"; supplement with fresh aquatic vegetables; access to grit
Gruiformes (eg, coots, gallinules, rails, cranes)	Commercial poultry, gamebird, waterfowl, or crane diets; can be supplemented with insects (eg, mealworms), minced rodents, and aquatic vegetables
Charadriiformes (eg, gulls, terns, plovers, sandpipers)	Mixture of dog food (ground or minced rodents if available), insects, and fish
Ciconiiformes (eg, herons, egrets, bitterns)	Minced or ground, whole rodents (skinned) for the first 10-14 days, then chopped rodents can be fed; or fresh or recently thawed fish at a rate of 30-60% of body weight daily; may need to supplement with vitamins (eg, E, B_1)
Falconiformes (hawks) and Strigiformes (owls)	Ground or minced, skinned, and beheaded adult rodents or plucked day-old chicks or quail rolled in bone meal (for falcons) for the first 2-10 days; thereafter, chopped whole animals (with some fur/feathers) can be fed until the bird is forming pellet well; then allow free access to food

a Although this outline is intended to provide general guidelines for the care of orphaned wildlife, the veterinarian is strongly encouraged to transfer these animals to experienced rehabilitators as soon as possible and/or to contact rehabilitators if questions arise. In addition, any individual working with wildlife should check with state and federal officials on permit requirements.

1 Evans RH. Care and feeding of orphan mammals and birds. In: Kirk RB (ed). *Current Veterinary Therapy IX: Small Animal Practice*. WB Saunders Co, Philadelphia, 1986. Pp 775-787.

2 Carpenter JW, Rupiper DJ. Personal communication. 1999.

Appendix 80. Classification of select antibacterials used in exotic animal medicine

Type	Antibacterial agent
• Natural penicillins[a]	Benzathine penicillin G Procaine penicillin G

• Extended-spectrum penicillins[a]
  Aminopenicillins
 	
  Antipseudomonal penicillins
    Carboxypenicillins
 	
    Piperazine penicillins
	Amoxicillin
	Ampicillin
	
	Carbenicillin
	Ticarcillin
	Piperacillin

• ß-Lactamase inhibitors Clavulanic acid	Amoxicillin-clavulanate Ticarcillin-clavulanate
• First-generation cephalosporins[a]	Cefadroxil Cefazolin Cephalexin Cephalothin Cephradine
• Third-generation cephalosporins[a]	Cefotaxime Ceftazidime Ceftiofur
• Macrolides[b]	Erythromycin Tylosin
• Tetracyclines[b]	Chlortetracycline Doxycycline Oxytetracycline Tetracycline
• Chloramphenicol[b]	Chloramphenicol
• Lincosamides[c]	Clindamycin Lincomycin
• Aminoglycosides[a]	Amikacin Gentamicin Kanamycin Neomycin Streptomycin Tobramycin
• Aminocyclitol	Spectinomycin[b]
• Nitroimidazole	Metronidazole[d]

Appendix 80. Classification of select antibacterials used in exotic animal medicine (cont.)

Type	Antibacterial agent
• Sulfonamides[b]	Sulfachlorpyridazine Sulfadiazine Sulfamethoxazole Sulfadimethoxine Sulfamethazine Sulfaquinoxaline Sulfathiazole Sulfisoxazole
• Trimethoprim[b]	Trimethoprim
• Trimethoprim-sulfa[a]	Trimethoprim-sulfadiazine Trimethoprim-sulfamethoxazole
• Quinolones	Nalidixic acid
• Fluoroquinolones[a]	Ciprofloxacin Enrofloxacin

[a] Bacteriocidal.
[b] Bacteriostatic.
[c] Bacteriostatic or bacteriocidal.
[d] Cidal vs amoebae, *Giardia*, *Trichomonas*, and most obligate anaerobes; inactive vs most aerobic bacteria or facultative anaerobes.

Appendix 81. General efficacy of select antimicrobial agents used in exotic animals

Gram ⊕ bacteria	Gram ⊕ bacteria (in general) • Lincosamides • Cephalosporins • Tetracyclines • Penicillins • Macrolides • Select aminoglycosides (gentamicin, kanamycin) • Chloramphenicol • Fluoroquinolones • Erythromycin
	Staphylococcus spp • Early-generation penicillins • Early-generation cephalosporins • Early-generation β-lactams • Macrolides • Select aminoglycosides (gentamicin, kanamycin) • Lincosamides • Fluoroquinolones • Chloramphenicol • Trimethoprim-sulfa
	Streptococcus spp • Cephalosporins • Penicillins • Early-generation β-lactams • Select aminoglycosides (gentamicin) • Macrolides • Lincosamides • Tetracyclines • Chloramphenicol • Fluoroquinolones • Trimethoprim-sulfa
	Clostridium spp and other anaerobes • Penicillins (amoxicillin-clavulanate) • Cephalosporins • Metronidazole[a] • Clindamycin • Lincomycin • Tetracyclines • Erythromycin • Chloramphenicol
Gram ⊖ bacteria	Enterobacteriaceae (in general) • Advanced-generation penicillins • Advanced-generation cephalosporins • Advanced-generation β-lactams • Fluoroquinolones • Trimethoprim-sulfa • Aminoglycosides (amikacin)

Gram ⊖ bacteria (continued)	*Campylobacter* • Erythromycin • Doxycycline • Chloramphenicol • Furazolidone • Gentamicin • Neomycin • Clindamycin
	Pasteurella spp • Sulfonamides • Penicillins • Erythromycin • Amikacin • Kanamycin • Fluoroquinolones • Trimethoprim-sulfa • Tetracyclines
	Pseudomonas (often resistant) • Aminoglycosides (frequently in combination with an advanced-generation β-lactam) • Advanced-generation β-lactam • Fluoroquinolones • Advanced-generation penicillins (carbenicillin, ticarcillin; frequently in combination with an aminoglycoside) • Advanced-generation cephalosporins (frequently in combination with an aminoglycoside) • Chloramphenicol
	Salmonella spp • Fluoroquinolones • Chloramphenicol • Advanced-generation penicillins • Trimethoprim-sulfa • Tetracyclines • Aminoglycosides
Chlamydia	• Tetracyclines • Enrofloxacin (vs some spp) • Erythromycin
Mycoplasma	• Tetracyclines • Macrolides • Enrofloxacin • Lincosamides • Chloramphenicol

[a] Effective vs most obligate anaerobes; inactive vs most aerobic bacteria or facultative anaerobes.

Appendix 82. Antimicrobial therapy used in exotic animals according to site of infection [a,1]

Site of infection	Antimicrobial agent

Bacteremia, septicemia
  Aerobic bacteria
 	
  Anaerobic bacteria
	Aminoglycoside with a penicillin or cephalosporin
	Enrofloxacin with amoxicillin
	Penicillins
	Chloramphenicol
	Clindamycin
	Metronidazole

Soft-tissue infection	Penicillins (ie, amoxicillin-clavulanate) Cephalosporins Clindamycin or metronidazole (vs anaerobes) Tetracycline Trimethoprim-sulfa Enrofloxacin Enrofloxacin with metronidazole (vs polymicrobial aerobic and anaerobic infections)
Respiratory tract	Penicillins Cephalosporins Tetracyclines Trimethoprim-sulfa Chloramphenicol Enrofloxacin (vs *Mycoplasma*, etc) Tetracycline (vs *Mycoplasma* and *Chlamydia*) Macrolides (vs *Mycoplasma*) Clindamycin (vs anaerobes) Metronidazole (vs anaerobes)
Alimentary tract	Trimethoprim-sulfa Enrofloxacin Cephalosporins Amoxicillin Tetracyclines Metronidazole (vs anaerobes) Neomycin
Skin	Amoxicillin-clavulanate Cephalosporins Erythromycin Enrofloxacin Trimethoprim-sulfa Lincomycin
Bone and/or joint	Cephalosporins Extended-spectrum penicillins Fluoroquinolones Aminoglycosides Lincosamides Penicillins with clindamycin (vs anaerobes) Third-generation cephalosporins with clindamycin (vs anaerobes)

Appendix 82. Antimicrobial therapy used in exotic animals according to site of infection (cont.)

Site of infection	Antimicrobial agent
Urinary tract	Penicillins (ampicillin, amoxicillin, amoxicillin-clavulanate) Cephalosporins (cephalexin, cefedroxil, cephazolin) Trimethoprim-sulfa Sulfisoxazole Enrofloxacin Tetracycline
Central nervous system	Chloramphenicol (encephalitis) Trimethoprim-sulfa Metronidazole (vs anaerobes) Fluoroquinolones (meningitis) Penicillins (in cases of inflammation) Third-generation cephalosporins
Reproductive tract	Chloramphenicol Trimethoprim-sulfa Enrofloxacin Amoxicillin-clavulanate Clindamycin (vs anaerobes)

[a] Definitive therapy should be based on bacterial culture and sensitivity and host species involved.

[1] Modified from: Allen DG, Pringle JK, Smith D. *Handbook of Veterinary Drugs.* JB Lippincott Co, Philadelphia, 1993; Pp 38-41; and Prescott JF, Baggot JD (eds). *Antimicrobial Therapy in Veterinary Medicine.* Iowa State University Press, Ames, IA, 1993.

Appendix 83. Antimicrobial combination therapies commonly used in exotic animals [a]

Drug	Synergistic or combination drug
Aminoglycoside[b] (amikacin, gentamicin)	Penicillins (carbenicillin, piperacillin, ticarcillin, amoxicillin, ampicillin), cephalosporins, trimethoprim-sulfa, lincomycin, metronidazole, fluoroquinolones
Amoxicillin	Clavulanate
Cephalosporin	Aminoglycosides,[b] clindamycin, fluoroquinolones, metronidazole, semi-synthetic penicillins
Clindamycin	Penicillins, third-generation cephalosporin, enrofloxacin
Fluoroquinolone (enrofloxacin, ciprofloxacin)	Aminoglycosides,[b] third-generation cephalosporin, extended-spectrum penicillins, clindamycin, metronidazole
Lincomycin	Spectinomycin, aminoglycosides[b]
Metronidazole	Amikacin, carbenicillin, cefazolin, cefotaxime, chloramphenicol, enrofloxacin, gentamicin, others as indicated
Penicillin (carbenicillin, piperacillin, ampicillin)	Aminoglycosides,[b] fluoroquinolones
Penicillin, early-generation	Aminoglycosides,[b] advanced-generation cephalosporin
Ticarcillin	Clavulanate
Trimethoprim	Sulfadiazine, sulfamethoxine
Tylosin	Oxytetracycline

[a] Indicated when synergy is advantageous in definitive therapy, to treat polymicrobial infections, to broaden empiric coverage, or to attempt to prevent the development of antimicrobial resistance.

[b] Generally amikacin, occasionally gentamicin, etc.

Appendix 84. Selected laboratories conducting avian and reptile diagnostic procedures [a]

Laboratory	Test/procedure	
American Histolabs 7605-F Airpark Rd Gaithersburg, MD 20879, USA (301) 330-1200	Surgical biopsies	
Animal Diagnostic Laboratory (AniLab) 5750 Executive Drive, Suite 102 Baltimore, MD 21228, USA (410) 788-8868	Avian: Reptiles:	*Aspergillus*, avian malaria *Cryptosporidium*
Animal Health Diagnostic Laboratory Michigan State University PO Box 30076 Lansing, MI 48909, USA (517) 353-1683	Avian:	Microbiology, *Chlamydia*, *Mycoplasma*, poxvirus, Pacheco's virus, other viruses, necropsy, histopathology, blood lead, other toxins
Antech Diagnostics 10 Executive Boulevard Farmingdale, NY 11735, USA (888) 397-8378	Avian: Reptiles:	Hematology, chemistries, microbiology, *Mycoplasma*, *Chlamydia*, psittacine beak and feather disease virus, polyomavirus, sexing Hematology, chemistries, microbiology, *Mycoplasma*, sexing (iguana)
APL Veterinary Laboratories 4230 S Burnham Avenue, Suite 250 Las Vegas, NV 89119, USA (702) 733-3791 (800) 433-2750	Avian: Reptiles:	Hematology, chemistries, pathology, aspergillosis, AGID serology (also other fungal diseases), *Chlamydia*, *Mycoplasma* and *Mycobac- terium* culture, TSH stimulation Similar to above
Avian Biotech International 4500 Shannon Lakes Plaza Unit 1, Suite 138 Tallahassee, FL 32308, USA (850) 893-5549 (800) 514-9672	Avian:	Sex determination (recombinant DNA), hematology, chemistries, polyomavirus, psittacine beak and feather disease virus, *Chlamydia*
Avian & Exotic Animal Clin Path Labs 3701 Inglewood Avenue, Suite 106 Redondo Beach, CA 90278, USA (310) 542-6556 (800) 350-1122	Avian: Reptiles:	Hematology, chemistries, bile acids, histopathology, cytology, microbiology, *Chlamydia*, *Mycoplasma*, parasitology, blood lead and zinc, iron assays Similar to above

Appendix 84. Selected laboratories conducting avian and reptile diagnostic procedures (cont)

Laboratory	Test/procedure	
Avian Genetic Sexing Laboratory 6551 Stage Oaks Drive, Suite 3A Bartlett, TN 38134, USA (901) 388-9548	Avian:	Sex determination (chromosome analysis; uses blood feather)
California Avian Laboratory 6114 Greenback Lane Citrus Heights, CA 95621, USA (916) 722-8428 (800) 783-2473	Avian: Reptiles:	Hematology, chemistries, cytology, histopathology, necropsy, microbiology, *Chlamydia, Mycoplasma,* parasitology, radiology consultation Similar to above
California Veterinary Diagnostic Laboratory System W Health Sciences Drive Davis, CA 95616, USA (530) 752-8700	Avian: Reptiles:	Histopathology, microbiology, parasitology, virology, serology Similar to above
Clinical Virology Laboratory Room A239 College of Veterinary Medicine University of Tennessee 2407 River Drive Knoxville, TN 37996, USA (423) 974-5643	Reptiles:	Ophidian paramyxovirus
Comparative Toxicology Laboratories College of Veterinary Medicine Kansas State University Manhattan, KS 66506, USA (785) 532-5679	General toxicologic analyses, pesticide screen, heavy metal screen, lead, mycotoxin screen	
Consolidated Veterinary Diagnostics 2825 KOVR Drive West Sacramento, CA 95605, USA (916) 372-4200 (800) 444-4210	Avian: Reptiles:	Hematology, chemistries, cytology, histopathology, microbiology, serology, parasitology Similar to above
Elliott Jacobson, DVM, PhD Department of Small Animal Clinical Sciences College of Veterinary Medicine University of Florida PO Box 100126 Gainesville, FL 32610, USA (352) 392-4700, Ext 5700	Reptiles:	Ophidian paramyxovirus

Appendix 84. Selected laboratories conducting avian and reptile diagnostic procedures (cont)

Laboratory	Test/procedure
Johne's Testing Center University of Wisconsin School of Veterinary Medicine Room 4230 2015 Linden Drive West Madison, WI 53706, USA (608) 265-6463	Avian: *Mycobacterium avium* culture

National Veterinary Services
  Laboratory
APHIS
USDA
PO Box 844
(Send specimens to 1800 Dayton St)
Ames, IA 50010, USA
(515) 239-8266
Note: Submission of samples requires
  approval by the federal
  Veterinarian-in-Charge of
  your area
	Avian: Microbiology culture and serology (aspergillosis, avian adenovirus, herpes, influenza, paramyxovirus, Pacheco's virus, poxvirus, reovirus, *Chlamydia, Mycoplasma, Mycobacterium, Salmonella,* Newcastle disease, etc), toxicology, parasitology
	Reptiles: Similar to above

Northwest ZooPath 18210 Waverly Drive Snohomish, WA 98296, USA (360) 668-6003	Pathology
University of Miami School of Medicine Division of Comparative Pathology PO Box 016960 (R-46) Miami, FL 33101, USA (305) 243-6928 (800) 596-7390	Avian: Hematology, chemistries, protein electrophoresis, histopathology, microbiology, serology *(Chlamydia, Aspergillus, Giardia, Cryptosporidium),* psittacine beak and feather disease virus, polyomavirus Reptiles: Hematology, chemistries, histopathology, microbiology
The Raptor Center University of Minnesota College of Veterinary Medicine 1920 Fitch Avenue St. Paul, MN 55108, USA (612) 624-4745	Avian: Aspergillosis ELISA
Research Associates Laboratory 5991 Meijer Drive Suite 24 Milford, OH 45150, USA (513) 248-4700	Avian: Psittacine beak and feather disease virus, polyomavirus, *Chlamydia* (DNA probe), sex determination (DNA probe)

Appendix 84. Selected laboratories conducting avian and reptile diagnostic procedures (cont)

Laboratory	Test/procedure	
Texas Veterinary Medical Diagnostic Laboratory Texas A&M University PO Drawer 3040 College Station, TX 77841-3040, USA (409) 845-3414 (Send specimens to 1 Sippel Rd, College Station, TX 77843, USA)	Avian: Reptiles:	*Chlamydia,* Pacheco's virus, polyomavirus, chemistries, necropsy, histopathology, cytology, microbiology, serology, toxicology Similar to above
Charles O Thoen, DVM, PhD Department of Microbiology, Immunology, and Preventive Medicine Veterinary Medicine Complex Iowa State University Ames, IA 50011, USA (515) 294-7608	Avian:	Tuberculosis ELISA (available for some species), lymphocyte blastogenic assays (LBA)
Veterinary Diagnostic Laboratory Oregon State University PO Box 429 Corvallis, OR 97339, USA (541) 737-6812	Avian: Reptiles:	Hematology, chemistries, pathology, microbiology, *Chlamydia, Mycoplasma* Histopathology, microbiology
Veterinary Medical Diagnostic Laboratory College of Veterinary Medicine University of Missouri PO Box 6023 Columbia, MO 65205, USA (573) 882-6811	General toxicologic analyses, pesticide screen, heavy metal screen, lead, mycotoxin screen	
Zoogen, Inc 1756 Picasso Avenue Davis, CA 95616, USA (916) 756-8089 (800) 995-2473	Avian:	Sex determination (recombinant DNA)

a   Similar services are generally offered at these laboratories for other exotic animals.

Appendix 85. Determining the basal metabolic rate of animals

The following information is provided so that drug dosages can be allometrically scaled for different species, and to assist in calculating metabolic needs for nutritional requirements and fluid therapy.

BMR (basal metabolic rate)
- BMR differs between species.
- The general equation to calculate BMR[a] is: $BMR = kW^{0.75}$

  BMR = kcal/kg/day
  k = kcal/kg constant
      (non-passerines = 78, passerines = 129, placental mammals = 70, marsupials = 49, reptiles at 37 °C = 10)
  W = weight in kg

- Other equations have been determined for passerine and non-passerine birds in relation to the daylight cycle. These cycles are termed "active phase" and "rest phase". However, results are similar to those obtained with the above formula.

Phase	Passerines	Non-passerines
Active phase	$BMR = (140.7)W^{0.704}$	$BMR = (91)W^{0.729}$
Rest phase	$BMR = (113.8)W^{0.726}$	$BMR = (72)W^{0.734}$

- Maintenance energy requirement (MER) = (kcal/day) = (1.5 x BMR)

In birds, the MER can then be adjusted for health status as follows[b]

Physical inactivity	$0.7-0.9 \times MER$
Starvation	$0.5-0.7 \times MER$
Hypometabolism	$0.5-0.9 \times MER$
Elective surgery	$1.0-1.2 \times MER$
Mild trauma	$1.0-1.2 \times MER$
Severe trauma	$1.1-2.0 \times MER$
Growth	$1.5-3.0 \times MER$
Sepsis	$1.2-1.5 \times MER$
Burns	$1.2-2.0 \times MER$
Head injuries	$1.0-2.0 \times MER$

[a] Sedgwick C, Pokras M, Kaufman G. Metabolic scaling: using estimated energy costs to extrapolate drug doses between different species and different individuals of diverse body sizes. *Proc Annu Conf Am Assoc Zoo Vet*: 249–254, 1990.
[b] Quesenberry KE, Mauldin G, Hillyer E. Review of methods of nutritional support in hospitalized birds. *First Conf Euro Comm Assoc Avian Vet*: 243–254, 1991.

Appendix 86. Allometric scaling of drugs used in animals

Although allometric scaling provides a means to calculate a drug dose in terms of an animal's basal metabolic rate (BMR; see Appendix 85), pharmacokinetically derived data are the preferred source of information for the dose and frequency. Allometric scaling can complement, or be an alternative to, empirical dosing and extrapolation from domestic animal and human dosing. Scaling does not guarantee that the dosage would be efficacious, nontoxic, safe, or correct. All allometrically scaled dosages, therefore, should be reviewed by the practitioner prior to administration. Use of a conventional dose is preferred over an allometric dose when the allometric dose seems disproportionate. The reader is referred to other sources of information concerning the use of allometric scaling.[1,2]

- BMR in kcal/day = kW$^{0.75}$
  - k = kcal/kg/day constant
    - (non-passerines = 78, passerines = 129, placental mammals = 70, marsupials = 49, reptiles at 37 °C = 10)
  - W = weight in kg

Example. The BMR needs to be calculated for the avian species for which a dosage is not known as well as for the species in which the drug is routinely used. For example, the dosage for enrofloxacin needs to be calculated for a 30 g canary patient (BMR_p) based on a model (known) dosage of 7.5 mg/kg q12h for an Amazon parrot (BMR_m) weighing 250 g.

1. Model BMR = BMR_m = (78 kcal/kg/day) (0.250 kg)$^{0.75}$ = 27.6 kcal/day
2. Model energy cost = kW$^{-0.25}$ = (78 kcal/kg/day) (0.250 kg)$^{-0.25}$ = 110 kcal/day
3. Model dose = 7.5 mg/kg
4. Model dose interval = q12h
5. Model treatment dose = (wt in kg) (dose) = (0.250 kg) (7.5 mg/kg) = 1.875 mg
6. BMR_m dose = (model treatment dose) / (BMR_m) = (1.875 mg) / (27.6 kcal/day) = 0.068 mg/kcal/day
7. Patient BMR = BMR_p = (129 kcal/kg/day) (0.030 kg)$^{0.75}$ = 9.3 kcal/day
8. Patient energy cost = kW$^{-0.25}$ = (129 kcal/kg/day) (0.030 kg)$^{-0.25}$ = 310 kcal/day
9. Patient treatment dose = (BMR_m dose) (BMR_p) = (0.068 mg/kcal/day) (9.3 kcal/day) = 0.63 mg
10. Patient dose = (patient treatment dose) / (wt in kg) = (0.63 mg) / (0.030 kg) = 21 mg/kg
11. Patient treatment interval
    = [(patient energy cost/model energy cost) / (model dose interval)]$^{-1}$
    = [(310 kcal/day /110 kcal/day)/(12 hours)]$^{-1}$ = 4.26 hours
12. Final dose = 21 mg/kg q4h

[1] Frazier DL, Jones MP, Orosz SE. Pharmacokinetic considerations of the renal system in birds: Part II. Review of drugs excreted by renal pathways. *J Avian Med Surg* 9:104-121, 1995.

[2] Jensen JM, Johnson JH, Weiner ST. *Husbandry and Medical Management of Ostriches, Emus and Rheas.* Wildlife and Exotic Animal TeleConsultants, College Station, TX, 1992.

Appendix 87. Common abbreviations used in prescription writing

a.c.	before meals	o.d.	right eye
a.d.	right ear	o.s.	left eye
ad lib	at pleasure	o.u.	both eyes
adm	administer	oz	ounce
aq	water	p.c.	after meals
a.s.	left ear	PO (p.o.)	per os
a.u.	both ears	prn (p.r.n.)	as needed
b.i.d.	twice a day	q. (q)	every
c.	with	q.d.	every day
cap(s)	capsule(s)	q4h	every 4 hours, etc
cc	cubic centimeter	q24h	once a day
disp	dispense	q.i.d.	four times a day
fl oz	fluid ounce	q.o.d.	every other day
g (gm)	gram	q.s.	a sufficient quantity
gr	grain	®	trademarked name
gtt(s)	drop(s)	SC (SQ)	subcutaneously
h (hr)	hour	Sig:	instructions to patient
h.s.	at bedtime	sol'n	solution
IM	intramuscularly	stat	immediately
inj	inject	susp	suspension
IP	intraperitoneally	tab(s)	tablet(s)
IV	intravenously	Tbs	tablespoon
kg	kilogram	t.i.d.	three times a day
lb	pound	tsp	teaspoon
mg	milligram	ut dict.	as directed
ml	milliliter		

Appendix 88. Common weight, liquid measure, and length conversions

Weights
- 1 milligram (mg) = 1000 micrograms (mcg or μg)
- 1 grain (gr) = 64.8 mg (≈65 mg)
- 1 gram (g) = 15.43 grains (≈15 grains) = 1000 mg
- 1 kilogram (kg) = 1000 g
- 1 ounce (oz) = 28.35 g (≈30 g)
- 1 pound (lb) = 454 g = 16 oz. = 0.45 kg
- 2.2 pounds = 1 kg

Liquid measures
- 1 drop = 0.05 (1/20) milliliter (ml)
- 1 cubic centimeter (cc) = 1 ml
- 1 liter (L) = 1000 ml
- 1 teaspoon (tsp) = 5 ml
- 1 tablespoon (Tbs) = 15 ml
- 1 fluid ounce (fl oz) = 29.57 ml (≈30 ml)
- 1 quart = 2 pints = 32 fl oz (≈0.95 L)
- 1 gallon = 4 quarts = 3.785 L
- 1 cup = 8 fl oz = 237 ml = 16 Tbs

Linear measures
- 1 millimeter (mm) = 0.039 inch (in)
- 1 centimeter (cm) = 0.39 in
- 1 meter (m) = 39.37 in
- 1 inch (in) = 2.54 cm
- 1 foot (ft) = 30.48 cm
- 1 yard (yd) = 91.44 cm

Appendix 89. Equivalents of Celsius (centigrade) (°C) and Fahrenheit (°F) temperature scales

°C	°F	°C	°F	°C	°F
0	32.0	17	62.6	34	93.2
1	33.8	18	64.4	35	95.0
2	35.6	19	66.2	36	96.8
3	37.4	20	68.0	37	98.6
4	39.2	21	69.8	38	100.4
5	41.0	22	71.6	39	102.2
6	42.8	23	73.4	40	104.0
7	44.6	24	75.2	41	105.8
8	46.4	25	77.0	42	107.6
9	48.2	26	78.8	43	109.4
10	50.0	27	80.6	44	111.2
11	51.8	28	82.4	45	113.0
12	53.6	29	84.2	46	114.8
13	55.4	30	86.0	47	116.6
14	57.2	31	87.8	48	118.4
15	59.0	32	89.6	49	120.2
16	60.8	33	91.4	50	122.0

Appendix 90. System of International (SI) Units conversion factors of clinical chemistries commonly used in exotic animal medicine [1]

Component	Conventional (USA) units	Conversion factor	SI Unit
Alkaline phosphatase	u/L	1.0	IU/L
ALT (SGPT)	u/L	1.0	IU/L
Albumin	g/dl	10	g/L
Ammonia (NH_4)	µg/dl	0.5871	µmol/L
Amylase	u/L	1.0	IU/L
AST (SGOT)	u/L	1.0	IU/L
Bilirubin	mg/dl	17.10	µmol/L
Calcium	mg/dl	0.2495	mmol/L
Carbon dioxide	mEq/L	1.0	mmol/L
Chloride	mEq/L	1.0	mmol/L
Cholesterol	mg/dl	0.02586	mmol/L
Cortisol	µg/dl	27.59	nmol/L
Creatine kinase	u/L	1.0	IU/L
Creatinine	mg/dl	88.40	µmol/L
Fibrinogen	mg/dl	0.01	g/L
Glucose	mg/dl	0.05551	mmol/L
Iron	µg/dl	0.1791	µmol/L
Lipase			
Sigma Tietz	u/dl	280	IU/L
Cherry Crandall	u/L	1.0	IU/L
Lipids, total	mg/dl	0.01	g/L
Osmolality	mOsm/kg	1.0	mmol/kg
Phosphate (as inorganic P)	mg/dl	0.3229	mmol/L
Potassium	mEq/L	1.0	mmol/L
Protein (total)	g/dl	10	g/L
Sodium	mEq/L	1.0	mmol/L
Thyroxine (T_4)	µg/dl	12.87	nmol/L
Urea nitrogen	mg/dl	0.3570	mmol/L[a]

[a] Urea.

[1] Modified from *The Merck Veterinary Manual* (7th edition, 1991), as adapted from The SI Manual in Health Care, Metric Commission, Canada, 1981.